Terence DuQuesne was born in Cambridge in 1942 and educated at Dulwich and Oxford. In 1964 he published an important study of source-materials for sexological research, *Catalogi Librorum Eroticorum*. He is the author of many articles and reviews on medical subjects, and also of a volume of poetry with translations from several languages. Terence DuQuesne is a Fellow of the Royal Society of Medicine and pharmacological consultant to Forum Publications Ltd.

Julian Reeves was born in 1937 in Derby. After taking a degree in history at Oxford, he studied medicine and qualified at Trinity College, Dublin. For some years he held appointments in psychiatry at hospitals in the Irish Republic, after which he set up practice in London. Julian Reeves served as an adviser on pharmacological matters – particularly on the non-medical use of drugs – to several voluntary agencies. Following his untimely death, the present volume was completed by the first-named author.

A Handbook of Psychoactive Medicines

tranquillizers – antidepressants – sedatives –
stimulants – narcotics – psychedelics

Terence DuQuesne and
Julian Reeves

Quartet Books
London Melbourne New York

First published by Quartet Books Limited 1982
A member of the Namara Group
27/29 Goodge Street, London W1P 1FD

Copyright © 1982 by J. T. DuQuesne

British Library Cataloguing in Publication Data

Du Quesne, J.T.
  A handbook of psychoactive medicines.
  1. Psychotropic drugs
  I. Title   II. Reeves, Julian
  615'.788   RM315

  ISBN 0-7043-2270-6
      0-7043-3393-7 pbk

Typeset by King's English Typesetters Limited, Cambridge
Printed in Great Britain by
King's English Bookprinters Limited, Leeds

Contents

Charts and Tables

Acknowledgements

Colleagues' and friends' faith in the value of this work has sustained the surviving author throughout the difficult period of its gestation. Some have helped by advising, criticizing and commenting upon the text at various stages, others less directly but no less significantly. In particular, the following should be signalized for their generous assistance:
Dr J A Atkinson; John Bagwell; David Ball, Editor of *Remedial Therapist*; Dr Colin Brewer; David Caleb, LlB; V S and Nicola Carrel; Dr Haydn Cash and Pfizer Ltd, Sandwich, Kent; Dr M C Charny; Mary Coplestone-Boughey; Dr R B Crail, Director of Weybridge Hospital; Dr Sharadindru Das Gupta of St Mary's Hospital, London; Dr David Delvin; Ralph Dwek, MPS; Edward A C Goodman, LlB; Candida Hershman; Dr Andrew Herxheimer of Charing Cross Hospital, London; Dr Arthur Hirsch; Dr Albert Hofmann, formerly of Sandoz AG, Basel; Professor John Hughes of Imperial College, London; the late Denys Irving; Professor Malcolm Lader of the Institute of Psychiatry, London; Dr Tim Liveright; Dr Christopher Lucas of Upjohn Scandinavia, Puurs, Belgium; Dr Martin Mitcheson of University College Hospital, London; Dr Ian Munro, Editor of *The Lancet*; Allen Paterson, Curator of the Chelsea Physic Garden; Dr Michael Rose of St George's Hospital, London; Dr I T Scoular and Reckitt & Colman Ltd, Kingston-upon-Hull; H Shemshem; Professor Bruno Silvestrini of the Instituto di Ricerca F Angelini, Rome; Chief Superintendent Charles Smith of the Metropolitan Police; Bing Spear of the Home Office Drugs Branch; Dr Peter Stonier and Hoechst Laboratories Ltd, Hounslow, Middx; and Eve Weston-Lewis.

The present writer's mother is owed an immense debt. Dwina Waterfield has given unstintingly of her love and her time, and has kindly supplied the illustrations for Annex 4. Michael Law, who, albeit unofficially, performed the services of agent and counsellor, has by his hard work and exacting standards provided constant encouragement. All those at Quartet Books who have been involved with the *Handbook* are owed profound thanks for their enthusiasm and their commitment.

Grateful acknowledgement must be given to the Librarian and staff of the Royal Society of Medicine, by whom no request – for bibliographical information, photocopies, for supply of sometimes abstruse books and dissertations – was not courteously and expeditiously fulfilled. The writer is grateful, too, for the assistance of the staff of the Nuffield Library, British Medical Association; to the librarians of the Wellcome Medical Institute, London; the Bodleian and Radcliffe Science Libraries, Oxford, and to those of the American Medical Association Library, Chicago.

Among the many pharmaceutical companies whose personnel have co-operated in this project, thanks are particularly expressed to: Astra Pharmaceutical Ltd, St Albans; Ayerst Laboratories Ltd, Farnborough; Bristol Laboratories Inc, Syracuse, NY; A H Cox Ltd, Brighton; Endo Laboratories Inc, Garden City, NY; Evans Medical Ltd, Speke; ICI Pharmaceuticals Ltd, Macclesfield; Kali-Chemie Pharma GmbH, Hanover; Lilly Research Laboratories Inc, Indianapolis; Lundbeck Ltd, Luton; May & Baker Ltd, Dagenham; Montedison (Farmitalia C Erba) Ltd, Barnet; Napp Laboratories Ltd, Cambridge; Nicholas Gesellschaft GmbH, Sulzbach/Taunus; Nordmark-Werke GmbH, Hamburg; Roussel Ltd, Wembley; Sandoz AG, Basel; Schürholz Arzneimittel GmbH, Munich; Smith Kline & French Laboratories Ltd, Welwyn Garden City; Théraplix SA, Paris; Upjohn Ltd, Crawley; USV Pharmaceutical Corporation, Tuckahoe, NY; Wander Ltd, Feltham; Winthrop Laboratories Ltd, Surbiton; and Wyeth Laboratories Ltd, Maidenhead.

For kind permission to reproduce copyright material, grateful thanks to:

Professor Leo Hollister, Department of Medicine, Stanford University, California; and Churchill Livingstone Ltd (Table 3: Guide To Dosage of a Standard Antidepressant: Amitriptyline);

Professor Max Hamilton, Department of Psychiatry, University of Leeds; the British Medical Association and the Editor, *Journal of Neurology, Neurosurgery and Psychiatry* (Table 1: A Rating Scale for Depression);

Dr Andrew Herxheimer, Department of Pharmacology, Charing Cross Hospital Medical School; and *Drug and Therapeutics Bulletin* (quotation on p.344);

Dr Albert Hofmann of Burg I L, Switzerland, formerly Research Director, Sandoz AG, Basel; and the Editor, *Indian Journal of Pharmacy* (quotation on pp.321-2);

Professor Stephen Curry, College of Pharmacy, University of Florida, Gainesville; and Professor Alan Richens, Welsh National School of Medicine, Editor of *British Journal of Clinical Pharmacology* (Fig. 1: Metabolism of Diazepam (Valium) and Related Tranquillizers);

Professor Ralph W Morris, Professor of Pharmacology, University of Illinois; and the Editor and Publishers, Skyline Publishers Inc, Portland, Oregon, publishers of *pharmIndex* (Table 6: Comparative Effects of Morphine and Other Potent Analgesics).

JTD

Introduction

This book, the result of almost a decade's research and collation, is essentially the first of its kind. While it is addressed chiefly to the layperson, the authors have become convinced that physicians and others will find the work useful. Although the *Handbook* was originally designed with the general reader in mind, the enthusiastic response to early drafts from GPs, nurses, social workers and other health professionals persuaded the present writers that for both groups a volume of its scope, style and format would be useful and could help fulfil an important need. The problems encountered in formulating a book which would be both acceptable to the medical worker and to the layman, though formidable, constituted a remarkable intellectual challenge. It is impossible to please everyone, however, and doubtless there are readers who will find defects of one sort or another herein.

Nevertheless, the authors have done their best to provide an accurate, unbiased, up-to-date, concise account of those medicines which influence mood or behaviour, in other words the compounds which act on the central nervous system. The layout of this book is such that the reader may easily identify whatever individual substance(s) or type of drug is of particular interest, and that it may be as readily used in the USA as in Britain or Continental Europe. In addition to Alphabetical Entries which consider each drug within the book's terms of reference, Essays are included to provide detailed accounts of six major classes of medicament: Antidepressants, Stimulants, Tranquillizers (Anxiety-Relieving Agents and Antipsychotic Drugs), Hypnotics (Sleep-Inducers) and Sedatives, Potent Analgesics, and Psychedelics or 'Hallucinogens'. These are accompanied by tabular Charts in which the significant characteristics of different compounds belonging to the same class can be conveniently compared, and which give data on side-effects, interactions with other drugs, precautions, abuse potential and other information. A number of Annexes have been added: among these are a guide to the identification of drug preparations, a Glossary of medical and other terms, and an account of the legislation on dangerous and restricted drugs. The Index is comprehensive, enabling the reader to locate information on specific compounds from proprietary (brand) and alternative names.

It has become almost a platitude to say that mood-altering medicines are overprescribed, and that altogether too many chemicals are taken. The great physician and jurist Oliver Wendell Holmes wrote at the turn of the century that, if all the drugs then available were thrown into the sea, it would be the better for mankind and the worse for the fishes. Nobody but a few eccentrics would hold such a view today, given the enormous contribution which has been made by antibiotics, sulphonamides and other life-saving medicines. But vast numbers of people are being treated (and in some cases treating themselves) unnecessarily and inappropriately with psychotropic drugs. A high proportion of these are said to suffer from some kind of psychological disturbance for which these substances are held to be suitable remedies. The scale of the problem can be indicated by epidemiological surveys of either whole populations or random samples of people in given places. An intensive examination of inhabitants of midtown Manhattan has revealed that 23.6% of these suffered from symptoms described as 'depressive'. The incidence of melancholic illness has been varously estimated as between 3.82% (Iceland) and 43.5% (Berlin) of the population in Western countries, depending of course on the criteria used to define depression.[1]* The overall prevalence of 'minor' psychiatric conditions – principally states of anxiety and tension – has lately been estimated, in a London borough, at 5.9% for men and 11.9% for women of a sample population (see also Essay II).[2] In the USA, almost half a million individuals are given annually some form of medical treatment for depression, representing some 15% of the adult population: perhaps surprisingly, the 15 to 34 age-group is that most heavily affected.[3] Most of these people receive psychotropic drugs.

Those who are extremely depressed may try to commit suicide, and the number of such attempts is often taken as a guide to the prevalence of psychological illness. In the USA more than 26,000 suicides are recorded each year, and perhaps five to eight times that number of unsuccessful attempts occur. With more and more patients being prescribed psychotropic agents (some of which intensify depression), these drugs are contributing increasingly to suicidal morbidity and mortality.[4] Antidepressants in particular, with their frequently underestimated toxic effects, now rank second only to the traditional barbiturate sleeping-pills as chemical means of self-annihilation. In the last year for which figures are available (1977), there were 234 deaths in the UK from antidepressant drugs, virtually all those concerned being tricyclic compounds of the amitriptyline type – the class most frequently prescribed – and a further 111 in which such compounds were implicated together with others: accounting for 12% of the annual total of approximately 3,000 deaths from noxious substances (barbiturates were involved in 24% of these

* References are to be found at the end of this introduction

cases).[5] Both the number and the proportion of lethal overdosages, accidental and deliberate, with psychotropic agents – antidepressants, tranquillizers, hypnotics – are rising at a disturbing rate.[6] And the motives of would-be suicides are interesting: in one representative sample of survivors the commonest reason given for making the attempt (65% of the respondents) was that 'the situation was so unbearable that [they] had to do something and didn't know what else to do'.[7]

So there are many very unhappy people in our society. How many of them should be diagnosed as 'over-anxious' or 'depressive' or 'phobic' – i.e. are the province of the physician or psychiatrist – is debatable, as is the use of such terms themselves unless very precise meanings are given (see Essay II). The subject of 'psychotic' illnesses – severe psychological disturbances – is particularly bedevilled by the inadequacy, arbitrariness and frequently the inappropriateness of the expressions which are the alienist's common currency (see also Essay VI). Whatever the ailment, or the label for it, the most regular mode of treatment includes (or consists entirely of) a prescription. It has been estimated that the tranquillizer diazepam alone (familiar as the branded preparation Valium) is taken by 14% of the population in the UK and USA, 15% in Denmark, 17% in France and Belgium, and so on.[8] Mood-altering drugs now account for about a quarter of all prescriptions issued on the National Health Service. In 1977 some 14 million prescriptions for sedatives, 21 million for tranquillizers, 7 million for antidepressants, and more than 30 million for other centrally-acting drugs (e.g. strong pain-killers, stimulants) were dispensed, at a 'wholesale' cost in excess of £75 million.[9]

In the USA more than 200 million such prescriptions are written each year, of which 60 million are for diazepam.[10] The reasons behind these staggering numbers and for the apparently inexorable increase in the prescribing of psychoactive medications are several. Among them one may cite the availability of a bewildering number of different compounds (marketed under proprietary or chemical names): for instance, more than twenty distinct major tranquillizers (neuroleptics or antipsychotics) are produced, and more than a dozen anxiety-relieving agents of the diazepam type (see Essay VI, opening remarks). Many if not most of these are virtual carbon copies of standard medicaments: a subject to which the authors will return. In the UK, both practitioner and patient are largely insulated from the real cost of a prescription by NHS charges which, currently at £1 per item, are still nominal. Neither are there effective sanctions against physicians who consistently prescribe the more expensive drugs. Repeat prescribing, whereby the patient simply telephones the GP's surgery for a further supply of this or that drug, has become the norm in many practices.[11]

Despite the availability of refresher courses and the publication of authoritative pharmacological books and journals, many practitioners remain woefully unaware of the attributes of substances which they so freely prescribe: or, if not ignorant, then irresponsible. There exist in every country the charlatans who will write prescriptions for almost anything, often for considerable pecuniary gain.[12] Much more common is the 'busy' GP working within the Health Service (or its equivalent), whose knowledge of the adverse effects (dependence risk, serious interactions with other compounds) appears to be negligible. The following brief case histories of patients referred to one of the authors (J.T.D.) during a one-month period are pertinent (see also Alphabetical Entries for accounts of the drugs mentioned):

CASE 1 A woman (nursing sister) who had suffered from ankylosing spondylitis (a condition of the vertebral and other joints, with abnormal ossification, characterized by severe inflammation and intermittent pain) was prescribed two pain-killers to be taken concurrently: DF-118 (dihydrocodeine) and Fortral (pentazocine). Within a few days she had become irrational, dysphoric, and was hallucinating and manifesting very severe anxiety ('paranoia'). Of the two analgesics, Fortral antagonizes the effects of narcotic-type agents (such as DF-118) and by itself can provoke bizarre mental states. The prescription of these two drugs at the same time could easily have led to even more unpleasant and dangerous reactions, e.g. withdrawal symptoms on Fortral administration if the patient had become dependent on DF-118. The Fortral was stopped immediately, the other compound gradually. In fact this patient gained more relief from a standard anti-inflammatory agent (indomethacin) than from either analgesic.

CASE 2 A 35-year-old man was prescribed two weeks' supply of a relatively high dose of lithium carbonate, to relieve recurrent depression, and asked to return for a second prescription when the tablets had been used up. Lithium is a very toxic drug: so much, indeed, that blood concentrations of the substance should be estimated at least once during the first week of treatment and regularly thereafter, because the margin between 'effective' and dangerous levels is narrow. Among the specific contra-indications for lithium is impaired kidney function. The patient attempted suicide by taking the entire 14 days' supply of tablets at once: he was discovered in time for treatment to be instituted. In this case the prescriber knew the patient's medical history, including the fact that there was significant kidney damage and that several previous attempts at suicide had been made. No arrangements had been made for blood tests. Because this drug is so toxic, many psychiatrists do not use it, or consider that its administration should be confined to patients with manic-depressive psychosis: its use in chronic depression may possibly be justified in some circumstances. But this case speaks for itself.

CASE 3   A woman of 39 had presented at a psychiatric clinic, suffering from severe anxiety. She was prescribed chlordiazepoxide (Librium) together with a high dose of tranylcypromine (Parnate). Within a few weeks she began to lose motivation, becoming unable to keep her job or manage her household, and complained of intense mental depression, profuse sweating, and gross weight gain. When first prescribed tranylcypromine (an antidepressant of the MAO-inhibitor type), she had not been issued with the standard treatment card (see Table 2) nor warned of the potentially lethal interactions between this drug and a range of commonly taken foods and beverages. The GP advised the patient to stop taking Librium, which she was unable to do.[13]

These are not isolated instances. Indeed, it was precisely because such cases were cropping up so regularly that the impetus for preparing this book was provided. The authors felt that, since nobody better qualified had undertaken a Handbook of this kind, they had a moral responsibility to do so. GPs and other practitioners rely for their information about drugs on a variety of sources, and the results of a recent survey are instructive. This large-scale study of UK doctors was intended to elicit the rank order of reference materials used by them: top of the list was *MIMS* (Monthly Index of Medical Specialties), a brief guide to branded preparations available for prescription. Yet *Drug and Therapeutics Bulletin*, arguably the most authoritative, up-to-date periodical describing new compounds and reassessing old ones, came only ninth in rank order of sources consulted.[14] Two enterprising London pharmacists have begun operating a card system to protect patients against prescribing errors: many such were reported, including the ordering of antibiotics to patients known to be allergic to them and of sugar-based liquid medicines for diabetics.[15] The number of persons in the UK requiring hospital treatment because of adverse drug reactions has been estimated currently to comprise between 10% and 25% of all admissions.[16] The problem is compounded by the fact that an increasing number, chiefly of older patients, are prescribed several medicines concurrently, often unnecessarily and dangerously.[17] That a high proportion of GPs are not adequately informed about even quite common interactions between drugs has been clearly demonstrated.[18]

On the subject of sources of information in this field, it should be pointed out that *MIMS*, while undeniably popular, is hardly an objective source of such data. Entries in this periodical for some of the most widely used medicaments are brief, and omit important details. A number may be considered misleading or unduly vague, for instance in certain headings for 'indications' when a given preparation may be prescribed. Still, since *MIMS* is apparently so useful to practitioners (as it is for very rapid checking of details such as dosage forms), one might suppose that patients could find it helpful too. On the cover of issues, till recently, were printed the words: '*MIMS* is an index of ethical preparations compiled monthly from details supplied by pharmaceutical manufacturing companies. *It is for use only by registered medical practitioners . . .*' (authors' emphasis).[19] On inquiry, one of the present writers was told by the (then) editor of the publication that 'we have to check that copies go out only to medically qualified people'.[20]

There exists a word for this phenomenon: Censorship. One wonders what the proprietors of *MIMS* have to fear. The non-medical reader who is interested in the medicines he or his associates take surely has a right to the kind of information which *MIMS* collates.

A volume which contains much relevant material is the annual *Data Sheet Compendium* produced by the Association of the British Pharmaceutical Industry (ABPI). Every British company that makes or distributes a medicinal product (Pharmacy and Prescription Only Medicines) must print a Data Sheet, and the *Compendium* collates these each year. These Sheets are often extended versions of the information given in *MIMS*, comprising accounts of therapeutic indications, side-effects, contra-indications and in certain cases useful additional information (e.g. suggestions for the treatment of overdosage with the preparation in question). A proportion of the Data Sheets provide excellent, balanced descriptions; but, as with *MIMS*, some of the entries are, to say the least, patchy. Certainly the serious researcher could not rely solely on the *Compendium*, because bias tends to creep in when commercial considerations are at work. And the annual should be seen at least partly as a means of promoting the drug products of the ABPI's member companies. In the case of particular compounds, such material as abuse potential and other undesirable characteristics are either obfuscated or minimized: for instance, the Data Sheet for a widely-abused narcotic pain-reliever coyly tells us that 'as with all potent analgesics, the possibility of addiction cannot be excluded and the usual precautions should be observed'.[21] Despite these strictures, the compendium does, as has been stated, possess some value. But this too has a circulation confined to members of the medical profession, and it is not possible to borrow the volume through the UK public library system, nor to buy it. Censorship, once again.

A 'new' *British National Formulary,* published early in 1981, was intended to remedy the chief defects of the works mentioned and provide an alternative source for GPs. It was supposed to include data on all pharmaceuticals produced in the UK, but signally fails to achieve this. And despite the imprimatur of the British Medical Association the work is in places tendentious and contains a quite remarkable number of errors.

The situation in the USA is somewhat different. There, *Physicians' Desk Reference,* the transatlantic counterpart of the *Data Sheet Compen-*

dium, may be purchased easily. But *PDR,* as it is known, is so detailed and technical in its drug descriptions that the lay-person may find difficulty in comprehending important points: also, like its British equivalent, the book is collated from material supplied by pharmaceutical companies and thus is not entirely dispassionate.[22] The standard reference texts of pharmacology are not only technical but often quite expensive. *Martindale's Extra Pharmacopoeia,* now in its 27th revision, is a work of remarkable scholarship and for a publication containing over 2,000 pages can hardly be considered overpriced at £30.[23] The American Medical Association's *Drug Evaluations,*[24] a valuable guide, costs about $100. And the new British *Pharmaceutical Codex,* which includes much useful information not only on medicines but on many related subjects, sells at £27.[25] There are less – as well as more – expensive sources, some of high quality; but most will be beyond the pocket of the general reader. None of the various cheap paperback guides to the field is adequate for anyone except with the most cursory interest.

PDR commendably includes some forty pages of photographs to help users identify the most commonly prescribed preparations. In the UK, the *MIMS Compendium,* which contained a similar guide, reproducing tablets and capsules, was discontinued some years ago.[26] The present author (J.T.D.) is frequently asked to identify solid-dose preparations, chiefly of psychotropic drugs. To do this is not always easy, because most tablets made in the UK are still white and round. Unbranded products in particular may be hard to recognize if they lack distinguishing marks. Most manufacturers of proprietary tablets and capsules do now provide some means of identification: a letter, number or symbol may be imprinted. Still, this may not be too helpful if one does not know the code employed: even the Metropolitan Police often find it difficult rapidly to recognize drug preparations in which there is illegal traffic. An international index of tablet imprints is published, but this is neither fully comprehensive nor does it contain illustrations.[27] Otherwise, the UK has only the *Chemist & Druggist* annual: this includes line-illustrations, but the identification guide is ridiculously incomplete and out-of-date. It is very cumbersome to use and preposterously expensive for what is offered.[28]

In view of these difficulties, Annex 4 provides a directory of markings on tablets and capsules. This is an index, accompanied by line-drawings, of solid-dose formulations of drugs prescribed in the UK within the terms of reference of this book. In general, pharmacists mark the containers in which tablets are dispensed with the generic (chemical) or brand name concerned. However, some practitioners strike out the letters NP (for *nomen proprium*) on NHS prescription forms if they do not wish the patient to know the nature of the medication. Further, prescriptions for restricted drugs (narcotic analgesics, amphetamine-type stimulants – soon barbiturates may be included) are dispensed in bottles which bear only such legends as 'The Tablets'.[29] This practice may cause problems in various situations, for instance in cases of overdosage, when it is of paramount importance to establish the type of drug taken as rapidly as possible.

A matter for serious concern is the fact that, according to one recent study, more than half the patients who are prescribed drugs do not understand what they are taking, why they need them, and how they should be taken.[30] The question of informed consent, which it is hoped this book will make easier to give or withhold, is of particular importance in the context of psychotropic medications which have potent central and other effects. Psychiatric patients are among the most vulnerable. Very severe adverse reactions may arise, notably when psychiatrists conduct a controlled trial: protocols for such studies often involve one group of patients who receive the active substance and another given inert tablets or injections (placebos).[31] An extensive survey of 200 long-term mental hospital inpatients has revealed that, even under accepted criteria for the use of 'antipsychotic' agents (see Essay VI), about half were receiving unnecessary or excessive medication.[32] The widespread administration of major tranquillizers to prisoners, often against their will, is at last causing questions to be raised in the appropriate places.[33]

Given the massive overprescribing of psychoactive agents, it may come as a surprise to non-medical readers that many practitioners are reluctant to give morphine or another suitable analgesic even for patients who are terminally ill.[34] The hospice movement is helping to correct this state of affairs, but such care is at present available only to a small minority.[35] Recent research has revealed that (in one sample) at least 65% of terminal cancer sufferers being treated at home and over 51% of those cared for in hospitals were denied adequate relief of pain.[36] This reflects what Colin MacInnes – who himself died of cancer without proper analgesia – correctly calls: 'a cruel and callous disgrace. This is the nonchalant attitude of the medical profession towards quite unnecessary suffering – so much so that the one place in the country where you can get least relief is a hospital itself.'[37] Given the will, it is always possible to provide the patient with a good night's sleep without pain and with relief in bed or chair during the daytime.[38] Nor is it only the dying who may legitimately require strong analgesics: the former Editor of the *Practitioner* has commented on the fact that the greater part of the population are penalized by many doctors, because of the latter's excessive concern with that small minority who might be predisposed to drug addiction[39] (see also Essay IV).

The word 'addiction' conjures up in the popular mind the image, fostered by the mass media, of a young person in some squalid place injecting heroin or some similar substance. While the scale of opiate dependency is considerable and increasing, a more appropriate *Leitmotiv* might be the anxious, bored housewife who 'goes running for the shelter / Of her mother's little helper'[40] – namely the yellow Valium tablet. Such iatrogenic (doctor-created) habituation is numerically, and in terms of seriousness, a greater problem – the drugs concerned including tranquillizers, barbiturates and other sleep-inducers, and amphetamine-type stimulants – than that posed by narcotic addiction.[41]

Of course the abuse of heroin and other opiates is a genuine and growing social problem. As that great pharmacologist the late Nathan Eddy wrote in this connection: 'Human desire cannot be legislated nor abolished by punishment.'[42] In the UK the number of opiate habitués notified to the Home Office has doubled during the past decade, with some 3,000 persons currently receiving drugs from Drug Dependency Units.[43] It has been evident for some time that this figure does not accurately reflect the real incidence of narcotic addiction in Britain[44] because many either do not present at treatment centres or supplement their legal supplies from the black market.[45] It has been unofficially estimated that only perhaps a quarter of such users are recorded in the Home Office statistics: what is certain is that the illicit traffic in hard drugs is growing at a rate of about 20% annually.[46] Opium cultivation for non-medical purposes continues virtually unchecked: Pakistan, Laos, Thailand and Burma (the 'Golden Triangle' area), and Afghanistan, Pakistan and Iran (the 'Golden Crescent'), ensure heroin supply for Western countries as well as the USA. Australia has also become a lucrative market.[47] In Britain, there are several disincentives for addicts to approach government clinics: partly because of cutbacks these are understaffed and waiting lists are excessively long.[48] And, even if one of these units takes on a new patient, he will almost certainly receive only a small quantity of a drug called methadone – a synthetic opiate at least as addictive as heroin itself – and will be obliged to collect his prescriptions daily from a designated pharmacy.[49] Perhaps a majority of notified addicts now supplement these with 'Chinese H': impure, adulterated and illegal heroin.[50] *Gesetz ist mächtig, mächtiger ist die Not* (Law is mighty: mightier is need).

Seizures by Customs officers and police of heroin amounted to about 3 kilogrammes in 1973 and 1974: by 1978 an extraordinary total of 61 kilos was seized in 350 raids. While the quantity was rather lower in the following year, at 45 kilos, almost double the number of seizures was made.[51] According to officers of the Drugs Squad at Scotland Yard, such confiscations represent only the tip of the iceberg; and it is reported that senior police are receiving five times more useful information on heroin traffic than they have officers to deal with it. In effect, this means that even known dealers may operate for years with relative impunity[52] (see further Essay IV). In the USA in 1980 there was an apparent drop in the incidence of narcotic addiction (more than 500,000 people), but the authorities believe that the numbers are again rising sharply: in part due to bumper opium harvests in the countries of the Golden Triangle, and also because the European market is saturated and higher prices are commanded in America. Opium is easy to convert into morphine for refining into heroin. With the European markets glutted, the price of heroin is decreasing in Germany, Italy, France and elsewhere, and the incidence of opiate dependency there, especially among teenagers, has been rising dramatically. International drug enforcement agencies report that they seize only 10% of the total heroin being imported, and that co-operation with some poppy-growing countries (Iran, Afghanistan) has for obvious reasons ceased. In 1980, over a ton of heroin was impounded in Europe, and the quantities confiscated are skyrocketing year by year.[53]

In Western society, habitués of narcotic drugs have become convenient scapegoats for a culture in which collective guilts are projected on to minorities. Thomas Szasz, in a stunningly perceptive book, has demonstrated how the addict (and the psychiatric patient) are today persecuted essentially as were witches and Jews in former ages.[54] Non-medical drug use of any kind is held to be in some way wrong. It is hardly a travesty of the Judaeo-Christian attitude, consolidated over centuries, that if something is pleasurable then it is probably also sinful. The appearance of the counter-culture stemmed in large measure from resistance to traditional views of this kind.[55]

The latter's application may be inferred from the way that British legislation on 'dangerous drugs' is enforced. During 1979 only 4% of offences against the Misuse of Drugs Act involved heroin, while 87% concerned cannabis. Annually, some 10,000 to 12,000 individuals are convicted for infractions of the law in respect of cannabis, the majority of cases being possession of small quantities of the substance.[56] And, while the opiates, barbiturates and many other indisputably dangerous drugs may be prescribed, a special licence from the Home Secretary is required by any physician intending to administer cannabis (q.v.),[57] whose therapeutic indications are slowly being realized,[58] and whose hazards have been grossly exaggerated.[59] Seizures of heroin, opium, amphetamines and other 'hard' drugs represent only a small fraction of these seriously dangerous agents which are illicitly imported, manufactured and distributed.[60]

So far as the evidently ineluctable rise in prescription of psychotropic drugs is concerned – the tranquillizers, anxiolytics, antidepressants, hypnotics, stimulants – it is the prescriber who must in the last analysis be accountable. But he is under extraordinary pressure, some of it at the subliminal level, to continue the trend. Much of this comes from certain of the pharmaceutical giants: he listens to the firms' representatives, sees the sophisticated and often misleading advertisements in the medical journals, happily accepts samples, promotional material and other propaganda. In addition he has to contend with increasing demands from patients.[61] The fact that many apparently new compounds are redundant, being minor chemical modifications of standard drugs, has already been signalized. In spite of this, yet more 'me-too' tranquillizers are being marketed, often at absurdly high prices.[62] While some of the multinational companies behave ethically, neither overselling their products nor abusing their power, others do both. And the regulation of their practices, long overdue, and particularly as these apply to the most vulnerable Third World countries, is only beginning.[63] The awesome reach of this power, and the devastating effects which it can bring, has been graphically illustrated by the case of Stanley Adams: a man who was imprisoned, financially ruined, and subjected to almost unbelievable suffering because, as a responsible citizen, he spoke out against price-fixing and other iniquities perpetrated by Hoffmann-La Roche (the manufacturers of Valium and Librium), his former employer.[64] Only after years of hardship is he at last being partially compensated.[65]

Voltaire wrote that 'the art of medicine consists of amusing the patient while nature cures the disease'. This could be regarded as a fair assessment of the position as it currently obtains. In psychiatry, as in other areas of medicine, it is well known that some conditions will improve, some remain stable, and some deteriorate irrespective of the administration of psychotropic drugs.[66] Of course there is a reverse to this coin. The advent of relatively selectively-acting antidepressants, anxiety-relieving agents and tranquillizers – for which the large pharmaceutical firms' R & D programmes are chiefly responsible – has meant the mitigation of suffering for a vast number of patients, and significant relief of symptoms in many cases without the distressing adverse effects or dangers of medicaments previously available. Treatment of psychiatric disorders, by most accounts, has been revolutionized by the introduction first of chlorpromazine (Largactil, Thorazine),[67] and more lately by long-acting injectable antipsychotic agents.[68] However, whether such therapy, which itself can provoke severe, insidious and sometimes irreversible side-effects, is desirable for the overwhelming majority of patients subjected to it, is a matter for debate (see also Essay VI).[69]

Ivan Illich has reminded us (1976) that in England every tenth night's sleep is drug-induced; that in the USA, compounds which affect mood comprise the fastest-growing sector of the pharmaceutical market; that dependence on prescribed tranquillizers has risen by 290% since 1962 (versus 23% for alcohol); that huge, excessive profits are made on these agents; that the drug houses spend $4,500 per physician each year to promote their products in America; and, not least, that according to the Food and Drug Administration, a fifth of the physicians who were researching new drugs had invented the data they sent to the pharmaceutical firms and pocketed the fees. Illich has been most vociferous in denouncing the 'expropriation of health' indicated by such facts.[70] He urges us to much greater self-reliance: if it hurts, do not immediately rush to the telephone for a doctor's appointment. He believes that perception of pain and modes of handling it are culturally conditioned, that experience of it is important philosophically, psychologically – indeed spiritually. And he cites the alleviation of pain (in the broad sense) by drugs as a prime example of this 'expropriation'.[71] The present writers believe that while Illich and his cohorts have taken the argument too far, in essence he is correct: *sunt lacrimae rerum.* Certainly intractable pain states should be relieved by whatever means are appropriate; and it has already been established that often this is not done, or done inadequately.

But suffering in most of its manifestations is transient and self-limiting. Tension, stress, apprehension, *Weltschmerz,* psychological distress – the very states so often mitigated by psychotropic drugs – are actually an intrinsic element of the human condition. To reach for the tablets whenever one of these states of malaise arises demeans the individual, causes attrition of his integrity; and in practical terms may pose more problems than it solves. Those who take potent substances such as lysergide (LSD) – or even cannabis – in a non-medical and therefore often illegal context may do so responsibly, and in a genuine spirit of inquiry. They may none the less fall into the same trap that is sprung on the patient whose reliance on prescribed tranquillizers has robbed him, not only of health, but of freedom of choice. An obvious question is: where does one draw the line between suffering with which the individual should deal alone; that which is amenable to treatment with reassurance and counselling; and that for which medication is appropriate? The authors have no simple answers: there are none. Instead readers, whether medical or lay-people, are invited at least to consider the matter carefully; to think before writing or accepting a prescription; to ascertain whether, if it is appropriate to take a certain type of drug, a suitable one has been or will be chosen; and to be alert for hazards, whether these involve likely adverse effects, interactions with other medicaments, dependence potential or any other important characteristic which might otherwise be overlooked. A few references from the recent clinical literature have, it is hoped, highlighted a few of the areas of most concern. Some might claim that information of the kind contained in this book is solely the province of the physician. But, even were there not such powerful compounds as are now available, or far less inappropriate and negligent prescribing than is the case, one should remember: it is the patient's – one's own – mind and body which is at issue. Thus one has not merely the right but the responsibility to discern how either or both may be affected. And it is the principal aim of the present work to make this process easier.

References

1. Helmchen, H., 'Häufigkeit depressiver Erkrankungen' in Hoechst AG Medizinische Abteilung (ed.): *Alival (Nomifensin): Symposium über Ergebnisse der experimentellen und klinischen Prüfung* (Schattauer: Stuttgart, 1977) 19–29; cf also references therein
2. Bebbington, P., Hurry, J. and Tennant, C., 'Recent advances in the epidemiological study of minor psychiatric disorders' *Journal of the Royal Society of Medicine* 73: 315–8 (1980)
3. Hollister, L.E., *Clinical Pharmacology of Psychotherapeutic Drugs* (Churchill-Livingstone: Edinburgh, 1978) 69
4. Brophy, J. J., 'Suicide attempts with psychotherapeutic drugs' *Archives of General Psychiatry* 17: 652–7 (1967)
5. Crome, P. and Newman, B., 'Fatal tricyclic antidepressant poisoning' *Journal of the Royal Society of Medicine* 72: 649–53 (1979); Office of Population Censuses and Surveys: *1977 Mortality Statistics* (HMSO: London, 1979) Table 9
6. Brewer, C., 'If speed kills, tricyclics massacre' *World Medicine* 11(12): 37–42 (1976)
7. Bancroft, J., Hawton, K., Simkin, S., Kingston, B., Cumming, C. and Whitwell, D., 'The reason people give for taking overdoses: a further inquiry' *British Journal of Medical Psychology* 52: 353–62 (1979)
8. Coleman, V.: *The Medicine Men* (Arrow: London, 1977) 84
9. Department of Health and Social Security: *Health and Personal Social Services Statistics for England . . . for 1977* (HMSO: London, 1980) Table 25; cf Robertson, H. A., Rogers, M. L. and Binns, T. B., 'The cost of prescribing' *Practitioner* 215: 773–81 (1975); Stern, R., 'Psychotropic drugs and behaviour therapy' *Practitioner* 225: 21–5 (1981)
10. Silverman, M. and Lee, P. R.: *Pills, Profits and Politics* (California University Press: Berkeley, 1974); Clark, M., 'The prisoners of pills' *Newsweek* 24 April 1978, 52
11. Parish, P. A., 'What influences have led to increased prescribing of psychotropic drugs?' *Journal of the Royal College of General Practitioners* 23 (Suppl 2): 49–57 (1973)
12. Edwards, J. G., 'Doctors, drugs and drug abuse' *Practitioner* 212: 815–22 (1974)
13. DuQuesne, J. T.: *Mind Drugs: a prospectus* (De Luxe: London, 1978) 12
14. Strickland-Hodge, B. and Jeqson, M. H., 'Usage of information sources by general practitioners' *Journal of the Royal Society of Medicine* 73: 857–62 (1980)
15. Shulman, S. and Shulman, J. I., 'Operating a two-card medical record system in general practice pharmacy' *Practitioner* 224: 989–92 (1980)
16. E.g. Ghose, K., 'Hospital bed occupancy due to drug-related problems' *Journal of the Royal Society of Medicine* 73: 853–6 (1980)
17. Pappworth, M. H., 'Suggestions for NHS savings' *World Medicine* 15(12): 39–58 (1980)
18. Petrie, J. C., Howie, J. G. R. and Durno, D., 'Awareness and experience of general practitioners of selected drug interactions' *British Medical Journal* I:

262–5 (1974); Salter, R. H., 'Hazards of sudden drug withdrawal' *Practitioner* 218: 871–3 (1977)

19. *MIMS* (Monthly Index of Medical Specialties) 22(12): cover (1980)
20. Rhenius V, personal communication (1978)
21. *ABPI Data Sheet Compendium 1980–81* (Datapharm: London, 1980) 208; cf 'Who is responsible for entries in *MIMS?*' *Drug & Therapeutics Bulletin* 19: 18–19 (1981)
22. *Physicians' Desk Reference,* ed.34 (Medical Economics: Oradell, NJ, 1980)
23. *Martindale's Extra Pharmacopoeia,* ed.27 by A. Wade (Pharmaceutical Press: London, 1977)
24. AMA Council on Drugs: *Drug Evaluations,* ed.4 (Publishing Sciences Group: Littleton, Mass., 1981)
25. *[British] Pharmaceutical Codex,* 11th revision (Pharmaceutical Society: London, 1979)
26. *MIMS Colour Index* (Haymarket Press: London, [1974]). *MIMS* has now begun to publish a new Index, appearing piecemeal
27. Collier, W. A. L.: *Imprex: index of imprints used on tablets and capsules,* ed.7 (Imprex Ltd: Cambridge, England, 1978)
28. *Chemist & Druggist Directory 1980* (Benn: Tonbridge, Kent, 1980) £20
29. For an account of the complex regulations on such matters, see Hay, C. E. and Pearce, M. E.: *Medicines and Poisons Guide,* ed.2 (Pharmaceutical Press: London, 1980) 23f
30. Cromie, B. W. 'Information given to patients about their medicines' *Journal of the Royal Society of Medicine* 73: 677–8 (1980)
31. Leff, J., 'Without informed consent' *Mind Out* 13: 5 (October 1975)
32. Fottrell, E., Sheikh, M., Kothari, R. and Sayed, I., 'Long-stay patients with long-stay drugs. A case for review: a cause for concern' *Lancet* I: 81–2 (1976)
33. Transcript of 'Holloway: The Inside Story': Thames Television (Thames Report) Editor, Michael Braham, 12 February 1981
34. Smith & Nephew Pharmaceuticals Ltd: *Management of Terminal Illness: the collected findings.* Postal Symposium no.1 (Smith & Nephew: Welwyn Garden City, Herts, 1973)
35. E.g. Crail, R. B., A pilot scheme in continuing care' *Practitioner* 224: 126–7 (1980); Twycross, R. G., 'Relief of terminal pain' *British Medical Journal* II: 212–5 (1975)
36. Parkes, C. M., 'Home or hospital? Terminal care as seen by surviving spouses' *Journal of the Royal College of General Practitioners* 28: 19–30 (1978)
37. MacInnes, C., 'Cancer ward' *World Medicine* 15(12): 35–7 (1980)
38. 'Narcotic analgesics in terminal cancer' *Drug and Therapeutics Bulletin* 18: 69–72 (1980); Twycross, R. G., 'Pain and analgesics' *Current Medical Research and Opinion* 5: 497–505 (1978)
39. Thomson, W. A. R.: *Herbs That Heal* (A. & C. Black: London, 1976) 76
40. Jagger, M. & Richard, K., 'Mother's Little Helper': track from The Rolling Stones, *Aftermath* LP (Decca, 1966)
41. For an excellent survey, see Jaffe, J. H., 'Drug addiction and drug abuse' in Goodman, L. S. and Gilman, A., (ed.): *The Pharmacological Basis of Therapeutics,* ed.5 (Macmillan: New York, 1980) 524ff; and cf now Kemper, N., Poser, W. and Poser, S., 'Benzodiazepin-Abhängigkeit' *Deutsche*

medizinische Wochenschrift 105: 1707–12 (1980), Petersson, H. and Lader, M. H., 'Withdrawal Symptons from clobazam' in Hindmarch, I. and Stonier, P. D.(ed.): *Clobazam* (London, 1981) 181–3 (=Royal Society of Medicine: International Congress & Symposium Series no. 43)

42. Eddy, N. B., 'Drug abuse and drug dependence' in Gordon, M. (ed.): *Psychopharmacological Agents,* vol.4 (Academic Press: New York, 1976) 11
43. 'Statistics of the Misuse of drugs in the United Kingdom, 1979' = *Home Office Statistical Bulletin* 11/80 (Surbiton, Surrey, 1980) Table 14. See now Ditton, J. & Speirits, K: *The Rapid Increase of Heroin-Addiction in Glasgow during 1981.* Diss. Glasgow, 1981.
44. Johnson, B. D., 'How much heroin maintenance (containment) in Britain?' *International Journal of the Addictions* 12: 361–98 (1977)
45. Hartnoll, R. L., Mitcheson, M. C., Battersby, A., Brown, G., Ellis, M., Fleming, P. and Hedley, B., 'Evaluation of heroin maintenance in controlled trial' *Archives of General Psychiatry* 37: 877–84 (1980)
46. *Statistics of the Misuse of Drugs: United Kingdom 1977* (Home Office: London, 1979) 5–9; ibid., *Supplementary Tables 1978–1979* (Home Office: Surbiton, Surrey, 1981) *passim*
47. Cf Hirst, D.: *Heroin in Australia* (Quartet: Melbourne, 1979) 10ff
48. Clark, D., 'Heroin horror in our midst' (London) *Observer* 4 April 1981, 11
49. Edwards, G., 'British policies on opiate addiction' *British Journal of Psychiatry* 134: 1–13 (1979)
50. Cf Blumberg, H. H., 'British users of opiate-type drugs: a follow-up study' *British Journal of Addiction* 71: 65–77 (1976)
51. 'Statistics of the misuse of drugs in the United Kingdom, 1978' = *Home Office Statistical Bulletin* 6/79; see also reference 46, above
52. Clark, *op. cit.*; Scotland Yard: C1-Drugs Section: personal communication, 1980
53. Morris, R. W., 'Use and abuse of narcotic analgesics and antagonists' *pharmIndex* 19(7): 11–16 (1977); Strasser, S., Brecher, D. and Reiss, S.,'Special Report: the booming drugs trade' *Newsweek* 9 February 1981, 10–19. Williams, D. A., 'Heroin: preparing for a new invasion' *Newsweek* 10 March 1980, 45
54. Szasz, T. S.: *Ceremonial Chemistry: the ritual persecution of drugs, addicts and pushers* (Routledge & Kegan Paul: London, 1975) *passim*
55. DuQuesne, J. T., 'Drug abuse' *Police Review* 89: 1966–9 (1981). Cf Reich, C.: *The Greening of America* (Random House: New York, 1970)
56. DuQuesne, J. T., 'Cannabis and the rule of law' *Lancet* II: 58 (1981)
57. *Misuse of Drugs Act, 1971* (HMSO: London, 1971) c.30; cf Rose, M., 'A legitimate case for prescribing marijuana?' *Medical News* 28 February 1980, 19
58. Lemberger, L., 'Potential therapeutic usefulness of marijuana' *Annual Reviews of Pharmacology & Toxicology* 20: 151–72 (1980)
59. For a balanced account, see 'Marijuana' *Medical Letter on Drugs & Therapeutics* 18: 69–70 (1976)
60. See reference 43, 1–5
61. Cf Mapes, R. (ed.): *Prescribing Practice and Drug Usage* (Croom Helm: London, 1980); Coleman, *op. cit.*
62. See e.g. 'Yet another benzodiazepine' *Drug & Therapeutics Bulletin* 18: 94–5 (1980); Tyrer, P., 'The benzodiazepine bonanza' *Lancet* II: 709–10 (1974);

and for examples of arbitrary differences in pricing between countries, see Jacoby, E. M. and Hefner, D. L., 'Domestic and foreign prescription drug prices' *Social Security Bulletin* 34: 15 (May 1971)

63. Agarwal, A., *op. cit.*, 'UN takes a stand on drugs' *New Scientist* 9 November 1978, 442–5; Yudkin, J. S., 'Pharmaceutical industry: golden goose or curate's egg?' *World Medicine* 14(9): 65–8 (1979)

64. Transcript of 'Reel Evidence – The Spy Who Caught A Cold', BBC Radio 4, 9 March 1980 (produced by Cogan, R.).

65. 'Stanley Adams: good guys finish last' *The Economist* 22 March 1980, 68–9

66. Stern, R., 'Psychotropic drugs and behaviour therapy' *Practitioner* 225: 21–5 (1981)

67. Kornetsky, C.: *Pharmacology: drugs affecting behavior* (Wiley/Interscience: New York, 1976) 86–90

68. Hollister, *op. cit.* 160–66

69. Berke, J.: *The Butterfly Man* (Hutchinson: London, 1977); cf also Packard, V.: *The People Shapers* (Futura: London, 1978) 40–60; Scheflin, A. W. and Opton, E. M. Jr: *The Mind Manipulators* (Paddington: New York, 1978) 417–25

70. Illich, I.: *Limits to Medicine: Medical Nemesis: the expropriation of health* (Marion Boyars: London, 1976) 69–70 and *passim*

71. Illich, *op. cit.* 133–54

How to Use this Book

This book contains detailed and up-to-date information on all the drugs which fall within its terms of reference. In Part One an alphabetical formulary gives information on the actions, uses, side-effects, abuse potential, contra-indications, and interactions with other medicines of all the sedative/hypnotic (sleep-inducing), tranquillizing, antipsychotic, anti-depressant and strong analgesic (narcotic) agents which are available for prescription currently in the United Kingdom and the United States. Data are also provided on psychedelics (hallucinogens) which, though they may not be prescribed, are under international legal restriction and some of which appear on the illicit drug market.

In Part Two, there are six Essays, each accompanied by a Chart, concerned with each class of psychotropic or mood-altering compounds. These contain more detailed knowledge of the relevant drug types, including comparisons of alternative medicaments for similar medical conditions, drug interactions, precautions and much additional material presented in the Charts in a form which is easy to assimilate.

Each Alphabetical Entry in Part One begins with the chemical name of the compound, with alternative names in parentheses where relevant. These conform to the British Approved Names system. Sometimes a drug is known in the USA differently from in the UK: for example, the potent analgesic PETHIDINE is called MEPERIDINE in the USA. Such alternative nomenclature is sometimes confusing, but all that is currently applicable may be found through use of the comprehensive Index of Brand Names and Alternative Names at the end of this book. If the individual drug is restricted under the UK Misuse of Drugs Act or corresponding American legislation, the legend **R** follows its official name. Entries are formulated with the use of five symbols, as below:

● This section is devoted to a general description of the relevant drug, the pharmacological class to which it belongs, its therapeutic actions and uses, and its principal side-effects. If several adverse reactions are listed, this does not imply that the patient is likely to experience all of them; simply that they may or may not occur commonly in some cases. If the substance has a potential for abuse and/or dependency, this is stated. Here 'dependency' means psychological or physical habituation. The term 'addiction' is employed only in accordance with the World Health Organization criteria for physical dependency: generally, this applies to drugs whose abrupt discontinuation after repeated use triggers off a clearly defined set of withdrawal symptoms. Addiction may develop to narcotics of the morphine type or to barbiturates; but not, strictly speaking, to certain other categories of psychotropic agents, e.g. amphetamines. There exist some drugs for which an intense craving may be experienced (cocaine is an example) but to which true addiction does not occur. Whether amphetamines are 'addictive' is at present a controversial question, but the weight of evidence suggests that they are not. Nevertheless prolonged abuse often leads to mental and physical deterioration. Reference in this section to other drugs described here is indicated by the use of capital letters. Thus: 'Anileridine is one of several derivatives of PETHIDINE.' This device obviates the need for frequent use of *q.v.* or some alternative means of cross-referencing.

▲ Here dosages are described. Unless otherwise stated, these are oral and for adults. The range of dose regimens given conforms in most cases to contemporary medical practice, but some practitioners may for different reasons prescribe more or less than the dosage indicated, depending on circumstances. For instance, in administering potent analgesics over long periods, as to terminal patients, tolerance may develop and individual patients may need much more of a drug (e.g. morphine) than a non-tolerant person. Variation in response to the same dose of many drugs by different patients may be considerable. If the relevant drug is prescribed for children or elderly or debilitated patients, dosage should be reduced accordingly by the physician. When maximum daily (or weekly) limits are stated, these are usually in accordance with manufacturers' recommendations or current usage as indicated in standard reference texts (e.g. *AMA Drug Evaluations,* ed.4, Littleton, Mass., 1981).

★ In this paragraph, brief data on precautions, contra-indications and interactions with other drugs are provided. Contra-indications refer to illnesses and conditions in which the medicament concerned should not be prescribed; or, if prescribed, only in exceptional situations. Mostly contra-indications are relative rather than absolute: for example, morphine and other narcotic analgesics are contra-indicated in cases of respiratory depression, because drugs of this type may provoke this or enhance it if it is already present. Nevertheless an opiate may be the only means of obtaining pain relief for someone suffering from inoperable lung cancer, when breathing may be impaired. It would, of course, be quite wrong to withhold pain-killers in such a case, but then careful monitoring is particularly necessary. Ultimately it is the practitioner's responsibility to make a judgment on the risk/benefit ratio for a particular medicine.

In a number of entries, pregnancy has been cited as a contra-indication to use of a drug. This does not mean that, when no such warning is given, the compound is safe at this time for women. As a rule, *all psychotropic drugs should be avoided during pregnancy,* especially during the first three months, unless the medical reasons are compelling. So far as children are concerned, only exceptionally are any mood-modifying drugs appropriate: among the few legitimate situations amitriptyline, the antidepressant, may be prescribed to control enuresis (bed-wetting), and diazepam (Valium) to stop sleepwalking or night terrors. The use of amphetamines and other stimulants in the childhood hyperkinetic syndrome (or 'attention deficit disorder'), a grossly overdiagnosed illness in any event, is contentious: the pros and cons are discussed in the relevant Essay.

Drug interactions have assumed a greatly increased significance now that so many individuals are receiving more than one type of medication (in some cases several drugs) concurrently. The most important of these are noted; some compounds are designated as 'inadvisable' for use at the same time as a particular psychotropic agent. The purpose of including such information for every drug is to tell the reader of potentially dangerous or inappropriate combinations about which many prescribers remain lamentably unaware: a simple example involves sedatives and sleep-inducers of the barbiturate type, which may reduce the effectiveness of oestrogen-containing contraceptive Pills. More serious instances – e.g. the danger of administering pethidine (meperidine) and other opiates to patients being treated with MAO-inhibitor antidepressants – are sometimes overlooked, and the patient is entitled to a warning.

➤ Here the reader is referred to one of the six Charts and Essays which describe in detail the categories of drugs which are the subject of this book. Fuller information on a given compound's characteristics will be found there, and the Charts enable the reader to compare the attributes (e.g. dependence potential) of different members of the same pharmacological class in a way that is readily assimilable. The inclusion of more comprehensive data on, for example, drug interactions in the Essays and Charts, to which cross-reference is easy, saves repetition in the Alphabetical Entries, which have been deliberately kept as concise as possible.

◆ This symbol stands for Presentations, that is the form(s) in which the compound is available in the UK and/or the USA. When pharmaceutical preparations are shown, this indicates that the drug in question has received the 'seal of approval' from official bodies, and generally means that it is considered therapeutically useful. Some preparations are marketed only in this way without brand names. This occurs particularly with standard items, e.g. *Morphine Sulphate Injection* BPC: Amps 10, 15 & 30 mg/1 ml, 30 mg/2ml. The great majority of psychoactive drugs, however, even if officially sanctioned, are marketed only under proprietary or brand names. Drugs prescribed under manufacturers' trade names are listed here, with details of maker's name, type of formulation (e.g.

tablets), and strengths. If you know only the brand name of a drug, look in the index at the back of this book. Compounds are listed here in alphabetical order of their proper (chemical) names, because often there are several branded preparations containing the same substance. Occasionally there are different chemical names for a drug in the UK and the USA. Alternative names may also be found in the Index.

The strengths of drug formulations are given in metric units (milligrammes, millilitres), which officially have replaced the old Imperial system (grains, drachms). Because some drugs are still prescribed by Imperial measures in the USA, we have included conversion of Imperial and Metric Units (Annex 1). A guide on how to decipher your prescription is provided in Annex 2.

The following abbreviations, many of them obvious, are employed in the Alphabetical Entries and elsewhere in the book:

Official Preparations

BPC = *(British) Pharmaceutical Codex,* ed.11. London, 1979
USP = *United States Pharmacopeia,* 20th revision. Rockville, Md., 1980

(Occasionally reference is made to preparations still available for prescription which have been deleted from the current editions of these standard works. In such cases the year of the latest pharmacopoeial entry is shown, e.g. *USP 1970*)

Dosage strengths

μg = microgramme (1 microgramme is 1/100 milligramme)
mg = milligramme
G   = Gramme (1 Gramme is 1,000 milligrammes)
ml = millilitre
L   = litre (1 litre is 1,000 millilitres)

Dosage forms

Tabs	=	Tablets (for oral administration; usually round or oblate spheroids)
Hypo Tabs	=	Hypodermic Tablets (for dissolving to make up an injection)
Sol Tabs	=	Soluble Tablets (usually for oral use, dissolved in a glass of water)
Subl Tabs	=:	Sublingual Tablets (to be held under tongue until dissolved)
Caps	=	Capsules (either two-part, bullet shaped, or continuous)
SR Tabs	=	Sustained-Release Tablets (specially made for prolonged action)
SR Caps	=	Sustained-Release Capsules (specially made for prolonged action)

Syr   = Syrup
Elix   = Elixir
Soln   = Solution
Susp   = Suspension   } these are concentrated
Draught   = Draught   } liquid preparations
Linct   = Linctus   } for oral administration
Tinc   = Tincture
Drops   = Drops

Amps	=	Ampoules (solutions of drugs in glass container for injection)
Dry Amps	=	Dry Ampoules (ampoules containing powder to be dissolved for injection)
Syrettes	=	Syrettes are syringes pre-filled with a single dose of drug
Vials	=	Vials (multi-dose glass, rubber-capped containers with liquid or powder for injection)
Ext	=	Extract (dry or liquid concentrate of a vegetable drug, e.g. opium)
Vitr	=	Vitrellae (glass capsules containing volatile liquid for inhalation)
Suppos	=	Suppositories (cone-shaped units for rectal administration)
Enema	=	Enema (large-volume liquid in container with nozzle for rectal insertion)
Pulv	=	Pulvis (bulk powder for making up into syrups etc.)

Part One

Alphabetical Formulary of Drugs

R restricted use (*see 'How To Use This Book', p. 17*)

● general description (*see pp. 17–18*)

▲ dosages (*see p. 18*)

★ precautions (*see pp. 18–19*)

➤ cross-reference to Essays and Charts in Part Two (*see p. 19*)

◆ presentations (*see pp. 19–20*)

Abbreviations (*see pp. 20–1*)

ACETOPHENAZINE

● Acetophenazine is a major tranquillizer or antipsychotic agent. It belongs to the phenothiazine class of drugs, of which CHLORPRO-MAZINE (Largactil, Thorazine) is the prototype. The compound is prescribed to control symptoms of severe mental illness, usually for psychiatric inpatients. It has been recommended to alleviate agitation, hyperexcitability and restlessness where such states are prominent features of schizophrenia and other psychotic conditions. Because acetophenazine is among the most potent drugs of its type, its use should be reserved for the most serious, often chronic, psychiatric disorders, and is unsuitable for treatment of minor emotional or psychological complaints. Common adverse effects include oversedation, lethargy, dry mouth, blurred vision, and symptoms which resemble those of Parkinson's disease. An insidious form of parkinsonism, known as tardive dyskinesia, may follow continuous administration of high dosages. Mental depression may occur or be intensified with this drug.

▲ There is considerable variation in the range of doses given, which must depend on the severity of the condition under treatment and on individual response. For outpatients, the range is 50–400 mg per day, and for hospital inpatients up to 1,500 mg daily, in divided doses.

★ Like other antipsychotics, this drug greatly enhances the effects of other agents which depress the central nervous system (CNS), including barbiturates and other sedatives and tranquillizers, narcotic pain-killers, and alcohol. Acetophenazine should be avoided in severe liver, kidney and cardiac complaints, respiratory insufficiency, during pregnancy and for administration to children. Known hypersensitivity to other phenothiazines will apply to this compound.

➤ For further information, see Essay VI and Chart VI(B): Antipsychotic Tranquillizers.

◆ USA:
Acetophenazine Maleate Tablets USP: available as
Tindal (Schering): Tabs 20 mg

ACETYLCARBROMAL (ACECARBROMAL)

● Acetylcarbromal is a muscle-relaxant and anxiety-relieving agent of moderate potency, with mild sedative action. Although it has been superseded by the benzodiazepine tranquillizers, such as diazepam (Valium), the compound is still available in Western Europe, usually in combination with other soporific drugs, under many brand names. Acetylcarbromal is an analogue of the obsolete bromide type of sedative and is generally similar to its parent drug CARBROMAL. Because of its relatively low toxicity, it has been considered suitable for use by the elderly and children. The compound is often used in conjunction with barbiturates for daytime sedation, but the combination is not recommended. Prolonged use may lead to insidious psychological and/or physical dependency, and because the drug is excreted slowly a buildup of toxic quantities in the tissues may occur.

▲ To promote sleep: usually 500 mg, but up to 1 G if necessary. Otherwise, 125–250 mg two or three times daily.

★ Adverse effects are infrequent if the agent is used only occasionally, but oversedation is common and this may impair reflexes. Confusion and stupor will indicate bromism, or potentially hazardous intoxication. If other CNS depressants, such as barbiturates, opiates, and alcohol are taken, special caution must be exercised. Contra-indicated in porphyria and in cases of known hypersensitivity; caution in severe respiratory ailments. Generally as for CARBROMAL.

➤ See under CARBROMAL.

◆ USA:
Paxarel (Circle): Tabs 250 mg
Sedamyl (Riker): Tabs 250 mg

ALLOBARBITONE (ALLOBARBITAL)

● This is one of the less popular of the intermediate-acting barbiturates, being similar in all important respects to AMYLOBARBITONE (AMOBARBITAL). Allobarbitone is available only in preparations which also contain one or more mild analgesics. There is now no justification for prescribing such combinations, partly because barbiturates antagonize the effects of pain-relieving drugs and also because, even if small doses are taken, prolonged use may easily lead to tolerance and psychological dependence. Physical addiction is a real hazard. Especially in the older patient, who suffers from chronic or intermittent pain, barbiturates, with or without concurrent analgesics, are not indicated: confusion, oversedation, and hangover are regular unwanted effects especially in this group. Adequate daily dosage of a single analgesic of the appropriate type and at the suitable dose level will obviate the need to 'buffer' simple pain-killers with any barbiturate.

▲ Of the preparations listed below, the usual dose is 1 or 2 tablets or capsules two or three times daily.

★ Contra-indicated in severe liver, kidney and respiratory illness, in porphyria, and in cases of known hypersensitivity to any barbiturate. Allobarbitone in any form is not advised for patients with a history of drug abuse. In addition to enhancing the actions of other central depressants (tranquillizers, opiates, and alcohol, among others), barbiturates should not be given concurrently with MAO-inhibitor antidepressants, certain anticoagulants, or with the contraceptive Pill.

➤ For further information, see Essay III and Chart III(A): Barbiturates.

◆ USA:

Dialog (Ciba): Tabs allobarbitone 15 mg, paracetamol (acetaminophen) 300 mg

Allylgesic (Elder): Tabs allobarbitone 15 mg, aspirin 150 mg, aluminium aspirin 100 mg, paracetamol (acetaminophen) 100 mg

Allylgesic with Ergotamine (Elder): Tabs allobarbitone 15 mg, aspirin 150 mg, aluminium aspirin 100 mg, paracetamol 100 mg, ergotamine tartrate 1 mg

ALPHAPRODINE R

● Alphaprodine is a narcotic analgesic derived from PETHIDINE (MEPERIDINE), to which it is similar in most respects. Although it has been tried for relief of postoperative pain, its short duration of action (½–1 hour) almost precludes its use for the majority of pain states. This compound is chiefly used in obstetrics, to relieve labour pains: for this purpose it is said to offer some advantages over the standard drug, pethidine, by depressing respiration less and by provoking fewer adverse effects. It is unclear whether these claims are justified. However, its brief action may make it more suitable than other opiates to relax the patient before diagnostic procedures such as bronchoscopy and cystoscopy; to relieve the acute pain of renal or biliary colic, which arises from gall- and kidney-stones; and in anaesthesia, as an adjunct to nitrous oxide. Common adverse effects are drowsiness, dizziness, euphoria or dysphoria, nausea, and constipation. Like other analogues of morphine and pethidine, this drug binds to receptor sites in the brain which are specific for opiate-type agents. Since alphaprodine, in common with almost all very potent analgesics, in some patients promotes a feeling of well-being (euphoria), it theoretically carries the risk of habituation and addiction characteristic of these compounds. Although few cases of such dependence have been reported, the hazard should be borne in mind if regular use of the drug is contemplated.

▲ Initially, up to 60 mg by subcutaneous or 30 mg by intravenous injection, depending on the clinical situation and other factors. Subsequently, one quarter of the original dose may be repeated after 20–30 minutes. The manufacturers recommend an upper limit of 240 mg per 24 hours. The drug may not be taken orally.

★ This compound increases the CNS and respiratory depressant effects of other drugs, such as barbiturates, tranquillizers and alcohol. Its use is not advised in cases of elevated intracranial pressure (e.g. in head injury), severe liver disorders, and respiratory distress. Alphaprodine must not be given concurrently with narcotic antagonists or partial antagonists except in emergency, nor with MAO-inhibitor antidepressants.

➤ For further information, see Essay IV and Chart IV: Morphine and Other Potent Analgesics.

◆ USA:
Alphaprodine Hydrochloride Injection USP: available as
Nisentil (Roche): Amps 40 & 60 mg/1 ml; Vials 600 mg/10 ml

AMITRIPTYLINE

● The first of the tricyclic antidepressants to be made commercially available, amitriptyline remains the most extensively prescribed of these compounds. It is indicated to relieve depressive conditions of various types, though it is by no means effective in all cases and may indeed exacerbate very profound depression. Unlike most other types of psychotropic agent, antidepressants of this class must be taken for between 3 and 6 weeks before relief of symptoms is apparent. However, amitriptyline may provoke other effects within 2–3 days. High doses tend to be sedative, and it has become customary for many practitioners to recommend a single daily dose at bedtime rather than the more conventional divided dosages. In addition to its antidepressive effect, the drug may be useful in treatment of asthma, in conjunction with inhaler bronchodilators; in childhood enuresis, or bed-wetting; and in psychotic illnesses, in combination with a major tranquilizer (antipsychotic). The use of antidepressant-tranquilizer combination products, which contain a fixed dose of each ingredient, is not pharmacologically sound. One of the most popular of these preparations is that containing amitriptyline with the antipsychotic perphenazine, which has been promoted to control symptoms of anxiety and tension, as well as depression, in general practice. This is usually not an appropriate treatment except in certain very severe psychological disturbances. The characteristic side-effects of tricyclic antidepressants – dry mouth, gastro-intestinal upsets, blurred vision, sedation, urinary hesitancy – are likely to be intensified by major tranquilizers. In recent years it has been shown that amitriptyline and similar antidepressants are much more toxic than was previously supposed, and they are very dangerous in overdosage. Pre-existing depression may be enhanced in some cases, with obvious hazards.

▲ Dosage must be tailored to meet individual requirements. At first, 75 mg per day is suggested, increasing over weeks to an average of 150 mg/day. The regimen is then adjusted upwards or downwards as appropriate, up to 300 mg/day.

★ Amitriptyline should not be used in cases of urinary retention, epilepsy, glaucoma, and severe liver disease. Very special caution in any form of cardiac complaint. Among the drugs to be avoided for concurrent use are amphetamines and all other appetite-suppressants; MAO-inhibitor antidepressants; and dosage of anticoagulants and anti-hypertensive drugs may require modification.

➤ For further information, see Essay II and Chart II: Antidepressants.

◆ UK:
Amitriptyline (Hydrochloride) Tablets BPC: 10, 25 & 50 mg
Amitriptyline (Hydrochloride) Injection BPC: Vials 100 mg/10 ml
Amitriptyline (Embonate) Elixir BPC: 10 mg/5 ml
Domical (Berk): Tabs 10, 25 & 50 mg
Lentizol (Warner): SR Caps 25 & 50 mg
Saroten (Warner): Tabs 10 & 25 mg
Tryptizol (MSD): Tabs 10, 25 & 50 mg; SR Caps 75 mg; Elix 10 mg/5 ml; Vials 100 mg/10 ml
— with PERPHENAZINE:
Triptafen (Allen & Hanbury): Tabs 25 + 2 mg; 10 + 2 mg; 25 + 4 mg; Syrup 25 + 2 mg/5 ml

USA:
Amitriptyline Hydrochloride Tablets USP: 10, 25, 50, 75 & 100 mg
Amitriptyline Hydrochloride Injection USP: Vials 100 mg/10 ml
Amitid (Squibb): Tabs 10, 25, 50, 75 & 100 mg
Amitril (Parke Davis): Tabs 10, 25, 50, 75, 100 & 150 mg
Elavil (MSD): Tabs 10, 25, 50, 75, 100 & 150 mg; Vials 100 mg/10 ml
Endep (Roche): Tabs 10, 25, 50, 75, 100 & 150 mg
SK-Amitriptyline (Smith Kline & French): Tabs 10, 25, 50, 75, 100 & 150 mg
— with PERPHENAZINE:
Etrafon (Schering): Tabs 25 + 2 mg; 10 + 2 mg; 25 + 4 mg
Triavil (MSD): Tabs 25 + 2 mg; 10 + 4 mg; 25 + 4 mg
See also under CHLORDIAZEPOXIDE (Limbitrol)

AMPHETAMINE (1-AMPHETAMINE) R

● Amphetamine is a highly potent stimulant of the central nervous system. On a weight-for-weight basis, it is slightly less effective than its dextro-isomer DEXAMPHETAMINE (DEXTROAMPHETAMINE), which is more frequently prescribed. Traditionally, amphetamine has been a remedy for obesity, because it reduces appetite. This action, however, is short-lived, wearing off almost completely within a few weeks. The energetic euphoria which amphetamine and related stimulants provoke makes these compounds widely abused. Whether physical addiction develops after repeated use is open to question, but tolerance develops quickly and psychological dependency occurs readily, not just in those who are commonly regarded as being 'predisposed' to drug abuse. Because of these risks, and the fact that chronic amphetamine use may induce a mental condition akin to psychosis, the therapeutic indications of amphetamine are limited. If the drug is prescribed in obesity, it should be for a few weeks only, and as an adjunct to strict diet and exercise: even then, alternative drugs are available with considerably less dependence potential. The use of amphetamine to relieve short-term depression is unjustified, not least because, as the action of the drug wears off, depressive states are experienced as part of the 'come-down'. The compound is still extensively prescribed in the childhood hyperkinetic syndrome, an overdiagnosed condition characterized by over-activity, poor attention span, and difficulty in learning. Administration of stimulants to relieve this condition is controversial and recent studies suggest that amphetamine may be of little benefit. The only genuine therapeutic application, according to some authorities, for use of the compound is in narcolepsy, a fairly rare ailment, sufferers from which are pathologically unable to remain awake despite normal amounts of sleep. Unwanted effects include nervousness, hyperexcitability, gastro-intestinal disturbances, and palpitations.

▲ In narcolepsy, the usual dose range is 2.5–10 mg two or three times daily. The last dose should be taken before 4 p.m.; otherwise sleep is likely to be disturbed.

★ Amphetamine should be avoided for patients who suffer from hypertension, heart disease, hyperthyroidism and severe kidney disorders, and in cases of insomnia, depression, anxiety and agitation. The agent should not be taken concurrently with tricyclic or MAO-inhibitor antidepressants; antipsychotic drugs, including lithium; reserpine and other drugs given to control hypertension; and alcohol.

➤ For further information, see Essay I and Chart I: Amphetamines. See also under DEXAMPHETAMINE

◆ UK:
Amphetamine Sulphate Tablets BPC: 5 mg (not available)
    USA:
Amphetamine Sulfate Tablets USP: available as
Benzedrine (Smith Kline & French): Tabs 5 & 10 mg, SR Caps 15 mg

AMYL NITRITE

● A volatile liquid, this compound is principally used in the emergency treatment of angina pectoris, though now much less often than previously: for this purpose it has been superseded by other cardiac drugs. Amyl nitrite is sometimes also given to control convulsions, such as those caused by strychnine or arsenic poisoning; to relieve asthmatic paroxysms; and in renal colic. The compound acts by dilating the blood-vessels, improving circulation and thus providing symptomatic pain relief. It has a more general stimulant action: this is shown by a transient but definite euphoria, associated with hot flushing, rapid heartbeat (tachycardia) and, if excessive quantities are taken, headache, sweating, watering of the eyes and coloured lights in front of the eyes may be experienced. The claim that amyl nitrite is an aphrodisiac has been discredited. Indeed, the drug, so far from improving sexual performance, may produce impotence immediately following usage. The formulation for this agent is unusual: it is presented in small glass capsules, called *vitrellae,* which are surrounded by cotton-wool. The vitrella is crushed between thumb and finger and the vapour inhaled. Effect is almost instantaneous, lasting some 3–5 minutes, after which dosage should be repeated as necessary. This extremely short duration of action limits the drug's usefulness.

▲ The contents of 1 or 2 vitrellae (0.2–0.6 ml) inhaled; repeat as necessary.

★ Amyl nitrite is highly inflammable. The drug should not be given to patients suffering from head injury, raised intracranial pressure or similar traumatic conditions, and is contra-indicated in glaucoma, as it raises pressure within the eye. Concurrent administration of other stimulants, e.g. AMPHETAMINE, is not advised except in emergency.

◆ UK:
Amyl Nitrite Vitrellae BPC: 0.2 & 0.3 ml
   USA:
Amyl Nitrite Inhalant USP: available as
Aspirol Amyl Nitrite (Lilly): Vitrellae 0.18 & 0.3 ml
Vaporole Amyl Nitrite (Burroughs Wellcome): Vitrellae 0.18 & 0.3 ml

AMYLOBARBITONE (AMOBARBITAL) and AMYLOBARBITONE SODIUM

● This typical member of the barbiturate class, which has an effective duration of activity of 6–8 hours, is prescribed both to promote sleep and for daytime sedation. For the latter indication preparations are available in which amylobarbitone is combined with simple analgesics: these are obsolete and may be dangerous, insofar as insidious dependency, psychological and/or physical, may develop with repeated use. Habituation is even more likely if the drug is taken regularly at hypnotic doses. The anticonvulsant action of barbiturates may be of benefit in preventing epileptic attacks, though more modern, safer anti-epileptic agents have been produced. Combination products which combine amylobarbitone with another barbiturate, such as quinalbarbitone in the widely available Tuinal capsule, are to be avoided, because the effects of each are duplicated. Preparations which contain amylobarbitone and dexamphetamine have no therapeutic justification: the addition of a barbiturate to potent stimulants of the amphetamine type, of which numerous tablets and capsules are marketed in the USA and elsewhere (though not in the UK), simply increases the risk of a dual dependency. The intention of such combination products is to mitigate the excitatory actions of the stimulant, as this might be prescribed in cases of obesity; but the result is usually a different kind of euphoria, which makes Dexamyl and similar products popular for illicit use. It is generally agreed that, like other barbiturates, amylobarbitone has such a high potential for abuse and dependency that it is unsuitable in the treatment of insomnia, for which other, less hazardous alternatives are available. Adverse effects are common, and include hangover, oversedation, impaired concentration, and paradoxical excitement. The sodium salt of amylobarbitone is more quickly eliminated from the system than the basic compound.

▲ As a hypnotic, 50–100 mg at bedtime. For daytime sedation, 15–50 mg two or (in exceptional cases) three times daily.

★ Amylobarbitone is contra-indicated in porphyria, severe liver and respiratory disorders; known hypersensitivity to any barbiturate; and for administration to individuals considered likely to abuse drugs. Patients who are thought to be suicide-prone should not be given barbiturates. Concurrent use with MAO-inhibitor antidepressants, oral anticoagulants, oral contraceptives, and alcohol may be dangerous.

➤ For further information on precautions and other aspects, see Essay III and Chart III: Barbiturates.

◆ NOTE: Preparations containing small doses of barbiturates in conjunction with other substances are listed in Table 4.

UK:

Amylobarbitone Tablets BPC: 15, 30, 50, 60, 100 & 200 mg

Amytal (Lilly): Tabs 15, 30, 100 & 200 mg

Amylomet (Larkhall): Tabs amylobarbitone 30 mg, emetine 0.2 mg; also amylobarbitone 100 mg, emetine 0.6 mg

Amylobarbitone Sodium Tablets BPC: 60 & 200 mg

Amylobarbitone Sodium Capsules BPC: 60 & 200 mg

Amylobarbitone (Sodium) Injection BPC: Dry Amps 250 mg/ml

Sodium Amytal (Lilly): Tabs & Caps 60 & 200 mg; Dry Amps 250 mg/1 ml & 500 mg/2 ml

Tuinal (Lilly): Caps amylobarbitone sodium 50 mg, quinalbarbitone (secobarbital) sodium 50 mg; also 100 + 100 mg

USA:

Amobarbital Tablets USP: 15, 30, 50 & 100 mg

Amobarbital Elixir USP: 22 mg/5 ml

Amytal (Lilly): Tabs 15, 30, 50 & 100 mg; Elix 22 mg/5 ml & 44 mg/5 ml

Amobarbital-D-Lay (Lemmon): SR Tabs 60 mg

Amesec (Lilly): Tabs & Caps amylobarbitone 25 mg, ephedrine hydrochloride 25 mg, aminophylline 130 mg

Aminophylline + Amytal (Lilly): Caps amylobarbitone 32 mg, aminophylline 100 mg

Ectasule (Fleming): Caps amylobarbitone 8 mg, ephedrine sulphate 15 mg; also 15 + 30 mg & 30 + 60 mg

Amobarbital Sodium Capsules USP: 65 & 200 mg

Sterile Amobarbital Sodium USP: Dry Amps 125, 250 & 500 mg

Amytal Sodium (Lilly): Caps 65 & 200 mg; Dry Amps 125, 250 & 500 mg; Suppos 200 mg

Tuinal (Lilly): as UK

NOTE: Numerous products which contain small amounts of amylobarbitone in combination with other, non-psychotropic agents, are marketed in the USA: only those listed above, however, are extensively prescribed.

See also under DEXAMPHETAMINE (DEXTROAMPHETAMINE)

ANILERIDINE R

● Anileridine is one of several derivatives of PETHIDINE (MEPERIDINE), which has been claimed to possess advantages over the parent drug. This compound, marketed only in the USA, is a powerful narcotic analgesic, and is administered for relief of labour pains and as an adjunct to general anaesthetics. Generally its effects closely resemble those of pethidine, though it is said to be less of a respiratory depressant, and like its prototype has a duration of effect of 2–4 hours following injection. Side-effects are typical of opiates, and may include sedation, nausea, headache, itching, and dizziness: mood changes (euphoria and dysphoria) do not seem to be marked. Nevertheless, because of its pharmacological profile anileridine should be considered potentially a drug of addiction, like morphine and pethidine. In common with other narcotic pain-killers, this compound is much more effective on a weight basis by injection than by mouth.

▲ Depending on the severity of the condition, and other factors such as individual idiosyncrasy, recommended doses are: 25–75 mg orally, every 2–4 hours. By intravenous or intramuscular injection, 25–100 mg at similar intervals.

★ This compound must be used with great caution when there is depression of vital functions (e.g. respiration), in cases of severe liver damage, in convulsive disorders, and in acute alcoholism. Tolerance to the analgesic effects of anileridine has been shown in a number of studies to develop quickly, and the risk of dependence should be borne in mind. The drug enhances the action of other CNS depressants, including barbiturates, tranquillizers, and alcohol. It should not be prescribed at the same time as MAO-inhibitor antidepressants; or narcotic antagonists or partial antagonists, except under close supervision, as withdrawal symptoms may be provoked.

➔ For further information, see Essay IV and Chart IV: Morphine and Other Potent Analgesics.

◆ USA:
Anileridine Hydrochloride Tablets USP &
Anileridine Phosphate Injection USP: available as
Leritine (Merck Sharp & Dohme): Tabs 25 mg; Amps 25 mg/1 ml & 50 mg/2 ml

APOMORPHINE

● This compound is a partial narcotic antagonist, i.e. it possesses some capacity to reverse the effects of morphine and similar 'agonists' and also a measure of opiate-like actions. In practice it has been found that apomorphine cannot be used as an analgesic because at doses that would be effective for pain relief a whole range of unacceptable adverse reactions occurs: rapid fall in blood-pressure (hypotension), dizziness, headache and depressed mood (dysphoria) are among these. Even small doses tend to make the patient nauseous, and it is for the drug's emetic action that it is given therapeutically. Poisoning with a number of drugs may be treated with apomorphine, provided that it is administered very soon after overdosage has taken place. As an antidote to opiate overdoses the compound is unsatisfactory, because it is liable to add to the respiratory depression already present in such cases. Historically apomorphine has been used as a sedative and in treatment of opiate addiction. The drug is seldom prescribed today because, except to provoke vomiting, more reliable and less toxic alternatives are available: for example, narcotic overdosage can be handled with NALOXONE, a pure antagonist of morphine-like agents with very few adverse effects, or with the partial antagonists LEVALLORPHAN and NALORPHINE.

▲ Since apomorphine is ineffective orally, it must be given by injection, usually by the subcutaneous route. As an emetic, the usual dose is 5–8 mg, preceded by 200–300 ml of water administered by mouth or via a nasogastric tube. Apomorphine is not stable in solution: solutions in ampoule form are manufactured in the UK but these have a short shelf-life and the colourless liquid turns green when unstable. In the USA hypodermic tablets are used instead: these are dissolved in sterile water.

★ Contra-indications include deep coma, shock, treatment of poisoning

with corrosive metals, and in convulsive states. Large doses may precipitate convulsions, cardiac arrest and death. Patients who have been
receiving morphine-like analgesics regularly should not be given apomorphine, as severe withdrawal reactions are likely to be provoked.

➤ For further information on narcotic antagonists, see Essay IV and
Chart IV: Morphine and Other Potent Analgesics.

◆ UK:
Apomorphine Hydrochloride Injection BPC: Amps 3 mg/1 ml
   USA:
Apomorphine Hydrochloride Tablets USP: Hypodermic Tabs 6 mg

APROBARBITONE (APROBARBITAL)

● Like AMYLOBARBITONE (AMOBARBITAL), the above-named
drug is characteristic of barbiturate hypnotics and sedatives. Because it is
presented only as a flavoured elixir aprobarbitone has superficial attrac-
tions for administration to children and the elderly. However, like all oral
barbiturates this one has a high potential for abuse and psychological
and/or physical habituation. The two groups of patients referred to are
particularly susceptible to the drug's regular adverse effects, such as
confusion, oversedation, hangover, and impairment of reflexes. Whether
for daytime or night sedation compounds of this type have been superseded by newer, safer remedies, including drugs of the benzodiazepine
class (e.g. TEMAZEPAM). The potential for suicidal use is higher for the
available liquid preparation than for tablet or capsule formulations of
barbiturates.

▲ For daytime sedation: 20–40 mg twice daily. Although the manufacturers may recommend a third or even a fourth daily dose this is seldom if
ever necessary. To promote sleep: 80–160 mg.

★ Aprobarbitone, like other barbiturates, is contra-indicated in porphyria, respiratory insufficiency, severe liver disease, and in cases of known
or suspected hypersensitivity to any barbiturate. The drug increases the
centrally depressant actions of tranquillizers, strong analgesics, and
alcohol. It should not be taken concurrently with MAO-inhibitor antidepressants, coumarin anticoagulants, or the contraceptive Pill.

➤ For further information on precautions, etc., see Essay III and Chart
III: Barbiturates.

◆ USA:
Aprobarbital Elixir USNF 1970: available as
Alurate (Roche): Elix 40 mg/5 ml

BARBITONE (BARBITAL) and BARBITONE SODIUM

● Barbitone and its sodium salt are, with PHENOBARBITONE, the longest-acting members of the barbiturate series of compounds. Effective duration of action may exceed 24 hours, and it is several days before a single dose of this drug is eliminated from the system. All barbiturates have a high potential for abuse and addiction: in the case of the long-acting ones these hazards are augmented by the fact that regular administration causes a build-up in the body of quantities of drug which may be toxic and even life-threatening. It is principally for this reason that barbitone use has declined sharply, and official preparations of the compound have been deleted from the major pharmacopoeias. Nevertheless, some prescribers continue to give barbitone as a soporific or daytime sedative, which with the risk of accumulation is even less acceptable than the administration of shorter-acting barbiturates such as AMYLO-BARBITONE (AMOBARBITAL). The only legitimate therapeutic role for barbitone is to prevent the occurrence of fits in epilepsy, though in this indication PHENOBARBITONE is preferred.

▲ In epilepsy, 150–300 mg not more than twice daily. To promote sleep: 200–450 mg. As a daytime sedative: 45–135 mg once or twice daily.

★ The typical side-effects of barbiturates are frequently experienced with barbitone: in particular, reflexes may be significantly slowed, and confusion and oversedation may give rise to dangerous situations. Barbitone is unacceptable, because of its slow rate of excretion, in severe liver or kidney disease, and in porphyria, and respiratory or cardiac insufficiency. Apart from barbiturates' tendency to increase the CNS depressant activity of other drugs, their effects on the liver are likely to alter response to anticoagulants, antidepressants, oral contraceptives and other agents. Despite the fact that barbitone appears on a schedule in US legislation which suggests that it is less dangerous than AMYLOBARBITONE and shorter-acting compounds, this is not so; and prolonged use should be avoided as it is just as likely to lead to dependency.

➤ For further information on drug interactions, warnings, etc., see Essay III and Chart III: Barbiturates.

◆ UK:
Barbitone Tablets BP 1970: 300 & 450 mg
Barbitone Sodium Tablets BP 1973: 300 & 450 mg
    USA:
unbranded Barbital Tabs (Lilly): 300 mg
Plexonal (Sandoz): Tabs barbitone sodium 45 mg, phenobarbitone sodium 15 mg, butalbital sodium 25 mg, scopolamine hydrobromide

0.08 mg, dihydroergotamine mesylate 0.16 mg; also 135 + 45 + 75 + 0.48 + 0.24 mg

BEMEGRIDE

● This drug is prescribed as a respiratory stimulant, whose sole clinical indication is in the treatment of barbiturate overdosage: here bemegride may be given in conjunction with other antidotes, by injection. Although the compound has more general central stimulant effects it has not been found liable to abuse. The US Food and Drug Administration has ruled that bemegride is ineffective in reversing the respiratory depressant and other features of barbiturate poisoning, but one of the present authors has found the drug of use in the treatment of mild cases, not only of overdosing with barbiturates, but with other hypnotics (e.g. METHA-QUALONE) also. Adverse effects are generally mild at recommended doses, though excessive dosage levels may cause twitching of the eyelids, fingers, and muscles, and in a few instances visual or auditory hallucinations and convulsions.

▲ 50 mg by intravenous injection, every 5–10 minutes until regular breathing is restored. The maximum recommended dose is 1 G. Now that more effective respiratory stimulants (e.g. nikethamide, Coramine) are available, bemegride has very limited usefulness.

★ Extreme caution must be exercised in cases of severe heart disease, and also if other stimulants of any sort are given concurrently.

◆ UK:
Megimide (Nicholas): Amps 50 mg/10 ml

BENACTYZINE

● This versatile and under-utilized compound has both antidepressant and anxiety-relieving properties. However, chemically it belongs to none of the classes associated with such actions. Benactyzine has been recommended to relieve phobias and obsessional states, some psychosomatic disorders such as 'nervous' eczema and other skin diseases, and certain types of asthma. At high doses there is some evidence that the drug is effective in controlling Parkinson's disease. Unfortunately benactyzine is no longer marketed as a single entity, but only in combination with the tranquillizer MEPROBAMATE. The latter seems to enhance its anxiety-relieving effect, and it lengthens meprobamate's short (3–5 hour) duration of action. While the sedative effect of meprobamate will be experienced almost immediately, the antidepressant activity of benactyzine will be apparent after 7–10 days. Dizziness, dry mouth, sleep disturbances, and other unwanted effects tend to occur at the beginning of therapy. In rare cases, the drug has at high doses produced depersonalization, euphoria, and other unusual psychological states. Some degree of dependency has been reported but this is uncommon. Most of the adverse reactions promoted by benactyzine are enhanced by the addition of meprobamate.

▲ Of the available Deprol preparation, 1 or 2 tablets 3 or 4 times daily, the dose raised gradually to 3 tablets twice or thrice daily, according to response. The compound is best taken after meals.

★ Particularly in conjunction with meprobamate, this drug may affect concentration. A black market in benactyzine has recently developed in the USA because of its supposed hallucinogenic activity, and the drug is known as DMZ: evidence for such effects is non-existent. Contra-indicated in severe neurotic and psychotic conditions; in glaucoma; known hypersensitivity; porphyria; and in patients who are to undergo ECT (shock) therapy.

➤ For further information on additional side-effects, warnings for meprobamate etc., see Essay VI and Chart VI(A): Tranquillizers.

◆ USA:
Deprol (Wallace): Tabs benactyzine 1 mg, meprobamate 400 mg

BENPERIDOL

● Benperidol is an antipsychotic tranquillizer closely related to HALOPERIDOL (Serenace, Haldol), the prototype of the butyrophenone class of drugs. These compounds are generally used to control the symptoms of very severe, psychotic mental disturbance. However, benperidol has been proposed by its manufacturers for the treatment of 'deviant', antisocial sexual behaviour, such as paedophilia (sexual desire for children), compulsive public exhibitionism and masturbation, and other acts considered socially unacceptable. The problem here is that there is apparently no evidence that the drug exerts a specific anti-aphrodisiac effect: rather, it has a more generalized damping-down action on the central nervous system, often provoking states of lassitude, apathy, fatigue and mental depression. Now whether exhibitionists, for instance, are 'psychotic' is questionable; and if they are not it appears to the present writers strange that so potent an antipsychotic agent is prescribed to control sexual behaviour. Neuroleptic tranquillizers of the haloperidol type, in addition to producing the effects described, commonly provoke a form of Parkinson's disease which patients are almost bound to find alarming. Pre-existing depression is frequently intensified by these drugs. Protracted use brings with it the risk of tardive dyskinesia, an insidious and in some cases irreversible severe form of parkinsonism, affecting motor and muscular co-ordination. Benperidol is not universally effective in suppressing sexuality; and if it is absolutely necessary to reduce or abolish libido, a hormonal compound recently developed, cyproterone (Androcur), may be more suitable. Given that many patients who are sexually 'deviant' are already in a state of depression, the likely psychological effects of benperidol, as of most antipsychotic medicaments, should be borne carefully in mind.

▲ The normal outpatient dose is 0.25–1.5 mg per day, usually in two doses. In hospital inpatients who are severely psychotic, up to 10 mg/day has been given.

★ Because benperidol at high doses tends to cause jaundice, it is recommended that regular blood-counts and liver-function tests be performed. Contra-indications include bone-marrow depression; convulsive disorders; and severe liver, kidney or cardiac complaints. This compound enhances the effects of other CNS depressants, including alcohol; it should not be given at the same time as amphetamines or other stimulants; pethidine, morphine and similar narcotics; or MAO-inhibitor antidepressants.

➤ For further information on warnings, contra-indications, etc., see Essay VI and Chart VI(B): Antipsychotic Tranquillizers.

◆ UK:
Anquil (Janssen): Tabs 0.25 mg

BENZOCTAMINE

● Benzoctamine combines some of the most useful attributes of the tranquillizers and of the antidepressants. In mild to moderate depression, especially when accompanied by tension and anxiety, the drug has been compared favourably with AMITRIPTYLINE and with other antidepressants of the tricyclic class. Hyperagitation and excitability are symptoms which apparently respond to treatment with benzoctamine, which is chemically much more closely related to the amphetamines than to other groups of psychotropic agents. This compound has muscle-relaxant and moderate sedative activity, and may be a useful remedy for 'nervous' insomnia. True antidepressant effects, if these do occur, will be experienced after about 7–10 days' treatment. Side-effects are generally mild: oversedation, dry mouth, and abdominal upsets have been reported, particularly at the beginning of therapy with this drug.

▲ Usually, 10–20 mg three times daily. A single nightly dose of 30–40 mg may help in cases of anxious insomnia. The recommended maximum daily dose is 60 mg.

★ Very severe depressive states may be intensified by benzoctamine, and the compound is ineffective in psychotic illness. It should be avoided by patients with severe liver or kidney disorders, and during pregnancy.

Concomitant use of amphetamines or other stimulants and of MAO-inhibitor antidepressants is contra-indicated.

> For further information, see Essay II and Chart II: Antidepressants.

◆ UK:
Tacitin (Ciba): Tabs 10 mg (hydrochloride)

BENZPHETAMINE R

● This amphetamine derivative is prescribed for its appetite-suppressant action in cases of obesity. Its prescription should be limited to a few weeks, as tolerance to this effect wears off quickly, and then given only as an adjunct to strict dieting and exercise. Although benzphetamine is no longer marketed in the UK, it appears on the schedules of Controlled Drugs, which indicates that it has some capacity for abuse. Most amphetamine derivatives, including this one, are central nervous system stimulants. Benzphetamine is not as potent as DEXAMPHETAMINE in this respect, but especially at high doses it does produce a qualitatively similar kind of energetic euphoria. Unwanted effects include restlessness, nausea, diarrhoea, tremor, sweating, and palpitations (tachycardia). In the USA, where the drug is available, its abuse potential has probably been underestimated.

▲ Average 12.5–25 mg twice daily. A third dose may be necessary in some cases: this should not be taken later than 4 p.m. if insomnia is to be avoided.

★ Contra-indicated in severe cardiac disorders, hypertension, hyper-thyroidism, and for use by patients who are agitated or hyperexcitable. Protracted use at high doses may lead to amphetamine-type dependency and paranoid-type mental states. Benzphetamine should not be prescribed for individuals with a history of drug abuse, and should be withdrawn slowly if dependence has developed.

> For further information on appetite-suppressants, see Essay I and Chart I: Amphetamines.

◆ USA:
Benzphetamine Hydrochloride Tablets USNF 1970: available as
Didrex (Upjohn): Tabs 25 & 50 mg

BROMISOVALUM (BROMISOVALERYL UREA)

● An analogue of CARBROMAL, bromisovalum was developed from the original, and now obsolete, bromide sedative/hypnotic agents. It is one of the oldest soporifics still available, and is still occasionally used for daytime sedation and to promote sleep. Its administration for relief of anxiety is no longer appropriate, as the less toxic and more selectively-acting minor tranquillizers fulfil this function. A disadvantage of bromisovalum is its short duration of action (2–4 hours). Attempts have been made to circumvent this by addition of similar, but longer-lasting, drugs such as ACETYLCARBROMAL to tablet formulations. Regular taking of the compound may lead to psychological and/or physical habituation, and tolerance develops readily. High doses administered repeatedly may cause rapid fall in blood-pressure (hypotension), confusion, and delirium.

▲ 150–350 mg 3–4 hourly for daytime use; as a hypnotic: 600–900 mg.

★ Accumulation of drug in the body, after regular use, may be dangerous. The compound should not be given in cases of severe respiratory illness, impaired liver or kidney function, and to persons known to be hypersensitive to bromisovalum or its analogues ACETYLCARBROMAL and CARBROMAL. The central and respiratory depressant effects of barbiturates, tranquillizers, opiate analgesics and alcohol are likely to be increased. Other precautions: as for BARBITURATES.

➤ For further information see Essay III and Chart III: Barbiturates.

◆ USA:
Isomel (Tutag): Caps bromisovalum 100 mg, acetylcarbromal 150 mg, paracetamol (acetaminophen) 300 mg
Tranquinal (Barnes-Hind): Tabs bromisovalum 250 mg, acetylcarbromal 130 mg, scopolamine hydrobromide 0.1 mg
Vannor (North American Pharmacal): Caps bromisovalum 100 mg, acetylcarbromal 150 mg, paracetamol (acetaminophen) 300 mg

BUFOTENINE **R**

● Bufotenine is a drug which is available neither for prescription in any country nor, so far as the present authors are aware, on the black market anywhere. Nevertheless, it is one of a small group of compounds which under US and British law are more stringently restricted than any other: it is theoretically accessible to researchers who must apply for a special licence to use or administer it. The group concerned comprises LYSERGIDE (LSD) and a number of its analogues. Bufotenine has been legally controlled probably because of its chemical similarity to DMT. These compounds are psychedelics, also known as hallucinogens and psychotomimetics. Bufotenine is an alkaloid found in *Piptadenia peregrina* and other plants native to Central and South America; it also occurs, rather astonishingly, in the secretions of the marine toad *Bufo marinus*. Its effects have been very little studied in man, but there seems no doubt that these are qualitatively similar to those produced by LSD. According to one study, in which volunteers received an intravenous injection of

bufotenine 8–16 mg, visual distortions, spatial and temporal disorientation, 'hallucinations' and other typically psychedelic reactions were
experienced. Why investigators choose the intravenous route when testing
these drugs, which have extraordinary and profound effects on perception, one fails to understand. Since the drug is apparently ineffective if
taken by mouth – like DMT it is substantially broken down by the
stomach acids – the alternatives are administration by injection or via a
mucous membrane. Indeed, the local people of parts of South America
take *Piptadenia* extracts by snuffing. If injection is the preferred mode,
intramuscular rather than intravenous administration will probably soften
the impact of the sensory overload: psychological effects will then be
apparent after 10–20 minutes. Studies of the compound's activity in
laboratory animals have yielded equivocal results. It is obvious that
bufotenine deserves further study. Advice on whether or how to take it is
at present academic, but if it should become available in the near future
the recommendations laid down for use of LYSERGIDE (LSD) should
apply.

> For an account of this class of drugs, see Essay V and Chart V:
Psychedelics.

BUPRENORPHINE

● Until about fifteen years ago, when a potent analgesic was required, a
narcotic 'agonist' such as MORPHINE or PETHIDINE (MEPERIDINE)
would be used as a matter of course; for although partial narcotic
antagonists like NALORPHINE, which reverses some of the effects of
morphine-like agents, were known to have pain-relieving activity, their
extremely unpleasant side-effects precluded their use. Then in the mid
1960s PENTAZOCINE was introduced: this was a partial narcotic
antagonist, i.e. if given to persons addicted to morphine or another
agonist, it would be likely to provoke withdrawal symptoms. Pentazocine
was found to relieve pain, though not the most severe states, with fewer
untoward effects than previous antagonists. It was further believed that
because the compound was an antagonist, it would *per se* not be liable to
abuse and addiction. Unfortunately there is now firm evidence that
pentazocine dependency does occur, though there are arguments about
the extent of this. The point is that research towards the ideal, potent,
non-addictive analgesic, which has been going on for many years, has
lately become concentrated on partial narcotic antagonists. Buprenorphine has been available for only three years in the UK, and has been
shown to be effective in alleviating postoperative pain, myocardial
infarction ('coronary thrombosis'), and to some extent in terminal cancer.
The research to date suggests that buprenorphine may be comparable to
morphine for pain relief, but with much less dependence potential.

Drowsiness, dizziness, and a light euphoria are the commonest reported side-effects, while large doses of the drug provoke nausea, vomiting, and respiratory depression. One clear advantage over conventional opiates is buprenorphine's long duration of action (6–8 hours), significantly greater than that of morphine. However, it is too early to make categorical statements regarding questions such as tolerance and capacity for abuse and addiction: as in the case of pentazocine, these may have been underestimated.

▲ Average adult dose: 0.3–0.6 mg by intramuscular or slow intravenous injection, repeated 6–8 hourly. At this writing only injectable formulations are available.

★ A significant snag with this drug is that, unlike other partial antagonists, buprenorphine cannot be antagonized by NALOXONE. Contra-indications include respiratory distress, severe liver ailments, and use during labour and in pregnancy. It should not be given concurrently with morphine or any similar opiate agonist.

➤ For further information, see Essay IV, Chart IV: Morphine and Other Potent Analgesics, and Addenda, p. 455.

◆ UK:
Temgesic (Reckitt & Colman): Amps 0.3 mg/1 ml & 0.6 mg/2 ml, Subling Tabs 0.2 mg

BUTALBITAL (ALLYLBARBITURIC ACID)

● This barbituric acid derivative is typical of the class of compounds, having sedative and hypnotic properties analogous to those of AMYLO-BARBITONE (AMOBARBITAL), similar adverse effects, and similar hazards of tolerance, abuse and dependency. The compound is not marketed in the UK, and in the USA is available only in tablet and capsule formulations which also contain the simple analgesics aspirin and paracetamol, usually with the gratuitous addition of caffeine. This combination of a barbiturate with analgesics is pharmacologically unsound, because sedatives of this type antagonize the effect of pain-relieving drugs. The continued availability of such products is surprising, as they have long been obsolete. If relief of chronic or intermittent pain is required, then analgesics of the appropriate type alone should be adequate. If in addition a sedative action is desired, there are now many alternatives to barbiturates. Continuous consumption of products of the kind listed here may easily result in insidious psychological and/or physical dependence, and adverse effects such as oversedation, confusion, and hangover, with consequent reflex impairment, may be expected.

▲ Manufacturers of the preparations available recommend 1–2 tablets or capsules two or three times daily.

★ The phenacetin component of these preparations is particularly undesirable, as this compound may damage the kidneys and cause anaemia. Because of the presence of butalbital, such products are contra-indicated in porphyria, severe liver or kidney disease, respiratory insufficiency, and known hypersensitivity to any barbiturate.

➤ For further information on precautions and interactions with other drugs, see Essay III and Chart III: Barbiturates (N.B. Table 4: Masked Barbiturates, pp.266–7).

◆ USA:
APC + Butalbital (Zenith): Tabs butalbital 50 mg, aspirin 200 mg, phenacetin 130 mg, caffeine 20 mg
Buff-A-Comp (Mayrand): Tabs butalbital 48.6 mg, aspirin 648 mg, caffeine 43.2 mg
Fiorinal (Sandoz): Tabs & Caps butalbital 50 mg, aspirin 200 mg, phenacetin 130 mg, caffeine 40 mg (also with codeine phosphate 7.5, 15 or 30 mg)

BUTAPERAZINE

● This is one of the most powerful antipsychotic drugs. It belongs to the phenothiazine class, of which CHLORPROMAZINE is the best-known member. Although not extensively used, butaperazine is sometimes prescribed to control aggression, hyperagitation and other symptoms of schizophrenia, usually for the psychiatric inpatient. While most compounds of this class produce or enhance mental depression, parkinsonian reactions, and anticholinergic effects such as dry mouth and blurred vision, butaperazine has the reputation of provoking these unwanted effects more often than other phenothiazines. This is a drug whose use should be reserved for the most severe forms of psychological disturbance, and it is unsuitable for treatment of minor emotional complaints. It is unlikely to possess any advantages over other antipsychotic agents of comparable potency.

▲ Outpatients: 10–30 mg per day, in 1 or 2 doses; hospitalized patients, up to a maximum of 100 mg daily, according to therapeutic response.

★ Butaperazine should be avoided in patients who are severely depressed; in bone-marrow depression; in cases of impaired liver function; and known sensitivity to any phenothiazine antipsychotic. Among the drugs to be avoided for concurrent use are antidepressants of the MAO-inhibitor class, some anti-hypertensive agents, and levodopa. The CNS-depressing actions of barbiturates, other tranquillizers, and potent analgesics, as well as of alcohol, will be increased.

➤ For further information, see Essay VI and Chart VI(B): Antipsychotic Tranquillizers.

◆ USA:
Repoise (Robins): Tabs 5, 10 & 25 mg

BUTOBARBITONE (BUTETHAL)

N.B. Not to be confused with butabarbital (SECBUTOBARBITONE)

● Butobarbitone will be familiar to older readers as the pink Soneryl tablet, which has been marketed in the UK for many years and remains one of the most popular hypnotics of the barbiturate class. The drug is prescribed primarily to promote sleep, and for this purpose a formulation also containing PROMETHAZINE is available. Its use, like that of other barbiturates, in conjunction with aspirin and other simple analgesics is today inappropriate, since the soporific may detract from the effect of these. More rational is a preparation comprising a hypnotic dose of butobarbitone and emetine, the main alkaloid of ipecacuanha: if more than the recommended dose of this is taken, vomiting will occur. The use of barbiturates in suicide is well-known and may be circumvented by prescription of one of these so-called 'barbemets'. However, regular taking of any barbiturate is inadvisable, partly because of the risk of dependency, and partly because oversedation, hangover and other unwanted effects are common. Alternative hypnotic drugs which lack the toxicity and abuse potential of butobarbitone and its analogues are available, and many practitioners feel that barbiturates should be avoided in the treatment of insomnia.

▲ Sleep: 50–200 mg at night. For use during the daytime, which is not indicated unless in exceptional circumstances, 30–60 mg two or at most three times daily.

★ Contra-indicated in severe respiratory and liver disorders and porphyria. Potentially serious interactions may arise between barbiturates and MAO-inhibitor antidepressants, oral anticoagulants, and oral contraceptives. Butobarbitone will increase the activity of other centrally depressant drugs, including alcohol.

➤ For further information, see Essay III and Chart III: Barbiturates.

◆ UK:
Butobarbitone Tablets BPC: 100 mg
Soneryl (May & Baker): Tabs 100 mg
Butomet (Larkhall): Tabs butobarbitone 100 mg, emetine O.6 mg
Sonalgin (May & Baker): Tabs butobarbitone 60 mg, paracetamol 375 mg, codeine phosphate 10 mg (deleted 1981)

Sonergan (May & Baker): Tabs butobarbitone 75 mg, promethazine hydrochloride 15 mg (deleted 1981)

BUTORPHANOL

● Butorphanol is the latest addition to a small class of strong analgesics which are chemically related to the conventional opiates but which are partial antagonists of morphine-like agents. Like BUPRENORPHINE and NALBUPHINE, this compound has been shown to have significant pain-relieving activity and is cautiously recommended by its manufacturers for relief of moderate to severe pain states. It partially antagonizes the effects of morphine and other 'agonists', such that if given to patients who are dependent on such drugs the compound will precipitate withdrawal symptoms. Butorphanol is assumed to have a low abuse and dependence potential. Its unwanted effects are somewhat different from those of the narcotic agonists and appear to arise less frequently. Sedation, nausea, and sweating have been commonly reported adverse reactions, and some patients find the drug strangely euphoriant, though not in the same way as morphine. Depressed respiration may occur with this as with all strong analgesics given at high dosage, but in the case of butorphanol (unlike buprenorphine) this can be reversed by the pure narcotic antagonist NALOXONE. It is too early to tell whether the compound will show significant advantages over standard opiates and whether or to what extent it may be dependence-producing.

▲ Butorphanol is at this writing available only in injectable form. An initial dose of 1–4 mg (average 2 mg) intramuscularly is recommended, depending on the patient's age, severity of pain and other factors; if the intravenous route is used, 0.5–2 mg. The drug's duration of effect is 3–4 hours after IM injection.

★ Contra-indicated in severe respiratory ailments and pregnancy; and not advised in myocardial infarction ('coronary thrombosis'), and severe liver or kidney disorders. This agent should not be given to patients receiving regular doses of morphine, pethidine, etc.

➤ For further information, see Essay IV and Chart IV: Morphine and Other Potent Analgesics.

◆ UK:
Stadol (Mead Johnson): Amps 2 mg/1 ml
     USA:
Stadol (Bristol): Amps 1 mg/1 ml, 2 mg/1 ml, & 4 mg/2 ml; Vials 20 mg/10 ml

BUTRIPTYLINE

● This compound is the most recently introduced of the tricyclic anti-depressants, whose prototype is AMITRIPTYLINE. It has been suggested that the newer agent is somewhat more effective in controlling anxiety and tension, when these accompany depressive states; but it is evidently not helpful in cases of psychotic depression. As with all antidepressants, if there is going to be any therapeutic benefit this will not be apparent for 2–4 weeks after commencement of treatment with this compound. Certain effects, such as sedation, dry mouth, difficulty in visual accommodation, and gastric disturbances may arise within 2–3 days of such treatment: these are usually dose-dependent. It is probable that butriptyline, like other related agents, intensifies very severe depression in some cases. The potential risks of attempted suicide with tricyclics, which may be additionally cardio-toxic, should be borne in mind.

▲ Initially, 25 mg three times daily, adjusted over 2–4 weeks, according to response, to an average of 75–150 mg/day. A single daily dose, taken at bedtime, may be appropriate. It is suggested that dosage should not exceed 150 mg per day.

★ The stated contra-indications include cardiovascular disease; epilepsy; enlargement of the prostate; urinary retention; and glaucoma. Butriptyline should not be prescribed at the same time as MAO-inhibitor antidepressants; certain anticoagulants and anti-hypertensive drugs; amphetamines and other stimulants; and alcohol.

➤ For further information, see Essay II and Chart II: Antidepressants.

◆ UK:
Evadyne (Ayerst): Tabs 25 & 50 mg

CANNABIS R

● *Cannabis sativa* (also called *C. indica*) is a bushy herb, growing in some places up to 12–14 feet high, which is either cultivated or grows wild in many parts of the world. The principal countries where it is harvested are India, Turkey, South and West African lands, and in Central America. The flowering tops of the plant, and to a lesser extent the leaves, exude a sticky resinous substance. This has been found to contain over 30 different alkaloids, of which the best known and most extensively studied is Δ^9-TETRAHYDROCANNABINOL (THC). Cannabis is used non-medically by an estimated 13 million people in the USA, 5 million in the UK, and millions more in other countries, Oriental and Occidental: in India and elsewhere it is taken medicinally. Among the forms in which cannabis is seen are *kif*, which resembles finely chopped green herbs, (from Morocco); *ganja* or *dagga,* a coarser, duskier material, in which the flowering tops may be intact (from the West Indies and Africa); and *charas* (or hashish), which is the concentrated resin. Marijuana usually refers to the herbal forms. Hashish comes in the form of a solid block, whose size, shape and colour depend on the country of origin. This is much more potent than most marijuana (e.g. *kif*), and may appear in palette-shaped, almost black masses (*charas* from India or Pakistan); in thin, light brown chewing-gum-sized, hard slabs (from Turkey); and in other forms. Hashish crumbles when heat is applied, and in this way is mixed with tobacco to form the 'joint' for smoking. Smoking is an effective mode of administration because the active ingredients are readily absorbed by the mucous membranes. Cannabis may also be taken orally. Onset of action is longer after consumption by mouth (½–1 hour) than when smoked (less than 5 minutes in many cases) but the herb may yield effects for a longer period (3–6 hours).

It has often been stated that the mood-altering action of cannabis is due to the presence of THC. In fact, other alkaloids contribute to the overall effect. Many researchers have regarded the cannabis euphoria ('being stoned') as a simple pharmacological activity, similar to that produced by alcohol. The nature and type of psychological effects depends partly on the relative concentrations of different alkaloids, e.g. *kif* tends to promote an action markedly different from that provoked by *charas*. Other factors to be considered in the cannabis experience include individual idiosyncrasy, prior mood, the circumstances obtaining, and familiarity or otherwise with the substance.

The intensity and duration of a cannabis 'high' vary considerably. Some of the psychological effects are, as any experienced smoker will confirm, extremely difficult to describe accurately. Among the commonest immediate actions are elation, profound relaxation and alteration of time perception. Sometimes dysphoria with nervousness and mildly 'paranoid' reactions occur, but these appear to be uncommon in regular users. 'Hallucinations' (optical alterations) are seen by a few but these tend to be transient. While one may feel a state of reverie, with fantasies flashing through one's head, it is often possible to 'come down' sufficiently (e.g. if disturbed) to talk and act coherently, even though one may wish to laugh and take nothing seriously. A good many cannabists claim that their creativity, whether in music, poetry, or the visual arts, is enhanced when they smoke. Attempts have been made to test this, but one suspects that few artists can achieve the appropriate mood under laboratory conditions. While cannabis is not an aphrodisiac, use of the substance may increase pleasures of many kinds. Long-term psychological effects are difficult to evaluate: it appears, however, that moderate consumption of cannabis over many years need not be attended by serious physical or psychological problems. Protracted use is stated by some workers to lead to an 'amotivational syndrome', i.e. a state of passivity and withdrawal from the world. It is probable that such reactions depend less on the drug itself than on the individual's pre-existing traits.

Physical effects are also many and varied. Increased heartbeat is common; possibly less so are slight eye inflammation, unsteadiness of gait, tremor, a degree of motor disco-ordination, urinary frequency, dry mouth, drowsiness and hunger (particularly a craving for sweetmeats). Use of cannabis by smoking may over years lead to bronchitis and emphysema, as is the case with tobacco. Acute panic reactions may be felt by inexperienced persons; these tend to be self-limiting. However, individuals who are already suffering from a behavioural disturbance may find the symptoms enhanced. No evidence has been adduced that in humans cannabis is harmful when taken during pregnancy: experimental animals, such as mice, fed with doses of cannabis far in excess of likely human consumption, have occasionally produced deformed offspring, but to extrapolate from these findings is at best questionable.

Whether the regular taking of cannabis over periods of months or years leads to tolerance has been disputed. Some researchers consider that not only does this not develop, but on the contrary that a phenomenon called 'reverse tolerance' occurs: this means that over time cannabists require less, and not more, drug to achieve the desired effect. Of course the situation with most psychotropic agents is just the opposite. The claim that cannabis is physically addictive, dormant for some years, has lately surfaced again. One report, for instance, concerned rhesus monkeys who were injected with THC 6–hourly for 3 weeks. On stopping the drug, some relatively trivial effects (e.g. increased teeth-baring) were noticed: the term 'abstinence syndrome' is clearly an exaggeration. One might further observe that the THC was given intravenously – a route of administration not used by humans and one which would produce uncharacteristically potent actions – and that extremely high doses (0.5 mg per kilo of body-weight) were used. The paper in question is Fredericks, A. B. and Benowitz, N. L., 'An abstinence syndrome following chronic administration of Δ^9-tetrahydrocannabinol to rhesus monkeys', *Psychopharmacologia* 71: 201–2 (1980). People may in fact smoke or ingest substantial quantities of cannabis daily for months or even longer and quite suddenly stop without the development of any perceptible withdrawal reactions.

The canard that experimental use of cannabis leads to opiate dependency (so-called 'escalation') is still believed by some medical practitioners who should know better. Adduced to support this theory is the fact that most narcotic addicts have previously tried cannabis: the argument runs that the person becomes dissatisfied with the marijuana 'high' and gravitates to hard drugs. First, the 'escalation' view illustrates the *post hoc, propter hoc* fallacy, e.g. that most cigarette smokers first took chocolate: no causal link has been established. More importantly, supporters of this hypothesis totally misunderstand the qualitative differences between the psychological effects of cannabis and those of opiates: while the former may raise the threshold of consciousness, spurring on the imaginative faculties, the narcotics obtund the senses. That both types of drug are illegal for non-medical purposes is hardly relevant, since the great majority of those who deal in cannabis refuse on principle to traffic in heroin and other hard drugs.

A term which crops up occasionally in the medical literature is 'cannabis psychosis'. Reports of such a phenomenon concern the supposed hazards of prolonged use, characterized apparently by paranoid ideas, delusions, confusion, severe panic and depersonalization (see Essay V: Psychedelics). No responsible researcher would deny that such reactions are sometimes found. But again a causal link is required: is the 'psychosis' actually due to cannabis or to other potentially important factors such as personality, environment, heredity – particularly a previous psychiatric history or a predisposition to psychological illness? Most of the characteristics of 'cannabis psychosis' would be regarded as normal, or at any rate unremarkable, symptoms by veteran users *who may have a quite different* Weltanschauung *and different criteria for illness from those of the psychiatrists who study them.* As far as chronic adverse effects from smoking cannabis are concerned, the *British Medical Journal* has cautiously observed, after reviewing the literature, that 'there is little evidence to suggest that adverse reactions in long-term users occur more often than in other comparable populations' (leader, 'Cannabis psychosis', II: 1092–3, 1976).

Turning now to the medical indications of cannabis, the present authors have prescribed for and monitored the effects of the substance in more than 50 healthy but anxious patients. For this purpose medicinal cannabis extract was given: a dark green, very viscous material prepared according to pharmaceutical specifications (*Cannabis Indica Extract*, BPC 1949). In addition to the usual physical and psychic reactions, more than 35 of the subjects noticed a significant anxiety-relieving and antidepressant action. These reactions, which were elicited through exhaustive questionnaires, appeared in many cases superior to those promoted by conventional anxiolytic and antidepressant agents.

The potential therapeutic applications of cannabis are now being intensively studied; but it should be remembered that for centuries the herb has held an important role in the Ayurvedic and Unani Tibbi schools of traditional medicine in India. Among the active alkaloids is cannabidiolic acid (CBDA), which has been shown to possess distinct antibiotic properties. Cannabis preparations were researched in considerable detail during the 1950s in Czechoslovakia: workers there demonstrated that such preparations, whether applied topically or given orally, relieved a number of bacterial infections with greater efficacy than penicillin and other standard antimicrobial agents. Zdeněk Krejčí reported that 'the bactericide effect of the hemp substances [was] experimentally proved on . . . organisms resistant to penicillin'. (Krejčí, Z., 'Antibakterielní Účin látek z Cannabis Indica L'*Acta Universitatis Palackianae Olomucensis* 6: 43–57 [1955].) Other researchers at Olomouc showed, in controlled trials involving thousands of patients, that alkaloids of cannabis were at least as successful, and in some cases much more so, than conventional antibiotics in sinusitis, otitis media, mouth ulcers and possibly also in tuberculosis. These studies, reported in the Czech journal referred to, have been almost totally ignored by subsequent investigators. An indication that this is so is the fact that at the only UK library to hold the periodical – the Bodleian, Oxford – the present author (J.T.D.) was obliged to cut open the volume's pages – indicating that this had not previously been consulted. The current British attitude was summed up at a recent symposium: during a 45-minute address on 'Cannabis: some growing points' one C. H. Ashton dismissed the potential medicinal benefits of cannabinoids in a few seconds, while the supposed hazards of marijuana were repeatedly rehearsed (Royal Society of Medicine: *Psychotropic Drugs in Perspective: Symposium,* London, December 1980).

The anti-anxiety and antidepressant effects of cannabis, as found by J.T.D. and J.J.R., have been confirmed in a number of subsequent studies of THC and a derivative, NABILONE, although it is fair to point out that some workers have been unable to replicate this research. Unpublished studies with another THC derivative, LEVONAN-TRADOL, appear to show unequivocally that this compound has anxiety-relieving attributes comparable with those of DIAZEPAM (Valium). While it is still experimental, there is scant doubt that levonantradol has other remarkable properties and is likely to become a valuable addition to the therapeutic armamentarium. This drug, more it seems than other cannabinoids, has been found also to represent a considerable improvement over standard anti-emetics such as PROCHLORPERAZINE, particularly in control of the nausea and vomiting so often provoked in patients receiving anti-cancer medication.

In addition, cannabis and analogues, according to several recent trials, are of benefit for asthma sufferers; in the treatment of glaucoma; to stimulate appetite; for relief of various types of pain, including that of advanced cancer; and perhaps also for their anticonvulsant properties. Most of this recent work comes from the USA. But now, despite intense bureaucratic and other difficulties, some studies are under way in the UK and elsewhere, and more are being planned. It is important that these be allowed to continue, for unquestionably there is far more research which should be conducted in the areas mentioned and in other fields which appear promising.

This is not the place to argue for or against the general legalization of cannabis. Possession of small quantities of the substance has been 'decriminalized' in Mexico and in several States of the Union. It may take some time before such a situation obtains in the UK. However, so far as cannabis use is concerned, the relevant legislation, especially the British, is in today's circumstances effectively unenforceable, so widespread has become the custom of marijuana smoking throughout the Western world. It is the considered judgment of the authors of this book that cannabis should at least be available to practitioners for prescription, and thus more accessible to researchers.

◆ UK:

Cannabis Indica Extract BPC 1949: soft, green extract (Ransom Ltd)

Cannabis Indica Tincture BPC 1949: green liquid containing cannabis extract (as above) 5 G, alcohol (90%) to 100 ml (Ransom Ltd)

➤ See also under Δ^9-TETRAHYDROCANNABINOL; LEVONANTRADOL; NABILONE

CARBROMAL

● As a sedative and muscle-relaxant of moderate potency, carbromal, like its analogue ACETYLCARBROMAL, used to be prescribed often. Its effects are essentially similar to those of the barbiturates. Currently the only preparations available contain the drug in combination with PENTOBARBITONE SODIUM, the most familiar being Carbrital, which has recently been deleted in the UK. The conjunction of two hypnotics with almost identical actions is inappropriate for a number of reasons: both carbromal and pentobarbitone have a high capacity for tolerance and habituation individually, and unwanted effects characteristic of each compound are likely to be intensified. Hangover, oversedation, ataxia, confusion and paradoxical excitement are not uncommon with the combination. While admittedly Carbrital is a highly efficacious aid in insomnia, it is extremely dangerous in overdosage, whether accidental or deliberate. In patients who are depressed, therefore, products of this kind are definitely contra-indicated. Similarly, the euphoriant action of carbromal with pentobarbitone makes these preparations popular among illicit drug users.

▲ One or two capsules at night.

★ Formulations of the type described should be avoided in porphyria, severe respiratory, liver and kidney disorders, and in cases of known hypersensitivity to either bromide-like agents or barbiturates. Physical addiction may result from repeated use of either carbromal or pentobarbitone. Potentially serious interactions may occur with other central depressants, oral anticoagulants, and oral contraceptives.

➤ See also under Essay III and Chart III: Barbiturates.

◆ USA:
Carbrital (Parke Davis): Caps carbromal 250 mg, pentobarbitone sodium 100 mg; also 125 + 50 mg; Elix carbromal 400 mg, pentobarbitone sodium 120 mg/5 ml
Carbropent (Blue Line): Tabs carbromal 250 mg, pentobarbitone sodium 100 mg

CARPHENAZINE

● Carphenazine is a potent antipsychotic tranquillizer of the CHLOR-PROMAZINE (Largactil, Thorazine) type. It is one of a wide range of compounds which are given to control the symptoms of psychotic illness, particularly schizophrenia, in cases where hyperagitation, excitability and aggressiveness are prominent. Adverse effects, which are frequent at higher dosages, include mental apathy, depression, parkinsonian reactions and anticholinergic effects such as dry mouth and blurred vision. Carphenazine should not be prescribed to severely depressed patients because their symptoms are likely to be enhanced; neither is this drug appropriate for treatment of minor emotional and psychological disturbances. Long-term use of large doses may result in tardive dyskinesia, a severe and perhaps irreversible form of Parkinson's disease.

▲ Outpatients: 50–150 mg per day; psychiatric inpatients: 75 mg to a maximum of 400 mg daily.

★ Among the contra-indications for phenothiazine antipsychotics, of which carphenazine is an example, are bone-marrow depression, severe cardiac, liver and kidney ailments, and convulsive disorders such as epilepsy. Interactions with other types of drug are several, these including amphetamine and other stimulants, lithium, oral anticoagulants, antidepressants and other agents which depress the central nervous system, such as barbiturates, other tranquillizers, and alcohol.

➤ For further information, see Essay VI(B) and Chart VI(B): Antipsychotic Tranquillizers.

◆ USA:
Carphenazine Maleate Tablets USP and
Carphenazine Maleate Solution USP: available as
Proketazine (Wyeth): Tabs 12.5, 25 & 50 mg; Oral Soln 50 mg/ml

CHLORAL HYDRATE

● Of the old-generation sedative and soporific drugs, chloral is probably the most acceptable in current medical usage. It has a reasonably low toxicity and a short duration of action, which may make it suitable for administration to the elderly and children. Usually chloral is prescribed as a standard pharmaceutical mixture, which despite some flavouring tastes extremely unpleasant. This problem can be overcome by giving sup-' positories, though now capsule formulations are marketed which contain the drug in liquid concentration. Repeated consumption of chloral has been shown to lead to psychic and in some cases physical dependency of the barbiturate type: the drug should thus not be taken over long periods. Chloral tends to provoke neausea, vomiting, and other gastro-intestinal disturbances in some patients: the compound's analogues TRICLOFOS and DICHLORALPHENAZONE are less likely to irritate the stomach. High doses may cause confusion, oversedation, and paradoxical excitement similar to that produced by barbiturates. It has been suggested that chloral is an effective adjunct to morphine and other opiate analgesics, but the evidence for this is not conclusive.

▲ 500 mg–1.5 G at night. For children, dosage must be adjusted according to age and/or body weight.

★ Chloral should not be given in gastro-intestinal complaints; in porphyria; and in severe liver, kidney and cardiac disorders. Great caution is necessary in cases of respiratory problems. The drug alters the metabolism of oral anticoagulants and increases the centrally depressant actions of other sedatives, tranquillizers, and alcohol.

➤ For further information, see Essay III and Chart III: Barbiturates.

◆ UK:
Chloral Hydrate Mixture BPC: 625 mg/5 ml
Chloral Elixir Paediatric BPC: 250 mg/5 ml
Noctec (Squibb): Caps 500 mg
   USA:
Chloral Hydrate Capsules USP: 250 & 500 mg, 1 G
Chloral Hydrate Syrup USP: 250 & 500 mg/5 ml
Aquachloral (Webcon): Suppos 300, 600 & 750 mg
Cohidrate (Coastal): Caps 500 mg
HS-Need (Hanlon): Caps 250 & 500 mg
Maso-Chloral (Mason): Caps 500 mg
Noctec (Squibb): Caps 250 & 500 mg; Syr 500 mg/5 ml
Oradrate (Coast): Caps 500 mg
Rectules (Fellows-Testagar): Suppos 600 mg & 1.2 G
SK-Chloral (Smith Kline & French): Caps 250 & 500 mg
Loryl (Kremers-Urban): Caps chloral hydrate 337.5 mg, phenyltoloxamine citrate 37.5 mg

CHLORDIAZEPOXIDE

● Better known under its proprietary name Librium, this was the first of the benzodiazepine series of tranquillizers to be introduced, and it is still among the most widely prescribed drugs in the world. Chlordiazepoxide is effective in alleviating anxiety states, tension, certain psychosomatic complaints, enuresis (bed-wetting) in children, and in some cases of alcoholic psychosis. Great attention has been focused lately on the fact that compounds of this class are tolerance-producing and that physical addiction may occur with prolonged treatment at high dosages. Many authorities believe these hazards to have been overstated, but unquestionably psychological dependency does develop fairly rapidly in some patients. Against this must be set the extremely low toxicity of the compound and its real therapeutic benefits. The commoner adverse effects, such as hangover, confusion, and oversedation, are in most instances transient and mild at appropriate dosage levels. Larger doses may produce serious physical and mental effects: among the latter, disinhibition has almost certainly been under-reported. This may manifest as unusual antisocial behaviour, provoked because of the drug's capacity to release inhibitions. The muscle-relaxant and anticonvulsant activity of chlordiazepoxide is also medically useful: in combination with clinidium, a powerful agent which reduces gut motility, it may be beneficial in symptomatic relief of peptic ulcer, the irritable colon syndrome and similar complaints. By injection the drug may be given to control seizures, though here it is not as effective as its analogue DIAZEPAM (Valium). In combination with the antidepressant AMITRIPTYLINE it is prescribed in mixed anxious/depressed states; but the available fixed-dose product Limbitrol is not recommended, because this precludes flexibility in assessing the required dose of each drug. There is no question that chlordiazepoxide is heavily overprescribed by busy practitioners, often to patients who would respond better to reassurance than to medication.

▲ The accepted range is 10–80 mg per day. The regular three-times-daily regimen is unnecessary because the drug has an inherently long duration of action. Thus a single bedtime dose will suffice in many cases.

★ Chlordiazepoxide is contra-indicated in severe respiratory distress; in cases of hypersensitivity to any benzodiazepine; for children (except to stop enuresis or somnambulism). Caution in myasthenia gravis, severe liver and kidney dysfunction. Effects of other CNS depressants will be enhanced.

➤ For further information, see Essay VI and Chart VI(A): Tranquillizers.

◆ UK:

Chlordiazepoxide Tablets BPC: 5, 10 & 25 mg
Chlordiazepoxide (Hydrochloride) Capsules BPC: 5 & 10 mg
Librium (Roche): Tabs 5, 10 & 25 mg; Caps 5 & 10 mg; Dry Amps 100 mg/2 ml
Libraxin (Roche): Tabs chlordiazepoxide 5 mg, clinidium bromide 2.5 mg
Limbitrol (Roche): Caps chlordiazepoxide 5 mg, amitriptyline 12.5 mg; also 10 + 25 mg

   USA:

Chlordiazepoxide Tablets USP: 5, 10 & 25 mg
Chlordiazepoxide Hydrochloride Capsules USP: 5, 10 & 25 mg
Sterile Chlordiazepoxide Hydrochloride USP: 100 mg/ml
Libritabs (Roche): Tabs 5, 10 & 25 mg
Librium (Roche): Caps 5, 10 & 25 mg; Amps 100 mg/2 ml & 250 mg/5 ml
A-Poxide (Abbott): Caps 5, 10 & 25 mg
Brigen-G (Grafton): Tabs 5, 10 & 25 mg
Chlordiazachel (Rachelle): Caps 5, 10 & 25 mg
Lo-Tense (Elder): Tabs 10 mg
SK-Lygen (Smith Kline & French): Caps 5, 10 & 25 mg
Screen (Foy): Caps 5, 10 & 25 mg
Tenax (Reid-Provident): Caps 10 mg
Zetran (Hauck): Caps 10 mg
Librax (Roche): Caps chlordiazepoxide 5 mg, clinidium bromide 2.5 mg
Chlornidium (Purepac): Caps chlordiazepoxide 5 mg, clinidium bromide 2.5 mg
Menrium (Roche): Tabs chlordiazepoxide 5 mg, conjugated oestrogens 0.2 mg; also 5 + 0.4 mg & 10 + 0.4 mg

CHLORMETHIAZOLE

● Chlormethiazole is chiefly prescribed for its tranquillizing and soporific effects, and has been recommended as a remedy for insomnia, particularly for elderly patients. This is perhaps because it is a relatively non-toxic drug at therapeutic doses and its rather short duration of action makes hangover unlikely. By injection the compound may be effective in controlling the repeated seizures of status epilepticus and other convulsive conditions. It has also been used in the treatment of acute withdrawal from alcohol and, with questionable success, to relieve narcotic withdrawal symptoms. Chlormethiazole's effectiveness is rather variable, and some practitioners dislike it. Tolerance may develop quickly if the drug is taken regularly, and physical dependency has been reported. Frequently found side-effects are tingling in the nose and sneezing; irritation of the eyes and abdominal upsets occur in some patients. A hazard which has recently been mentioned is the taking of large doses of the drug by ex-alcoholics some weeks or months after withdrawal: after such an interval some of the tolerance to its effects will have been lost, and toxic delirium may result. It is difficult to assess the incidence of habituation to chlormethiazole, but some authorities believe that this is not uncommon.

▲ To promote sleep: 1–2 G at night. For daytime use, 500 mg–1 G three or four times daily.

★ Chlormethiazole is not recommended in cases of severe liver disorders. It may be dangerous in conjunction with alcohol and will increase the CNS-depressing effects of other tranquillizers, hypnotics, and narcotics.

➤ For further information see Essay VI and Chart VI(A): Tranquillizers.

◆ UK:
Heminevrin (Astra): Tabs & Caps 500 mg; Syr 250 mg/5 ml; Injection-Infusion 8 mg/ml (Tabs deleted 1981)

CHLORMEZANONE

● This is a mild sedative agent with muscle-relaxant properties. It may be useful in some cases of anxiety and tension unresponsive to other therapy. Chlormezanone is useful in controlling muscular spasm and is sometimes prescribed in conjunction with simple analgesics such as aspirin to relieve inflammatory pain, e.g. in arthritic conditions. At doses of 200–400 mg, the drug has been shown not to impair reflexes in tasks such as driving, according to one study. However, these subjects were young men, and it is probable that the elderly are more susceptible to this agent's central effects. Although adverse effects are said to be usually mild and transient, flushing, skin rashes, nausea, lethargy, constipation and loss of appetite have been reported. If such reactions persist dosage should be reduced or the drug discontinued. Jaundice may occur with repeated use.

▲ On average, 200–400 mg three times daily is recommended.

★ Chlormezanone should not be given during pregnancy, nor concurrently with antipsychotic tranquillizers of the CHLORPROMAZINE type or MAO-inhibitor antidepressants.

◆ UK:
Trancopal (Winthrop): Tabs 200 mg
Lobak (Winthrop): Tabs chlormezanone 100 mg, paracetamol 450 mg
    USA:
Fenarol (Winthrop): Tabs 100 & 200 mg
Trancopal (Winthrop): Caps 100 & 200 mg

CHLORPHENTERMINE R

● Although this amphetamine-like stimulant appears on the schedules of restricted drugs in the UK, chlorphentermine is no longer available there. The drug is prescribed as an adjunct to diet and exercise in the treatment of obesity, since it reduces appetite. This effect, however, wears off within a few weeks. Because of this fact, and also because it has a moderate abuse potential, prescription of chlorphentermine should be strictly short-term. The substance was derived from AMPHETAMINE and shares many of the characteristics of this class of drugs, including stimulation of the central nervous system. While chlorphentermine is less potent than amphetamine or dexamphetamine in this regard, it still tends to produce an energetic feeling of euphoria. At even moderate doses some individuals experience restlessness, palpitations, agitation, and other amphetamine-like reactions. Psychological dependence is not uncommon.

▲ 65–130 mg daily, generally in two doses, the latter being taken before 4 p.m.: otherwise insomnia may occur.

★ Like other stimulants of this type, chlorphentermine should not be given in hypertension, severe cardiac ailments, hyperthyroidism, urinary retention, glaucoma, and its use is inadvisable by agitated or anxious patients. Among possibly serious interactions with other drugs are concomitant use with MAO-inhibitor or tricyclic antidepressants, antipsychotics, some anti-hypertensive agents, and alcohol.

➤ For further information, see Essay I and Chart I: Amphetamines.

◆ USA:
Chlorophen (Robinson): Tabs 65 mg
Pre-Sate (Warner-Chilcott): SR Tabs 65 mg

CHLORPROMAZINE

● This agent was the first major tranquillizer of the phenothiazine series to be introduced, and it is still the most extensively used. It is, or should be, principally indicated to control the symptoms of schizophrenia and other severe psychological disturbances. At much lower doses the drug is prescribed as a sedative and anti-emetic and to enhance the pain-relieving effects of opiate analgesics. For the latter purpose it is normally given by injection, and this may be appropriate also for premedication before surgery. There is a tendency to administer chlorpromazine to relieve minor psychological problems, such as anxiety and tension states: this is often inappropriate, partly because alternative medicaments (e.g. benzodiazepine tranquillizers) are available and additionally because, like other phenothiazines, the compound may provoke mental depression or intensify this if it is already present. Further, except at extremely small dosage levels, oversedation, lassitude, anticholinergic effects (abdominal upsets, blurred vision, dry mouth), and parkinsonian reactions – disturbances of motor or muscular co-ordination – may be produced. Undoubtedly there exist several proper therapeutic applications for the drug, particularly in controlling agitation, hyperexcitability and aggressiveness in patients suffering from severe mental illnesses. Long-term administration of substantial doses in some cases provokes a condition known as tardive dyskinesia, a severe form of Parkinson's disease.

▲ The dosage employed depends on the condition being treated, on age and other factors. In severe psychological illness, the range is 50–400 mg per day for outpatients and up to (exceptionally) 1,500 mg for inpatients. To control or prevent vomiting, much smaller quantities are required: 5–25 mg.

★ Chlorpromazine should be used only with utmost caution in severe cardiac, liver, kidney or respiratory complaints, and is contra-indicated in convulsive disorders. Contra-indicated for concurrent administration with amphetamines and other stimulants, certain anti-hypertensive drugs, and anti-diabetic agents. Chlorpromazine increases the central depressant effects of barbiturates, other tranquillizers, potent analgesics, and alcohol.

➤ For further information, see Essay VI(B) and Chart VI: Antipsychotic Tranquillizers.

◆ UK:
Chlorpromazine (Hydrochloride) Tablets BPC: 10, 25, 50 & 100 mg
Chlorpromazine (Hydrochloride) Elixir BPC: 25 mg/5 ml
Chlorpromazine (Hydrochloride) Injection BPC: 25 mg/ml
Chlorpromazine (Hydrochloride) Suppositories BPC: 100 mg
Largactil (May & Baker): Tabs 10, 25, 50 & 100 mg; Elix 25 mg/5 ml; Susp 100 mg/5 ml (embonate); Oral Conc 10 & 25 mg/ml; Amps 25 mg/1 ml & 50 mg/2 ml; Suppos 100 mg
   USA:
Chlorpromazine Hydrochloride Tablets USP: 10, 25, 50, 100 & 200 mg
Chlorpromazine Hydrochloride Syrup USP: 25 mg/5 ml
Chlorpromazine Hydrochloride Injection USP: 25 mg/ml
Chlorpromazine Hydrochloride Suppositories USP: 25 & 100 mg
Thorazine (Smith Kline & French): Tabs 10, 25, 50, 100 & 200 mg; SR Caps 30, 75, 150 & 200 mg; Syr 25 mg/5 ml; Amps 25 mg/1 ml & 50 mg/2 ml; Vials 250 mg/10 ml; Suppos 25 & 100 mg
Chlorzine (Mallard): Vials 250 mg/10 ml
Klorazine (Myers-Carter): Vials 250 mg/10 ml
Komazine (Hyrex): Vials 250 mg/10 ml
Promachel (Rachelle): Tabs 10, 25, 50, 100 & 200 mg
Promachlor (Geneva): Tabs 10, 25, 50, 100 & 200 mg

Promapar (Parke Davis): Tabs 10, 25, 50, 100 & 200 mg
Promaz (Keene): Vials 250 mg/10 ml
Sonazine (Tutag): Tabs 10, 25, 50, 100 & 200 mg

CHLORPROTHIXENE

● Chlorprothixene is a major tranquillizer, or antipsychotic drug, the first of the thioxanthene series. This fact is significant because antipsychotics of the other two principal classes, the phenothiazines such as CHLORPROMAZINE and butyrophenones like HALOPERIDOL, have a strong tendency to exacerbate mental depression. Thus, in treating severe mental disturbances, there was and is a risk of intensifying such symptoms which occur frequently in psychoses. Chlorprothixene and its new analogues (e.g. FLUPENTHIXOL) therefore have noteworthy advantages over the more commonly prescribed major tranquillizers belonging to the other classes. Thioxanthenes are often as effective as phenothiazines in reducing agitation, hyperexcitability, hallucinations and other features of schizophrenia and some other psychotic and severely neurotic conditions. Chlorprothixene may provoke lassitude and drowsiness, but is less apt to produce the more undesirable side-effects of antipsychotic medication. Parkinsonian effects, for instance, occur less often. As in the case of more popular neuroleptic agents, it is appropriate to warn against the use of this compound in the therapy of minor psychological problems, although severe anxiety states may well respond to treatment with the drug.

▲ For psychiatric outpatients, an average daily dose is 30–45 mg daily in divided doses. For hospitalized patients, a maximum of 400 mg per day is suggested. Dosage levels will depend on the severity of the illness and on individual response.

★ Great caution in severe cardiac, liver or kidney disorders, in convulsive conditions such as epilepsy, and in known hypersensitivity to antipsychotics. Interactions with other drugs follow the pattern of the phenothiazines, but the potential hazards of concomitant medication may not be so great: concurrent use of amphetamines and other stimulants is to be avoided, and care must be exercised if oral anticoagulants, certain antihypertensive drugs, and other CNS-depressant agents are to be administered concurrently.

➤ For further information, see Essay VI(B) and Chart VI: Antipsychotic Tranquillizers.

◆ UK:
Taractan (Roche): Tabs 15 & 50 mg
   USA:
Chlorprothixene Tablets USP
Chlorprothixene Oral Suspension USP &

Chlorprothixene Injection USP: available as
Taractan (Roche): Tabs 10, 25, 50 & 100 mg; Oral Susp 100 mg/5 ml;
Amps 25 mg/2 ml

CLOBAZAM

● This compound is one of the most recent additions to an already overcrowded market, namely benzodiazepine tranquillizers of the DIAZEPAM (Valium) type. It is unclear whether clobazam offers other than marginal advantages over diazepam in the treatment of anxiety and tension. The assertion that clobazam is less sedative than comparable tranquillizers of the same class at therapeutic dosage has yet to be confirmed by much clinical experience. Although a two- or three-times-daily dose regimen has been proposed by the manufacturers, the compound may just as well be taken at night in a single dose: its duration of effect will in most cases persist through most if not all of the subsequent day, and adverse effects such as sedation, unsteadiness, impaired reflexes may be circumvented. In addition, if tension and anxiety tend to insomnia, this drug like other benzodiazepines will help promote sleep if the total daily dosage is taken at bedtime. Tolerance and psychological dependency may develop with prolonged use. Clobazam is extremely expensive in relation to its supposed benefits. Physical habituation in some cases has now been documented.

▲ The usual range is 10–60 mg daily, taken in divided doses or as described above at night.

★ Contra-indicated in myasthenia gravis, severe respiratory problems, and hypersensitivity to tranquillizers of this type. The effects of clobazam are potentiated by other drugs which depress the central nervous system, i.e. other tranquillizing agents, barbiturates, opiates, and alcohol.

➤ This compound appears to be typical of diazepam-type drugs: its actions, and other more detailed data, are described in Essay VI and Chart VI(A): Tranquillizers.

◆ UK:
Frisium (Hoechst): Caps 10 mg

CLOMIPRAMINE

● Clomipramine, like other tricyclic antidepressants, is an analogue of AMITRIPTYLINE and IMIPRAMINE. It is prescribed to control depressive states of various types, and may be helpful in treating obsessional and phobic anxiety and depression. If such therapeutic benefit is going to occur, the drug must be taken for 2–4 weeks before symptoms begin to be relieved. In common with related antidepressants, dry mouth, blurred vision, urinary hesitancy, and sedation are regularly encountered side-effects, particularly at the beginning of treatment. If depression is already very severe, it may be intensified. The potential of antidepressants for lethal overdosage should be borne in mind, as the number of such cases is considerable and increasing annually.

▲ 25–100 mg daily in most cases; for more severe psychological disorders, up to 150 mg daily. A single dose at night may suffice, once the optimum response has been determined.

★ Contra-indicated in severe cardiac conditions, liver disorders and convulsive states. Utmost caution in glaucoma, urinary retention, and enlargement of the prostate. Clomipramine should not be prescribed at the same time as antidepressants of the MAO-inhibitor type, amphetamines and other stimulants and appetite suppressants, and oral anticoagulants.

➤ For further information, see Essay II and Chart II: Antidepressants.

◆ UK:
Anafranil (Geigy): Caps 10, 25 & 50 mg; Syr 25 mg/5 ml; Amps 25 mg/2 ml & 100 mg/8 ml

cis-CLOPENTHIXOL DECANOATE

● Clopenthixol is one of the most recently introduced depôt antipsychotic agents. The drug is esterified in a vegetable oil base, so that a single, deep intramuscular injection of it will act for two to four weeks. The convenience of this type of formulation in controlling schizophrenic and other psychotic symptoms is obvious, whether on an in- or outpatient basis. Earlier depôt preparations of major tranquillizers, such as FLUPHENAZINE DECANOATE (Modecate, Prolixin), belong to the largest chemical class of antipsychotics, the phenothiazines. One of the particular risks with these is their tendency to provoke mental depression or to intensify this if it is already present. The thioxanthene group of drugs, to which clopenthixol and the better-known FLUPENTHIXOL belong, do not have this disadvantage, and indeed there is some evidence that they mitigate depression as well as anxiety, aggressiveness, hyperexcitability and other features of psychotic illness. Side-effects of the thioxanthenes also tend to be fewer and less troublesome than those produced by the more commonly-used phenothiazines of the CHLORPROMAZINE (Largactil, Thorazine) type: apathy, drowsiness, and lassitude may be experienced with clopenthixol, and in some cases anticholinergic reactions (dry mouth, abdominal upsets) and parkinsonism occur. Long-acting antipsychotics of this class have been in use for a relatively short time, so it is not yet clear whether protracted administration of them is likely to cause tardive dyskinesia, a severe form of Parkinson's disease which long-term use of phenothiazines often provokes. The convenience of long-acting antipsychotic injections is such that some practitioners may be less careful than they should be in monitoring the patient's progress. Clopenthixol should not be prescribed in other than severe psychological illnesses.

▲ The recommended average dose is 200–400 mg (1–2 ml) every 2–4 weeks, given by deep intramuscular injection. Dosage should be titrated according to response.

★ Contra-indicated in severe cardiac, liver and kidney diseases; acute intoxication with alcohol, barbiturates, or opiates; parkinsonism and other convulsive disorders; and for patients who cannot tolerate oral antipsychotic drugs. Not recommended for concurrent use with amphetamines or MAO-inhibitor antidepressants.

➤ For further information, see Essay VI and Chart VI(B): Antipsychotic Tranquillizers.

◆ UK:
Clopixol (Lundbeck): Amps 200 mg/1 ml

CLORAZEPATE

● This compound belongs to the crowded benzodiazepine class of tranquillizers, whose best-known examples are DIAZEPAM (Valium) and CHLORDIAZEPOXIDE (Librium). Clorazepate is often highly effective in controlling anxiety and tension states, and may combat insomnia. Since, like most diazepines, this compound is intrinsically long-acting, a single dose taken at bedtime will suffice, in most patients, to promote sleep and to exert its anxiolytic effects through the following day. Certainly more than two daily doses are quite unnecessary. It is uncertain whether clorazepate confers benefits which may not be obtained by the far cheaper diazepam, but the former is preferred by many practitioners. The present writers have found that, at approximately equipotent doses, clorazepate appears more effective for some patients. Oversedation, confusion, and disinhibition are among the more often reported side-effects, but these are seldom troublesome at appropriate doses. Long-term administration of any benzodiazepine should be eschewed unless in exceptional cases, because there exists some risk of tolerance and psychological habituation.

▲ 7.5–45 mg at night, or in two daily doses. The suitable dose for any particular patient must be ascertained empirically: a single 15 mg capsule may be sufficient for many sufferers from anxiety, while others may require up to 60 mg per day.

★ Like other compounds of the diazepam class, clorazepate is contra-indicated in myasthenia gravis, severe respiratory difficulties, and in known hypersensitivity to any benzodiazepine tranquillizer. The drug enhances the CNS-depressant actions of other tranquillizers, barbiturates, other hypnotics, opiates, and alcohol.

➤ For further information see Essay VI and Chart VI(A): Tranquillizers.

◆ UK:
Tranxene (Boehringer Ingelheim): Caps 15 mg (dipotassium)
    USA:
Tranxene (Abbott): Caps 3.75, 7.5 & 15 mg; SR Tabs 11.25 & 22.5 mg (dipotassium)
Azene (Endo): Caps 3.25, 6.5 & 13 mg (monopotassium)

CLORTERMINE

● Clortermine is the most recent addition to the ranks of appetite-suppressants derived from AMPHETAMINE. The compound was heavily promoted on its introduction in the USA a few years ago as a new drug, more effective (it was claimed) than previous anti-obesity agents. However, it is in chemical structure so close to CHLORPHENTERMINE that only careful examination will tell the two apart. Similarly, in terms of pharmacological effect, clortermine appears to be almost identical: both drugs, in common with most amphetamine derivatives, have some central stimulant activity and so may provoke mild to moderate energetic euphoria, and exert their appetite-curbing effect in the same way. The latter wears off within a few weeks of regular use. So clortermine should be prescribed on a shut-ended basis only, as an adjunct to exercise, dieting and other measures which may be appropriate. Because the drug is longer-acting than its analogues, a single daily dose only will be required. Habituation and abuse should be regarded as a genuine hazard. Over-stimulation, insomnia, palpitations, and anxiety are frequent unwanted effects of virtually all amphetamine-like agents.

▲ 50–100 mg at breakfast-time: no further dose is required. If any quantity of the drug is taken after lunch-time, insomnia may occur.

★ Clortermine should be avoided in hypertension, glaucoma, hyper-thyroidism, and cardiac or cardiovascular disease. It should not be prescribed for patients who are prone to anxiety or agitation, or for those with a history of drug abuse. Concomitant use of antidepressants (tricyclic and MAO-inhibitor), major tranquillizers (antipsychotics), certain anti-hypertensive agents and alcohol is inadvisable.

> For further information, see Essay I and Chart I: Amphetamines.

◆ USA:
Voranil (USV): Tabs 50 mg (hydrochloride)

COCAINE R

● Cocaine is the principal alkaloid of the bush *Erythroxylon coca,* which grows in parts of Bolivia and Peru and the leaves of which have been chewed by local people for many centuries. It was not until the 1880s, however, that cocaine was isolated and used medicinally. Its effects as a powerful stimulant and local anaesthetic were made known by Sigmund Freud and Karl Köller in 1884. Freud saw the drug almost as a panacea: he was so enthusiastic about it that he invited many of his friends to try it and himself became dependent upon it. Cocaine produces a type of euphoria which is difficult to describe: in some respects this is similar to the central stimulation promoted by AMPHETAMINE, but is more pervasive, including a sense of warmth, increased energy, and an extra-ordinary feeling of wellbeing. Taken by mouth, cocaine is relatively ineffective, being broken down rapidly, but after snuffing or injecting the drug it provides an almost immediate 'high'. The pure drug may be seen as a white powder or as glistening, transparent micro-crystals. The hydro-chloride salt, which is used in medicine, is highly hygroscopic and will be dissolved in half its own weight of water. Solutions of the drug are not stable, so for many purposes these are freshly prepared. The principal legitimate applications of cocaine are in ear, nose and throat surgery as a surface anaesthetic; to lower intra-ocular pressure and produce dilatation of the pupils as eye-drops; and as an ingredient in the 'Brompton cocktail', an elixir containing DIAMORPHINE or MORPHINE and cocaine, for relief of terminal pain. The benefits of concurrently adminis-tered opiates and cocaine have been established over many years by tradition. However, Ronald Melzack and his colleagues have recently found that addition of the latter to analgesic mixtures does not enhance their pain-relieving potency. 'Ratings of confusion, nausea and drowsiness . . . showed that there was no significant difference between the Bromp-ton mixture and morphine administered orally' (*Canadian Medical Association Journal* 120:435 [1979]). The symptoms referred to are those commonly found following administration of morphine-like drugs, which addition of cocaine is supposed to lessen. However, Melzack does not comment on the euphoriant effects of the combination, about which there can be no doubt at all. Until 1968 when the Drug Dependency Clinics were set up in the UK, opiate addicts obtained prescriptions for cocaine as well as morphine or heroin, for the purpose of injecting both drugs together. The mixture produces an almost indescribable euphoria, and so it was extremely popular. Then, chiefly because a few practitioners were overprescribing these drugs, it became unlawful for a doctor to prescribe cocaine or heroin, uniquely, except for relief of organic pain or injury. It was belatedly realized that, although cocaine use led almost immediately (within a few minutes, very often) to intense craving for a further dose, the drug was not physically addictive, i.e. that on its abrupt discontinuation no clear withdrawal symptoms appear, even in persons who have taken it regularly for prolonged periods. Today only a tiny handful of people are 'registered' for cocaine. Despite the drug's resurgent popularity in some circles, it has a number of harmful effects. Chronic sniffing may destroy the septum between the nostrils; long-term use may provoke delusions, hallucinations, formication (a feeling that insects are crawling on the skin), and other severely disturbed states which resemble AMPHETAMINE psychosis. The claim that chronic cocainism destroys brain cells has not been established, but undoubtedly this has severe behavioural and social ill-effects. Even a single small dose may cause hyperagitation, restlessness, tremors, tachycardia (fast heartbeat), hypertension, nausea, and vomiting, among other reactions. An expression applied to heroin – 'it's so good, don't even try it once' – is apt here. For most therapeutic purposes cocaine has been superseded by more modern drugs, for example lignocaine (lidocaine), for local anaesthesia.

▲ As little as 10 mg of cocaine crystals may provoke psychological effects: this quantity may cover only a couple of cubic millimetres.

★ Contra-indicated in hypertension, severe cardiac disease, thyrotoxicosis. Cocaine should be avoided for concurrent administration of anti-hypertensive drugs, tricyclic and MAO-inhibitor antidepressants, and amphetamine-like stimulants. Habituation may arise within days or weeks of regular use of the drug in any form. Prolonged use of eye-drops may cause eye damage. Hypersensitivity is not uncommon.

➜ For an account of amphetamine psychosis, see Essay I and Chart I: Amphetamines.

◆ UK:
Cocaine Hydrochloride BPC: crystals for solution
Cocaine (Hydrochloride) Eye-Drops BPC: 2% and 4%
Cocaine (Hydrochloride) and Homatropine Eye-Drops BPC: each 2%
Mydricaine (APF formula): Amps cocaine hydrochloride 6 mg, atropine sulphate 1 mg, adrenaline tartrate 0.1 mg/0.3 ml (for ocular injection)
    USA:
Cocaine Hydrochloride USP: powder for solution
Cocaine Hydrochloride Tablets for Topical Solution USP: 8 & 15 mg
see also under DIAMORPHINE

CODEINE R

● Codeine is well known as a pain-killer of moderate potency, as a cough suppressant, and as a remedy for diarrhoea. For these indications a vast number of compound preparations are marketed: while in the USA these are prescription-only, many of them may be supplied over the counter in the UK. Simply to list the available preparations which contain a certain quantity of codeine, whether with other analgesics such as aspirin and paracetamol, or with ephedrine and other agents as cough-syrups, would occupy an excessive amount of space in this book. Therefore only pure codeine formulations, which are all restricted as Controlled Drugs in the USA, are described below under Presentations. In the UK only injectable codeine is thus restricted, while pharmaceutical codeine linctus may be bought without a prescription. The analgesic effect of the drug (methyl-morphine) probably lies in the fact that 10% of it is metabolized to MORPHINE in the body. Earlier authorities have overestimated codeine's analgesic effectiveness, but it is still useful for mild to moderate pain states, whether alone or in conjunction with aspirin and other compounds. On the other hand, in the UK at least, its dependence potential has been understated. While this in no way compares with that of morphine and other potent narcotics, codeine addiction does occur and is usually, but not always, therapeutic in origin. If the drug is taken repeatedly, tolerance develops and on abrupt discontinuation of supply a withdrawal syndrome may appear: this is less intense than that associated with morphine or heroin but it may be extremely unpleasant nonetheless. At recommended dosages codeine does not ordinarily produce euphoria, though if taken by injection this may occur. Unwanted reactions include in a few cases drowsiness and lethargy (at high doses), and allergic responses have been reported. Relatively, the drug is more toxic than morphine, and it is particularly important not to exceed the correct dose. Codeine is prescribed by some practitioners, who do not wish to give restricted drugs, to relieve very severe pain, such as that of inoperable cancer: this may be effective in a few cases but generally a far more potent analgesic is then required.

▲ Orally, 10–60 mg three or four times daily; by injection, 30–120 mg.

★ Caution in severe respiratory ailments, and severe liver and kidney disorders. Preferably, codeine should not be given concurrently with MAO-inhibitor antidepressants. It will potentiate the effects of other centrally depressant drugs.

➤ For a comparison with other analgesics, and further information, see Essay IV and Chart IV: Morphine and Other Potent Analgesics.

◆ UK:
Codeine Phosphate Tablets BPC: 15, 30 & 60 mg

Codeine (Phosphate) Linctus BPC: 15 mg/5 ml
Codeine (Phosphate) Syrup BPC: 25 mg/5 ml
unbranded Codeine Phosphate Amps 60 mg/1 ml
   USA:
Codeine Phosphate Tablets USP: 15, 30 & 60 mg
Codeine Phosphate Injection USP: Amps 15, 30 & 60 mg/1 ml
Codeine Sulfate Tablets USP: 15, 30 & 60 mg
Terpin Hydrate and Codeine Elixir USP: codeine phosphate 10 mg, terpin
hydrate 85 mg/5 ml

CYCLOBARBITONE

● Cyclobarbitone is typical of the intermediate-acting barbiturates, such
as AMYLOBARBITONE (AMOBARBITAL). This compound is prescribed almost exclusively to promote sleep. As with other drugs of its
class prolonged use may lead to the onset of tolerance and psychological
and/or physical dependency. Although cyclobarbitone is commonly
regarded as being one of the most, if not the most, short-acting oral
barbiturate, its duration of action is such that even a moderate bedtime
dose is likely to be followed by a hangover. Oversedation, confusion, and
impairment of reflexes are particular hazards in elderly patients, though
such reactions are not exclusive to them. It is believed by most practitioners that barbiturates are unsuitable, chiefly because of their abuse and
dependence potential, as hypnotics, having been replaced by the less toxic
and more selectively-acting benzodiazepines of the DIAZEPAM (Valium) and NITRAZEPAM (Mogadon) type. Certainly regular use of
cyclobarbitone and its analogues as aids to sleep should be discouraged.

▲ 100–400 mg at night. It is important to note that, although intermediate-acting barbiturates have essentially the same effects, these often differ
in potency on a weight basis. Therefore, 200 mg of cyclobarbitone ≡
100 mg amylobarbitone.

★ The compound is contra-indicated in porphyria, severe respiratory and
liver ailments, and in cases of hypersensitivity to any barbiturate. It
should be avoided for concomitant use with oral anticoagulants, the
contraceptive Pill, antipsychotic tranquillizers, and alcohol.

➤ For further information on interactions, etc., see Essay III and Chart
III: Barbiturates.

◆ UK:
Cyclobarbitone (Calcium) Tablets BPC: 200 mg
Phanodorm (Winthrop): Tabs 200 mg
Cyclomet (Larkhall): Tabs cyclobarbitone calcium 200 mg, emetine
0.6 mg

DEANOL

● Deanol is a central nervous system stimulant of moderate potency, whose closest analogue is perhaps PROLINTANE. While not itself an amphetamine derivative, deanol has an action which is not dissimilar. It has been prescribed in the treatment of acute depression and chronic fatigue and has been tried as an alternative to AMPHETAMINE or METHYLPHENIDATE in controlling the hyperkinetic syndrome in children, on whom stimulants have a paradoxical, calmative effect. The American Medical Association has stated, cautiously, that this compound may be useful in learning problems, making concentration easier, possibly for the hyperkinetic or hyperactive child. A number of studies have been carried out to assess the drug's benefit in this indication and, with one exception, these do not support the claim. It has been said that the full therapeutic effect of deanol takes some days, or weeks, to appear. There is a suggestion that the drug may help relieve the tardive dyskinesia, a form of Parkinson's disease, which can occur after prolonged treatment with major (antipsychotic) tranquillizers of the CHLORPROMAZINE type. Further investigations of the compound are needed before its potential benefits can be confirmed. Side-effects, usually mild and transient, include itching, slight headache, weight loss, and insomnia: these are dose-related. Deanol appears to have only a very slight abuse and dependence capacity.

▲ Adults: 25–50 mg two or three times daily; children, up to 300 mg/day.

★ Large doses of deanol have been found to provoke seizures in some patients: thus the drug is contra-indicated in convulsive disorders. Concurrent administration of amphetamine-like stimulants and antidepressants is not advised.

➤ For further information, see Essay I and Chart I: Amphetamines.

◆ USA:
Deaner (Riker): Tabs 25 & 100 mg (acetamidobenzoate)

DESIPRAMINE

● This drug is an antidepressant of the tricyclic group and is similar in most particulars to IMIPRAMINE. It is used to control various forms of depressive illness and may be helpful in anxiety states. Claims have been advanced that desipramine is superior to other tricyclics in the treatment of severe melancholia. However, caution must be exercised because in some patients extremely profound depression may be intensified. In common with other antidepressive agents of its class, desipramine must be taken for two to four weeks before therapeutic effects will be experienced if they do occur. Drowsiness, dizziness, dry mouth, gastro-intestinal disturbances and appetite changes are among the drug's adverse reactions. The potential of tricyclic antidepressants for suicidal use has been, and is still, greatly underestimated by some practitioners.

▲ 75–300 mg daily, generally in divided doses; after stabilization, a single nightly dose may suffice.

★ Desipramine should not be prescribed to patients with severe heart disease, enlargement of the prostate, urinary retention, glaucoma, or convulsive disorders. Concurrent use of MAO-inhibitor antidepressants, amphetamine and other stimulants and appetite-suppressants, and certain anti-hypertensive medicaments, is inadvisable.

➤ For further information, see Essay II and Chart II: Antidepressants.

◆ UK:
Desipramine (Hydrochloride) Tablets BPC: available as
Pertofran (Geigy): Tabs 25 mg
   USA:
Desipramine Hydrochloride Tablets USP &
Desipramine Hydrochloride Capsules USP: available as
Norpramin (Merrell-National): Tabs 25 & 50 mg
Pertrofrane (USV): Caps 25 & 50 mg

DEXAMPHETAMINE (DEXTROAMPHETAMINE) R

● Dexamphetamine, known in the USA as dextroamphetamine, is the most extensively prescribed of its class of central nervous system stimulants: it is also second only to METHYLAMPHETAMINE (METH-AMPHETAMINE) in potency. Because of the energetic type of euphoria which it produces, the drug is much abused and there is in almost every Western country an extensive illicit market. Tolerance to most of its effects sets on rapidly, often within weeks, and although it is not settled whether chronic dexamphetamine use gives rise to true addiction, psychological habituation most certainly occurs with prolonged use. In the UK, prescription of this and related compounds to reduce appetite in obesity has dwindled because of a self-imposed ban among practitioners. But in the USA dexamphetamine and its analogues are still often supplied for this purpose, despite the fact that the drug's appetite suppression lasts only a short time and regardless of the high risk, even in patients not predisposed to drug abuse, of dependency. It has become popular to prescribe amphetamines, and this medicament in particular, to control the childhood hyperkinetic syndrome, as it appears to exert a paradoxical, calming effect in pre-adolescents. The use of powerful stimulants in therapy of an overdiagnosed, and insufficiently defined, condition such as the hyperkinetic or hyperactive state is controversial, having vocal supporters and equally articulate antagonists. Only in the treatment of narcolepsy, a fairly rare disorder characterized by the patient's chronic falling asleep during the daytime despite normal nocturnal sleep, is administration of dexamphetamine generally regarded as acceptable and proper. In the absence of any known cure for this ailment, the drug at least provides symptomatic relief. Like other sympathomimetic agents, dexamphetamine may cause loquaciousness, restlessness, anxiety, depression, palpitations, sweating, and other effects associated with strong central stimulants. Repeated use of large quantities may provoke a phenomenon referred to as amphetamine psychosis: this may be indistinguishable in many respects from spontaneous paranoid states.

▲ Usually 2.5–15 mg daily, depending on the medical indication, age of patient, severity of the condition under treatment. Much larger doses may be needed in narcolepsy.

★ Contra-indicated in glaucoma, hypertension, hyperthyroidism, agitation or depression, and cardiovascular disease. Utmost caution in liver and kidney ailments. Antidepressants and antipsychotic tranquillizers are among the types of drug which should not be taken at the same time as dexamphetamine.

➤ For further information, see Essay I and Chart I: Amphetamines.

◆ UK:
Dexamphetamine Sulphate Tablets BPC: 5 mg
Dexamed (Medo): Tabs 5 mg
Dexedrine (Smith Kline & French): Tabs 5 mg
Durophet (Riker): SR Caps 1- & dexamphetamine resinate 7.5, 12.5 & 20 mg
Durophet-M (Riker): SR Caps 1- & dexamphetamine resinate 12.5 & 20 mg, methaqualone 40 mg (deleted 1981)
    USA:
Daro (Fellows-Testagar): SR Caps 15 mg (hydrochloride)
Dextroamphetamine Phosphate Tablets USP: 5 mg
Dextroamphetamine Sulfate Tablets USP: 5 & 10 mg
Dextroamphetamine Sulfate Elixir USP: 5 mg/5 ml
Dexedrine (Smith Kline & French): Tabs 5 mg; Elix 5 mg/5 ml; SR Caps 10 & 15 mg
Dexampex (Lemmon): Tabs 5 & 10 mg, SR Caps 15 mg
Diphylets (Tutag): SR Caps 10 & 15 mg
Ferndex (Ferndale): SR Tabs 5 & 15 mg
Oxydess (North American Pharmacal): Tabs 5 & 10 mg
Robese-Forte (Rocky Mountain): SR Tabs 15 mg
Spancap (North American Pharmacal): SR Caps 10 & 15 mg
Tidex (Allison): Tabs 5 mg
Biphetamine (Pennwalt): SR Caps 1- & dexamphetamine resinate 7.5, 12.5, 20 mg

Delcobese (Delco): Tabs 1- & dexamphetamine adipate 5, 10 15 & 20 mg; SR Caps 10, 15 & 20 mg

Dexamyl (Smith Kline & French): Tabs dexamphetamine sulphate 5 mg, amylobarbitone (amobarbital) 32 mg; SR Caps 10 + 65 mg, & 15 + 97 mg

Dextrobar (Lannett): Tabs dexamphetamine sulphate 5 mg, amylo-barbitone 32 mg

Eskatrol (Smith Kline & French): SR Caps dexamphetamine sulphate 15 mg, prochlorperazine maleate 7.5 mg

Obetrol (Obetrol): Tabs dexamphetamine sulphate & saccharate each 5 mg, amphetamine sulphate, amphetamine aspartate each 5 mg (also half-strength)

Obotan (Mallinckrodt): SR Tabs 17.5 & 26.25 mg (tannate, equiv. 5 & 7.5 mg)

Ro-Trim (Rocky Mountain): Caps dexamphetamine sulphate 15 mg, atropine sulphate 0.6 mg

Trimex (Mills): Caps dexamphetamine sulphate 15 mg, amylobarbitone 60 mg, thyroid extract 180 mg

see also under AMYLOBARBITONE (AMOBARBITAL)

DEXTROMORAMIDE ℞

● Dextromoramide is one of the most powerful of the narcotic analgesics, a synthetic compound related to METHADONE. It is pre-scribed in severe pain states, such as postoperatively and in terminal cancer cases. Like most potent opiates this drug has significant respiratory depressant effect: its use is not advised during labour. It has been estimated that 5–10 mg of dextromoramide is equivalent to 10 mg of morphine, each taken orally. This medicament may also be given by injection and as rectal suppositories. Estimates of the incidence and severity of side-effects vary, but some patients experience nausea, vomiting, constipation, drowsiness, dizziness or other reactions charac-teristic of narcotic agents. Addiction potential for dextromoramide is similar to that for MORPHINE and METHADONE, i.e. this is high in persons predisposed to drug abuse, but of course in terminal patients it does not matter. The number of British 'notified' addicts using the compound has been increasing in recent years: its black-market avail-ability is limited, and it is considered somewhat less desirable than heroin or morphine: this is undoubtedly in part because dextromoramide is not so euphoriant as other opiates.

▲ Initially, 5–10 mg orally or by subcutaneous injection, repeated within 4–5 hours. Dosage is dependent on pain severity, individual response, etc.

★ Should be avoided if possible in severe respiratory distress and severe liver dysfunction. Concomitant use of MAO-inhibitor antidepressants and barbiturates is not advised. Caution with other central-depressant agents.

> For further information, see Essay IV and Chart IV: Morphine and Other Potent Analgesics.

◆ UK:
Dextromoramide (Tartrate) Tablets BPC &
Dextromoramide (Tartrate) Injection BPC: available as
Palfium (MCP): Tabs 5 & 10 mg; Amps 5 & 10 mg/1 ml; Suppos 10 mg

DEXTROPROPOXYPHENE (PROPOXYPHENE)

● This is a pain-relieving agent whose potency is approximately equivalent to that of CODEINE and thus lies midway between simple analgesics such as aspirin and the opiates. It is most often prescribed in preparations which also contain paracetamol (acetaminophen) and aspirin. Even at high doses dextropropoxyphene seldom has more than mild and transient psychological effects. Dependency on the drug, however, has been under-recorded. The compound is more effective in injectable form: such products, however, are used in continental Europe but not in the UK or USA. Nausea, drowsiness, loss of appetite and allergic skin rashes sometimes occur if high doses are given. Dextropropoxyphene provides some relief of opiate withdrawal symptoms, an indication which we believe has hitherto been overlooked: a number of patients have been successfully withdrawn from diamorphine (heroin) by one of the present writers, with the milder drug substituted for periods of up to 7 days. The capacity of preparations containing propoxyphene in conjunction with paracetamol for suicidal use (e.g. Distalgesic) should be borne in mind: such overdosages are difficult to treat.

▲ 65–200 mg orally, every 4–6 hours, according to the severity of the condition being treated. The napsylate salt appears to be more effective for analgesia than the hydrochloride.

★ Caution in respiratory depression and severe liver disorders. This drug should never be prescribed concurrently with the anti-parkinsonian agent ORPHENADRINE, and central stimulants should not be administered in cases of overdosage.

> For further information, see Essay IV and Chart IV: Morphine and Other Potent Analgesics.

◆ UK:
Depronal-SA (Warner): SR Caps 150 mg (hydrochloride)
Cosalgesic (Cox): Tabs dextropropoxyphene hydrochloride 32.5 mg, paracetamol 325 mg
Distalgesic (Dista): Tabs as *Cosalgesic*

Dextropropoxyphene (Napsylate) Capsules BPC: available as
Doloxene (Lilly): Caps 65 mg
Distalgesic-Soluble (Dista): Sol Tabs dextropropoxyphene napsylate (HC1 equiv.) 32.5 mg, paracetamol 325 mg
Dolasan (Lilly): Tabs dextropropoxyphene napsylate 100 mg, aspirin 325 mg
Doloxene-Compound (Lilly): Caps dextropropoxyphene napsylate 65 mg, aspirin 375 mg, caffeine 30 mg
Napsalgesic (Dista): Tabs dextropropoxyphene napsylate 50 mg, aspirin 500 mg
(N.B. napsylate doses are hydrochloride equivalents)
    USA:
Propoxyphene Hydrochloride Capsules USP: 32 & 65 mg
Propoxyphene Hydrochloride and APC Capsules USP: as *Darvon-Co*
Propoxyphene Hydrochloride and Acetaminophen (Paracetamol) Tablets USP: 65 & 650 mg
Darvon (Lilly): Caps 32 & 65 mg
Dolene (Lederle): Caps 65 mg
Harmar (Zemmer): Caps 65 mg
Progesic (Ulmer): Caps 65 mg
Pro-Pox (Kenyon): Caps 65 mg
Propoxychel (Rachelle): Caps 65 mg
Ropoxy (Robinson): Caps 65 mg
Scrip-Dyne (Scrip): Caps 65 mg
SK-65 (Smith Kline & French): Caps 65 mg
S-Pain-65 (Saron): Caps 65 mg
Dolene-AP65 (Lederle): Caps dextropropoxyphene 65 mg, paracetamol 650 mg
Darvon-Co (Lilly): Caps dextropropoxyphene 65 mg, aspirin 227 mg, phenacetin 162 mg, caffeine 32.5 mg.
The following containing the same ingredients at the same strengths:
Dolene-Co (Lederle), *Doraphen-Co* (Cenci), *ICN-65-Co* (ICN), *Myospaz* (Dunlap), *PC-65* (Archer), *Poxy-Co* (Sutliff & Case), *Propoxyphene-Co* (Wollins), *Proxagesic-Co* (Tutag), *Repro-Co* (Reid-Provident), *Scrip-Dyne-Co* (Scrip), *SK-65-Co* (Smith Kline & French), *S-Pain-CPD* (Saron)
Propoxyphene Napsylate Tablets USP: 100 mg
Propoxyphene Napsylate Oral Suspension USP: 50 mg/5 ml
Propoxyphene Napsylate and Acetaminophen (Paracetamol) Tablets USP: as *Darvocet-N*
Propoxyphene Napsylate and Aspirin Tablets USP: as *Darvon-N + ASA*
Darvon-N (Lilly): Tabs 100 mg; Susp 50 mg/5 ml
Darvocet-N (Lilly): Tabs propoxyphene 50 mg, acetaminophen 325 mg
Darvon-N + ASA (Lilly): Tabs propoxyphene 100 mg, aspirin 325 mg

DIAMORPHINE (HEROIN) R

● Diamorphine is a controversial drug. It is unusual in that British practitioners, according to a special statute which also applies to COCAINE, may prescribe it 'only for the treatment of organic desease or injury', i.e. not to opiate addicts. A few psychiatrists who work at Drug Dependency Clinics are theoretically exempted from this regulation, but in practice heroin prescription has been drastically curtailed even there, and the great majority of notified addicts receive METHADONE instead: the latter compound is a synthetic narcotic, usually given orally, to 'maintain' opiate habitués, and is just as addictive. In the USA diamorphine may not be prescribed at all as it is not considered therapeutically useful. Some British physicians maintain that heroin has distinct advantages over MORPHINE in the relief of the most severe pain states, such as myocardial infarction ('coronary thrombosis') and inoperable cancer. Small doses have an excellent cough-suppressant activity. As an analgesic, diamorphine 5 mg is generally considered equivalent to 10 mg of morphine. It is claimed to provoke fewer unwanted reactions than morphine at comparable doses, although it is definitely shorter-acting (3–4 hours against 4–6): nausea, sometimes vomiting, loss of appetite, vertigo, dizziness, drowsiness, constipation and mood changes occur commonly after administration of both medicaments, and indeed are characteristic of the opiates in general. The assertion that heroin depresses respiration less than morphine seems to have substance. The mood changes produced by diamorphine are enjoyed by some (euphoria) and found disagreeable (dysphoria) by others, and perhaps more patients find it dysphoriant than euphoriant. It is because some so greatly like the dreamy, warm, self-sufficient sensation which the drug provokes in them that repeated doses are taken, tolerance develops, and physical dependence may arise. The enormous and ever-increasing illicit traffic in heroin attests to its popularity among certain people who are regarded as being predisposed to opiate abuse. It is interesting, however, that cancer patients can often be maintained on a constant dose of the drug for months, and if it is no longer needed the compound in many instances may be withdrawn without difficulty, i.e. that even prolonged use does not necessarily result in addiction. Certainly if heroin has been used for many weeks, it should be discontinued gradually. The real point is that the hazards of diamorphine use, medical or non-medical, have been exaggerated both by the mass media and by the more ignorant members of the medical profession. Of course the incidence of illicit use is high, not just among young people with 'personality disorders', but by some balanced and intelligent individuals. In some cases addiction arises following medical treatment but more often by introduction to such drugs in other settings. The facile condemnatory attitudes towards heroinism which are still prevalent should be re-examined. There is evidence that persons who gravitate to heroin 'abuse' are not simply ill, but that they may have an inherent deficiency of endorphins, the 'natural opiates' found in the brain to which, at the molecular level, drugs of the morphine type bind. The criminal activity associated with heroin addiction is not surprising, since the drug is impossible to obtain legally and black-market prices have skyrocketed. That many heroin users are shabby, prone to infection and physically run-down is a function of the way the drug is used, and not of its direct effects. Thus, if adulterated drug is injected without proper aseptic injection techniques, the results may be anticipated. Certainly a number of opiate users have inadequate personalities and take heroin as a psychological crutch to insulate them from the unpleasantness of the real world. This is far from the whole story, as we have tried to show. Onset of physical dependency occurs much less quickly than is generally believed: only after two to three months' repeated use of diamorphine will even moderately severe withdrawal reactions be experienced. Heroin, in the therapeutic context, may be given orally, but this is considerably less effective than by injection. The drug is not stable in solution, and for this reason hypodermic tablets have been employed. Recently ampoules containing a bolus of the opiate, which has been freeze-dried, have been introduced: addition of the required quantity of sterile water makes these ready to use and convenient.

▲ 5–20 mg, orally or by subcutaneous or intramuscular injection, depending on the patient's age, the severity of the condition, and other variables. Some individuals, e.g. terminal cancer sufferers, may require single doses of up to 100 mg. To relieve intense pain, the drug should be given 3–4 hourly.

★ Contra-indicated in severe respiratory insufficiency, delirium tremens, and severe head injuries. Diamorphine is to be avoided with MAO-inhibitor antidepressants, antipsychotic tranquillizers, barbiturates and, generally, alcohol. Caution with all other CNS depressants. Concomitant use of pure or partial opiate antagonists (e.g. PENTAZOCINE) is contra-indicated except in opiate overdosage.

➤ For further information, see Essay IV and Chart IV: Morphine and Other Potent Analgesics.

◆ UK:
Diamorphine Hydrochloride BPC: Hypodermic Tabs 10 mg
Diamorphine Hydrochloride Injection BPC: Amps 10 & 60 mg/1 ml (liquid), Amps 10, 15 & 30 mg/2 ml (freeze-dried)
Diamorphine (Hydrochloride) Linctus BPC: 3 mg/5 ml
Diamorphine and Cocaine Elixir BPC ('Brompton Cocktail'): diamorphine hydrochloride 5 mg, cocaine hydrochloride 5 mg, alcohol (90%) and flavourings/5 ml

Diamorphine and Terpin Elixir BPC 1973: diamorphine hydrochloride
3 mg, terpin hydrate 15 mg, alcohol (90%), flavourings/5 ml
see also under COCAINE

DIAZEPAM

● Under the brand name Valium, diazepam is familiar to most house-
holds and for several years now has been the most often prescribed drug
of any kind, both in the USA and in the UK. In the latter country it is
estimated that the cost of diazepam prescriptions is of the order of £6
million annually. This compound and CHLORDIAZEPOXIDE (Librium) were the prototypes of the benzodiazepine class of anxiety-relieving
tranquillizers and possess the characteristics of this series of drugs in
general, having calmative, muscle-relaxant and anticonvulsant actions.
Diazepam is chiefly given to alleviate tension and anxiety states, and for
some patients has antidepressive effects also. It may also be prescribed to
induce sleep: a single dose, equivalent to the total recommended daily
dosage, may be effective for this purpose and can continue its anxiolytic
activity through the following day. In alcoholic withdrawal, diazepam
relieves agitation, tremor, and delirium and may be given in conjunction
with other drugs, as it may not be sufficiently potent to overcome these
reactions on its own. There is evidence that diazepam may be a useful
adjunct to standard anticonvulsant drugs (e.g. phenytoin, Epanutin) in
epilepsy. By intravenous injection the compound provides excellent
premedication before dental, surgical and investigative procedures, and
controls the repeated fits of status epilepticus. Adverse effects include
oversedation, confusion, unsteadiness of gait, and vertigo: these are dose-
related. Even quite low quantities of the drug may impair reflexes, and it
is important that patients be warned about this hazard. High doses,
especially if taken regularly, may provoke paradoxical excitement and
disinhibition, a state analogous to that produced by excess of alcohol: the
usual social inhibitions having broken down, antisocial and sometimes
violent behaviour has been reported with increasing frequency. As
'mother's little helper' diazepam is unquestionably overprescribed. Repeated use is likely to lead to tolerance and psychological and occasionally to
physical dependency: therefore, unless there are compelling reasons,
long-term administration of the drug is not advised. It is worthwhile to
note that diazepam is more effective taken orally than by intramuscular
injection.

▲ Dosage must be established by empirical means, as individual
response to the drug is so variable. The usual range is 4–40 mg daily.
Because of the drug's inherently long duration of action, a single dose
taken at night may be the most appropriate regimen for many patients:
certainly three-times-daily dosage is unnecessary. When diazepam is given

by intravenous injection, it should not be mixed in the same syringe with any other drug, as precipitation will occur; further, the injection should be delivered extremely slowly. Although the manufacturers recommend use of veins in the antecubital fossa (bend of the elbow), we do not recommend this, as accidental intra-arterial injection is more likely to occur than if other sites (e.g. back of the hand) are used.

★ Contra-indicated in severe respiratory difficulties, known hypersensitivity to any benzodiazepine; caution in severe liver and kidney disorders, myasthenia gravis, concurrent administration of other CNS depressants (e.g. barbiturates, other tranquillizers, including antipsychotic agents, opiate analgesics, and alcohol). Not advised for children except short-term use to control night terrors and somnambulism, nor during pregnancy or lactation. The action of the anticonvulsant phenytoin may be affected, that of thyroxine (thyroid hormone) enhanced. Caution is required in cases of concomitant administration of the cardiac drugs digoxin and warfarin.

➤ For further information, including an account of the Committee on Review of Medicines' recent recommendations, see Essay VI and Chart VI(A): Tranquillizers, and Addenda, p. 455.

◆ UK:
Diazepam Tablets BPC: 2, 5 & 10 mg
Diazepam Capsules BPC: 2 & 5 mg
Diazepam Elixir BPC: 2 mg/5 ml
Diazepam Injection BPC: Amps 5 mg per ml
Atensine (Berk): Tabs 2, 5 & 10 mg
Diazemuls (KabiVitrum): Amps 10 mg/2 ml (emulsion)
Evacalm (Unimed): Tabs 2 & 5 mg
Sedapam (Duncan, Flockhart): Tabs 2 & 5 mg
Solis (Galen): Caps 2 & 5 mg
Valium (Roche): Tabs 2, 5 & 10 mg; Caps 2 & 5 mg; Elix 2 mg/5 ml; Amps 10 mg/2 ml & 20 mg/4 ml; Suppos 5 & 10 mg
　　USA:
Diazepam Tablets USP: 2, 5 & 10 mg
Diazepam Injection USP: 5 mg per ml
Valium (Roche): Tabs 2, 5 & 10 mg; Amps & Syrettes 10 mg/2 ml; Vials 200 mg/10 ml

DIBENZEPIN

● Dibenzepin is an antidepressant of the tricyclic type and in many particulars is similar to AMITRIPTYLINE and IMIPRAMINE. The medicament has not enjoyed a wide commercial success, but some practitioners consider it useful in severely neurotic and psychotic states, and it may be beneficial in controlling the mood-swings of manic-depressive illness. Side-effects, such as sedation, dry mouth, blurred vision, sweating and gastro-intestinal upsets are dose-related and more likely to be troublesome at the beginning of therapy. The above reactions can arise within 2–3 days of starting the drug, while if it is going to be effective in relieving depression dibenzepin must be taken regularly for between two and four weeks: only then will benefit be apparent. The potential suicidal use of this, as of other tricyclic antidepressants, should be considered by the prescriber. Blood tests are advised at intervals before the patient is stabilized on a given dose.

▲ Usually 80 mg three times daily, increasing gradually over 2–3 weeks. Dosage is then adjusted according to response.

★ In common with related drugs, dibenzepin should not generally be used in cases of glaucoma, urinary retention, prostatic enlargement, or severe cardiac disease. It should not be used with MAO-inhibitor antidepressants, amphetamines, any other stimulant or appetite-suppress-ant, or certain anti-hypertensive drugs.

➤ For further information, see Essay II and Chart II: Antidepressants.

◆ UK:
Noveril (Wander): Tabs 80 mg (hydrochloride)

DICHLORALPHENAZONE (DICHLORALANTIPYRENE)

● This compound is a sedative and hypnotic with actions and uses almost identical to those of CHLORAL HYDRATE. Dichloralphenazone is preferred by many because it is less likely than chloral to irritate the lining of the stomach. Because of its relatively low toxicity dichloralphenazone is considered a suitable medicament for promoting sleep in children and in elderly patients. Hangover, oversedation, confusion, and paradoxical excitement may suggest that the dose is too high: the elderly are particularly susceptible to such reactions. Tolerance and psychological (in some cases physical) dependency have been noted but the latter is uncommon. Repeated use over a prolonged period is undesirable. Dichloralphenazone has been claimed to enhance the analgesic effects of both mild and opiate pain-relieving agents. It has a rapid onset of action.

▲ 650 mg–2 G at night. Dosage should be adjusted for children.

★ Contra-indicated in porphyria, severe liver and kidney disorders, and known sensitivity to chloral. This drug enhances the activity of tranquilliz-ers, barbiturates, alcohol and other compounds which depress the central nervous system.

➤ For further information, see Essay III and Chart III: Barbiturates.

◆ UK:
Dichloralphenazone Tablets BPC &
Dichloralphenazone Elixir BPC: available as
Welldorm (Smith & Nephew): Tabs 650 mg; Elix 225 mg/5 ml
Paedo-Sed (Pharmax): Elix dichloralphenazone 200 mg, paracetamol
100 mg/5 ml; Sachets, each equivalent to 5 ml of Elixir
Midrid (Carnrick): Caps dichloralphenazone 100 mg, paracetamol
325 mg, isometheptene mucate 65 mg
   USA:
Midrin (Carnrick): as *Midrid*, UK

DIETHYLPROPION (AMFEPRAMONIUM)

● With the decline in the prescription of AMPHETAMINES themselves, certain of their derivatives which have a less powerful central
stimulant effect have become popular. Among these is diethylpropion,
known on the continent of Europe as amfepramonium. Like other
amphetamine analogues, this compound will exert an appetite-depressing
action for only a limited period: as tolerance develops fairly quickly with
these drugs effect on food consumption becomes negligible within a few
weeks. The drug should be given only for a limited period of time to obese
patients, and then as an adjunct to strict dieting and exercise. Large doses
of diethylpropion cause restlessness, agitation, excitability and other
reactions typical of sympathomimetic agents. Habituation is a risk if the
drug is taken repeatedly.

▲ Diethylpropion is most often prescribed as delayed-release tablets, a
single dose of which, taken at breakfast, will act throughout the day. The
usual dosage range is 50–150 mg daily. If the compound is taken in divided
doses, take not later than 4 p.m. to avoid insomnia.

★ Not recommended in cases of hypertension and severe cardiac or
cardiovascular disorders. The medicament should not be prescribed at the
same time as antidepressants (tricyclic or MAO-inhibitor) or antipsychotic tranquillizers.

➤ For further information, see Essay I and Chart I: Amphetamines.

◆ UK:
Tenuate (Merrell): Tabs 25 mg (deleted 1981); SR Tabs 75 mg (hydro-
chloride)
Apisate (Wyeth): SR Tabs diethylpropion hydrochloride 75 mg, thiamine
hydrochloride 5 mg, riboflavine 4 mg, pyridoxine hydrochloride 2 mg,
nicotinamide 30 mg (B vitamins)
   USA:
Diethylpropion Hydrochloride Tablets USP: 25 mg
Nu-Dispoz (Coastal): Tabs 25 mg

Ro-Diet (Robinson): Tabs 25 mg; SR Tabs 75 mg·
Tenuate (Merrell): Tabs 25 mg; SR Tabs 75 mg
Tepanil (Riker): Tabs 25 mg, SR Tabs 75 mg

DIETHYLTHIAMBUTENE **R**

● This compound is prescribed to anaesthetize animals in veterinary medicine: in the UK it is chiefly used in connection with surgical procedures on dogs, but in tropical countries diethylthiambutene is delivered as a tranquillizing dart, fired from a special gun, to sedate rhinoceros and other large mammals. Why, the reader may inquire, is such a drug included in this book? Firstly, it is one of two opiate analgesics (the other being ETORPHINE) of considerable potency, whose legal use is confined to veterinary applications, which are restricted under the UK Misuse of Drugs Act and corresponding legislation in other countries. Then again, diethylthiambutene is pharmacologically interesting in that its molecule is considerably larger than those of morphine and similar narcotics, and it was believed that this fact made it, for biochemical reasons, less likely to be abused. Unfortunately this proved not to be the case: soon after the introduction in Japan during the 1950s of preparations of the compound for analgesia in humans, a near-epidemic of diethylthiambutene misuse and dependency occurred. Experiments in ex-addicts have shown that 40–60 mg of the drug is equivalent to 15 mg of morphine by subcutaneous injection. Withdrawal symptoms are apparently less marked than those following abrupt discontinuation of morphine. At a time when the number of breakings-in to pharmacies by addicts is increasing, it is worth observing that thiambutene may be taken. Because it is unstable in solution, it is presented in the form of hypodermic tablets for administration by veterinarians.

➤ For further information, see Essay IV and Chart IV: Morphine and Other Potent Analgesics.

◆ UK:
Diethylthiambutene (Hydrochloride) Solution Tablets for Injection BPC, BVetC:
Themalon (Burroughs Wellcome): Hypo Tabs 50 mg

DIHYDROCODEINE **R**

NB Do not confuse with HYDROCODONE (dihydrocodeinone)

● Although dihydrocodeine was introduced early in the century, and subsequently used as a cough suppressant, it was not until the 1950s that the compound was prescribed on a large scale. While seldom given in the

USA, oral preparations of dihydrocodeine are among the most extensively prescribed of analgesics in the UK: in the opinion of many the drug completely bridges the gap between mild pain-relievers such as paracetamol and the potent opiates (morphine and its congeners). The fact that only injectable formulations are under special legal restriction is undoubtedly a factor in the compound's popularity among British practitioners. In addition to a pure tablet product, there are available also preparations in which dihydrocodeine is combined with aspirin or paracetamol. At usual analgesic doses most of the adverse effects associated with MORPHINE or CODEINE have been reported, generally in a mild form: among these dizziness, drowsiness, nausea, and at higher doses respiratory depression. It has been estimated that the drug has considerably less potential for abuse and addiction than morphine and analogues, because except following large oral doses or injection euphoria is not often experienced. Nevertheless, it is probable that this characteristic has been understated. Dihydrocodeine is unlikely to be effective in controlling the most severe pain states, for which it is frequently prescribed. Although workers at Lexington have found subcutaneous doses of the medicament to be 'morphine-like' in psychological effect (i.e. 150 mg ≡ morphine 20 mg), dihydrocodeine does not completely suppress the morphine or heroin abstinence syndrome.

▲ 30–90 mg orally, every 3–5 hours; up to 100 mg per dose by intramuscular or subcutaneous injection. The drug must not be given intravenously.

★ Caution in impaired respiratory or liver function, asthma, delirium. Not for administration concurrently with MAO-inhibitor antidepressants.

➤ For further information, see Essay IV and Chart IV: Morphine and Other Potent Analgesics.

◆ UK:
Dihydrocodeine (Tartrate) Tablets BPC &
Dihydrocodeine (Tartrate) Injection BPC: available as
DF-118 (Duncan, Flockhart): Tabs 30 mg; Elix 10 mg/5 ml; Amps 50 mg/ 1 ml
Onadox-118 (Duncan, Flockhart): Tabs dihydrocodeine 10 mg, aspirin 300 mg
Paramol-118 (Duncan, Flockhart): Tabs dihydrocodeine 10 mg, paracetamol 500 mg
    USA:
Synalgos-DC (Ives): Caps dihydrocodeine bitartrate 16 mg, promethazine hydrochloride 6.25 mg, aspirin 194.4 mg, phenacetin 162 mg, caffeine 30 mg

DIMETHYLTRYPTAMINE (DMT) **R** and DIETHYLTRYPTAMINE (DET) **R**

● These are two psychedelic or 'hallucinogenic' agents with a virtually identical activity. They are among the active alkaloids of the Central and South American shrubs *Piptadenia peregrina* and *P. macrocarpa*, though the substances have been isolated from other plants. Powdered extracts and decoctions have been used, generally in the form of snuff, for religious purposes by the indigenous populations of Mexico and neighbouring countries for many centuries. Dimethyltryptamine itself appears as very soluble light brown crystals which have a translucent sheen. The drug is not available for prescription but occasionally appears on the illicit market for psychedelic compounds. In terms of qualitative effects, DMT and DET resemble LYSERGIDE (LSD), though duration of action is much shorter (½–1 hour). All forms of perception may be radically altered, 'sensory overload' may occur, and the phenomenon of depersonalization is as likely with these alkaloids as with LSD. Because DMT is poorly absorbed from the gut, it is taken as snuff or by injection: intravenous use is contra-indicated. On account of the almost indescribable intensity of the reactions provoked by psychedelic drugs, these should be taken only under medical supervision. Doses of 50–100 mg are likely to promote profound psychological effects. DMT's activity is decreased by pre-treatment with antidepressants of the MAO-inhibitor type.

➤ For warnings and other important information, see Essay V and Chart V: Psychedelics.

DIPHENHYDRAMINE

● This is one of the most popularly employed antihistamine drugs, being a constituent in an enormous number of cough syrups and elixirs. There are so many of these, which generally contain small quantities of the drug, that they are not listed here. On its own the drug is not only useful in allergic rhinitis, asthma, and other conditions requiring administration of an antihistamine, but also because it has sedative properties. Diphenhydramine is indeed marketed in several European countries as an over-the-counter remedy for insomnia. For this purpose it is relatively non-toxic and may be effective especially for children and the elderly, who tolerate more powerful hypnotics less readily. Even quite low doses may cause drowsiness and impair reflexes: the reader might well be advised to note whether diphenhydramine is present in a cough suppressant or expectorant, whether purchased or prescribed. Allergic reactions to the compound sometimes occur. Diphenhydramine is a component of the highly dangerous hypnotic Mandrax (METHAQUALONE).

▲ To relieve cough, 12.5–25 mg three or four times daily; as a soporific, 50–100 mg.

★ The effects of other drugs which have CNS-depressant activity, such as barbiturates, tranquillizers, opiates and alcohol, are likely to be potentiated. Diphenhydramine should not be given concurrently with antidepressants of the MAO-inhibitor type. See also under METHAQUALONE.

◆ UK:
Diphenhydramine Capsules BPC: available as
Benadryl (Parke Davis): Caps 25 mg
    USA:
Diphenhydramine Hydrochloride Capsules USP
Diphenhydramine Hydrochloride Elixir USP &
Diphenhydramine Hydrochloride Injection USP: available as
Benadryl (Parke Davis): Caps 25 & 50 mg; Elix 12.5 mg/5 ml; Amps 10 mg/1 ml; Vials 100 mg/10 ml & 300 mg/30 ml

DIPHENOXYLATE

● Technically, diphenoxylate is an opiate, a derivative of PETHIDINE (MEPERIDINE), and as such is included in the schedules of Controlled Drugs internationally. However, preparations which contain small quantities of the drug for oral administration, in conjunction with atropine, are exempted: only very high doses of diphenoxylate, taken by injection, induce even slight euphoria and may be habituating. In fact the only preparations available are tablets and an oral solution. These combine the drug with atropine and are effective in controlling diarrhoea and motion sickness. Diphenoxylate has recently been tried as an opiate substitute in withdrawal from heroin and similar narcotics, with questionable success. The combination of this compound with the antibiotic neomycin is often given in severe diarrhoea, but since this complaint is usually precipitated by viral infection antibiotics are not often effective. A small proportion of patients exierience nausea, vertigo, itching, skin rashes or other unwanted effects. Numbness of the extremities has been recorded. Diphenoxylate preparations should be given on a short-term basis only.

▲ Initially, 5–10 mg; then 2.5–5 mg 4–6 hourly thereafter.

★ Caution in liver and severe abdominal disease, especially in severe colitis. The drug enhances the actions of opiates, barbiturates and other central depressants.

➤ For further information, see Essay IV and Chart IV: Morphine and Other Potent Analgesics.

◆ UK:
Lomotil (Searle): Tabs diphenoxylate hydrochloride 2.5 mg, atropine sulphate 0.25 mg; Soln 5 ml ≡ 1 tab; also with *Neomycin* 250 mg
Reasec (Janssen): Tabs as *Lomotil* (deleted 1981)
    USA:
Diphenoxylate Hydrochloride and Atropine Sulfate Tablets USP &
Diphenoxylate Hydrochloride and Atropine Sulfate Oral Solution USP:
Lomotil (Searle): Tabs diphenoxylate 2.5 mg, atropine sulfate 0.25 mg
Colonil (Mallinckrodt) &
SK-Diphenoxylate (Smith Kline & French): as *Lomotil*

DIPIPANONE R

● Dipipanone is a potent narcotic analgesic derived from METHADONE: like that drug it has a high potential for abuse and physical dependency. The available British preparation Diconal, a tablet which also contains the anti-emetic cyclizine, is a useful oral alternative to MORPHINE: it provokes less intense adverse effects, although nausea, vomiting, dizziness, confusion and other reactions characteristic of the opiates do occur. The extent to which dipipanone produces euphoria has in the past been underestimated. In recent years Diconal tablets have become much sought after on the illicit market. Non-medical addiction to the drug is increasing at an alarming rate: whereas in 1970 there were only 40 dipipanone addicts notified to the British Home Office, by 1978 the figure had reached 296. In medical practice, the drug has been shown to be less effective than morphine and other analogues such as LEVOR-PHANOL in controlling the most severe pain states: perhaps it is more useful for postoperative pain relief than in other indications.

▲ 10–20 mg four-hourly is an average regimen. In very severe protracted pain, higher doses may be necessary.

★ Caution in severe liver, kidney and respiratory ailments. Not recommended for children, nor for use during pregnancy. Contra-indicated for concomitant administration with barbiturates and MAO-inhibitor antidepressants. Potentiation of other drugs which depress the CNS. Patients who have been receiving this drug should not be suddenly switched to partial opiate antagonists such as PENTAZOCINE.

➤ For further information, see Essay IV and Chart IV: Morphine and Other Potent Analgesics.

◆ UK:
Diconal (Burroughs Wellcome): Tabs dipipanone hydrochloride 10 mg, cyclizine hydrochloride 50 mg

DOM (2,5-DIMETHOXY-4-METHYL-AMPHETAMINE: STP) R

● This compound, as its chemical name indicates a derivative of amphetamine, first appeared on the illicit drug scene in the USA a decade ago. DOM has been categorized by most researchers with the psychedelic agents such as LYSERGIDE (LSD). In fact, in terms of physical and psychological effects, the compound is more amphetamine-like than LSD-like. Both drugs exert an extremely intense effect and produce perceptual distortions, including depersonalization in some cases. The qualitative differences between them are difficult to describe but important. While lysergide may be of interest to the serious-minded individual delving into altered states of consciousness, DOM, like PHEN-CYCLIDINE ('angel dust'), seldom if ever provokes the insights or sparks the creativity which many claim for LSD. Furthermore, like other strong amphetamine derivatives, the former drug is habituating and even a few doses may lead to a form of 'amphetamine psychosis', which is characterized by paranoid delusions. Usually such reactions are self-limiting, and the current difficulty in obtaining illicit supplies of DOM, while probably transient, is welcome. The closest analogue to this chemical is METHYLAMPHETAMINE, and there is dispute as to whether it should be described as a psychedelic. The effects of a single dose of DOM often last in excess of 24 hours. At various times samples have been taken of powders which purport to contain DOM or some other 'hallucinogen', but in the event these frequently turn out to be illegally-manufactured amphetamine or phencyclidine.

➤ A fuller account will be found in Essay V and Chart V: Psychedelics.

DOTHIEPIN (DOSULEPINE)

● Dothiepin shares most of the attributes of other tricyclic antidepressants, such as AMITRIPTYLINE and IMIPRAMINE. The drug may be effective in alleviating depressive conditions of varous types and grades of severity, but must be taken regularly for 2 to 4 weeks before relief of symptoms begins. Dothiepin is among the most sedative of this class of compounds, and a single nightly dosage may be more suitable for some patients than the usual twice- or thrice-daily regimens. Adverse reactions, which tend to occur during the early part of treatment and are related to dosage, include anticholinergic effects (dry mouth, hesitancy in urination, blurred vision, gastro-intestinal disturbances), as well as drowsiness, dizziness, and rapid fall in blood-pressure. The potentially toxic effects of tricyclic antidepressants on the heart have only recently been recognized, and even at therapeutic doses changes in heart rhythm can occur. Great caution is required if dothiepin is administered to patients with very severe depression, as this is in some cases intensified. The potential use of this type of antidepressant for suicidal purposes should be noted by the prescriber.

▲ In the range of 75–150 mg, either in divided doses or as a single bedtime dose: a convenient tablet formulation is available for taking prior to sleep.

★ Contra-indicated in glaucoma, urinary retention, hypertrophy of the prostate. Special caution is to be observed in cases of cardiac and cardio-vascular disease. Dothiepin should be avoided concomitantly with MAO-inhibitor antidepressants, amphetamines and other stimulants and appe-tite-suppressants, and certain drugs prescribed to lower blood-pressure.

➤ For further information, see Essay II and Chart II: Antidepressants.

◆ UK:
Dothiepin (Hydrochloride) Capsules BPC: available as
Prothiaden (Boots): Caps 25 mg; Tabs 75 mg

DOXAPRAM

● Doxapram is a central nervous system stimulant which has been given after surgical anaesthesia to quicken respiration and general recovery after operation, and has also been used in treatment of overdosage with depressant drugs. The compound is delivered by intravenous injection, and a single dose has a duration of effect of only a few minutes: further doses may then be required. Many anaesthesiologists consider administra-tion of doxapram inadvisable, because of its narrow margin of safety at therapeutic doses; and that in the treatment of opiate overdose, other, more specific antidotes such as NALOXONE are preferable. However, certain partial narcotic antagonists (e.g. BUPRENORPHINE) which are given for pain relief are not antagonized by naloxone, and doxapram may then be indicated. Side-effects which have been observed are many and in certain instances serious. Fast heartbeat (tachycardia), hypertension, nausea, restlessness, coughing, muscular twitching and even convulsions may follow administration of high doses. Combination of doxapram (1.5–2.0 mg/kg body-weight) with MORPHINE, according to one study, caused much less reflex coughing, fewer breathing problems and less expectoration than did morphine given alone.

▲ Initially 0.5–2.5 mg per kilogram of body-weight, intravenously, repeated after 5 minutes as required. Injections of doxapram must not be mixed with any alkaline solution in the same syringe or infusion set.

★ Among the principal contra-indications are epilepsy and other convul-sive ailments, cerebral oedema (raised pressure), hyperthyroidism, phaeochromocytoma, and pre-existing respiratory distress. The drug is unsuitable in barbiturate poisoning, and should not be given with amphetamines or amphetamine-like drugs or MAO-inhibitor antidepressants. Doxapram stimulates adrenaline production.

➤ For further information, see Essay I and Chart I: Amphetamines.

◆ UK:
Doxapram (Hydrochloride) Injection BPC: available as
Dopram (Robins): Amps 100 mg/5 ml; Infusion Bottles 1 G/500 ml
   USA:
Doxapram Hydrochloride Injection USP: available as
Dopram (Robins): Vials 200 mg/20 ml

DOXEPIN

● This compound is essentially similar to DOTHIEPIN, in that both have antidepressant and a certain anxiety-relieving activity. Doxepin, however, is much less sedative than dothiepin, which may be an advantage or a disadvantage according to the case being treated. Like other tricyclic antidepressants, the prototype of which is AMITRIPTYLINE, the drug will yield psychological benefits only if taken at least once daily for 2 to 4 weeks. Even then it is not effective in all depressive states: if these are of extreme severity their intensity may be increased. Doxepin appears to provoke fewer adverse reactions than some other comparable medicaments, but the characteristic dry mouth, abdominal upsets, difficulty in visual accommodation, and urinary hesitancy, are not uncommon, especially at the commencement of therapy. The possibility of cardio-toxicity should be considered with doxepin as with other tricyclic compounds, and the hazard of lethal overdosage noted. Although doxepin has been prescribed in schizophrenia and other psychotic conditions, evidence that its use in these very profound mental disturbances may be beneficial is inconclusive.

▲ Average 10–100 mg daily, according to response and the severity of symptoms. Daily dosage should not exceed 300 mg.

★ Because this drug sometimes produces parkinsonian reactions (such as are commonly associated with antipsychotic tranquillizers) its administration is not advised in convulsive states; nor in glaucoma, urinary retention, hyperthyroidism, or enlargement of the prostate gland. Extreme caution in heart disease. Concurrent use of MAO-inhibitor antidepressants, and amphetamines and similar stimulants and anorexiants, is contraindicated.

➤ For further information on interactions, warnings, etc., see Essay II and Chart II: Antidepressants.

◆ UK:
Doxepin (Hydrochloride) Capsules BPC: available as
Sinequan (Pfizer): Caps 10, 25 & 50 mg
   USA:
Doxepin Hydrochloride Capsules USP &
Doxepin Hydrochloride Oral Solution USP: available as
Sinequan (Pfizer): Caps 10, 25, 50 & 100 mg; Oral Soln 10 mg/1 ml
Adapin (Pennwalt): Caps 10, 25 & 50 mg

DROPERIDOL

● Droperidol belongs to the butyrophenone class of antipsychotic tranquillizers and has actions similar to those of HALOPERIDOL. However,
its clinical indications are more specialized. On its own the drug is
prescribed to control hyperagitated and manic states in manic-depression
and other psychoses. At low dosages it has been given to control very
severe nausea and as an adjunct to opiates in premedication, generally by
injection. Together with the short-acting narcotic analgesic FENTANYL,
droperidol is administered in the surgical technique of neuroleptanalgesia:
this is a system whereby the patient is enabled to remain conscious,
although pain-free, while a surgical operation or procedure (e.g. bronchoscopy) is carried out. The tranquillizer considerably enhances the
analgesic and other actions of fentanyl. So far as the compound's use in
psychiatry is concerned, this should be reserved for only the most
intractable cases, which do not respond to other medication. Droperidol
at the required dose levels tends to provoke a variety of unpleasant
unwanted effects, such as parkinsonism, oversedation, mental depression,
and alterations in the blood picture.

▲ In psychotic states, 5–20 mg daily, orally, in single or divided daily
doses. For neuroleptanalgesia, see under FENTANYL.

★ Contra-indicated in severe liver disease, convulsive disorders, and
known hypersensitivity to antipsychotic agents. Utmost caution in kidney
and cardiac dysfunction; also in respiratory insufficiency. Should not be
given concomitantly with antidepressants (particularly of the MAO-
inhibitor class), amphetamine and related drugs, and some antihypertensive agents.

➤ For further information, see Essay VI(B) and Chart VI: Antipsychotic
Tranquillizers.

◆ UK:
Droleptan (Janssen): Tabs 10 mg; Amps 10 mg/2 ml; liq 1 mg/1ml
   USA:
Droperidol Injection USP: available as
Inapsine (McNeil): Amps 5 mg/2 ml & 12.5 mg/5 ml; Vials 25 mg/10 ml
see also under FENTANYL

EPHEDRINE

● The principal alkaloid of the plant *Ephedra vulgaris,* ephedrine has many medical applications. It is probably most often used in hay fever, rhinitis, and asthma (to relieve nasal congestion and control spasm of the bronchial muscles); as a central stimulant in narcolepsy and as an antidote to overdosage from sedatives and analgesics (obsolete); and, rarely, to prevent hypotension during spinal anaesthesia. Other uses include enuresis (bed-wetting) in children, symptomatic relief of weakness in myasthenia gravis, and in the form of eye-drops to dilate the pupils. Ephedrine is an ingredient of numerous cough syrups and expectorants, often in conjunction with DIPHENHYDRAMINE and other antihistamines. Except at low doses, the drug may provoke headache, nausea, palpitations, restlessness, dizziness, and acute (though transient) mental depression as its effect begins to wear off. Generally, adverse reactions resemble those of AMPHETAMINES and are not necessarily less severe. The high incidence of some of the above-mentioned side-effects tends to militate against abuse of the compound, although occasionally cases of amphetamine-type dependency have been reported in the literature.

▲ The appropriate dose will depend on the ailment being treated. For most purposes, 15–50 mg three or four times daily.

★ Ephedrine, unlike other central stimulants, may be given cautiously with MAO-inhibitor antidepressants in narcolepsy: this combination has been found effective in some cases. It should be avoided if possible in hypertension, thyrotoxicosis, cardiac ailments, prostatic hypertrophy, and in cases of agitation and depression. Ephedrine is potentiated by tricyclic antidepressants, and concurrent use with digitalis may disturb cardiac rhythm.

➤ For further information, see Essay I and Chart I: Amphetamines.

◆ UK:
Ephedrine Hydrochloride Tablets BPC: 15, 30 & 60 mg
Ephedrine Hydrochloride Elixir BPC: 15 mg/5 ml
unbranded ephedrine hydrochloride Amps 30 mg/1 ml
    USA:
Ephedrine Sulfate Tablets USP: 25 & 50 mg
Ephedrine Sulfate Capsules USP: 25 & 50 mg
Ephedrine Sulfate Injection USP: 20, 25 & 50 mg per ml
Ephedrine Sulfate Nasal Solution USP: 1% & 3%
Ephedrine Sulfate Syrup USP: 20 mg/5 ml
Ephedrine Sulphate and Phenobarbital Capsules USP: 21 + 15 & 50 + 30 mg
Ephedrine & Amytal (Lilly): Caps ephedrine sulfate 25 mg, amylobarbitone (amobarbital) 50 mg

Ephedrine & Seconal (Lilly): Caps ephedrine sulfate 25 mg, quinalbarbitone (secobarbital) sodium 50 mg
NB The very large number of compound ephedrine preparations is such that, for reasons of space, they are not listed here
see also under AMYLOBARBITONE

ETHAMIVAN

● A central and respiratory stimulant, ethamivan has been given in the treatment of barbiturate and carbon dioxide retention, and has been proposed as a remedy in chronic disease of the lungs. Whether administered orally or by injection, the drug is short-acting (10–30 minutes following intravenous use) and tends to produce a range of undesirable effects, including cough, tremors, twitching, sneezing, itching and, at high doses, convulsions and severe cardiac irregularities. The American Food and Drug Administration has ruled that ethamivan is ineffective and, with the introduction of safer and more effective alternatives, obsolescent.

▲ Injection: 2–5 ml of a 5% solution intravenously, repeated at intervals or infused continuously.

★ Contra-indicated in coma, epilepsy, and respiratory failure precipitated by a convulsant drug (e.g. antipsychotic tranquillizers), and when antidepressants of the MAO-inhibitor class have been prescribed.

◆ UK:
Ethamivan Elixir BPC 1973: 5% in purified water
Clairvan (Sinclair): Oral Soln 50 mg/1 ml; Amps 100 mg/2 ml

ETHCHLORVYNOL

● As a sleep-inducing agent of moderate potency, ethchlorvynol is a useful medicament unrelated to the barbiturates. It begins to act quickiy after ingestion and promotes 5–7 hours' sound sleep in many patients: its low toxicity is noteworthy. Unfortunately the drug is no longer marketed in the UK but is produced in the USA as capsules which contain the drug in liquid form. While ethchlorvynol is well tolerated in most cases, some individuals experience hangover, dizziness, confusion, blurred vision, or gastric upsets, and paradoxical excitement may follow administration of large doses. Rarely, a form of jaundice and an optical complaint (amblyopia) have been known to occur, as well as hypersensitivity reactions such as skin rashes. Adverse effects are less likely to arise if the drug is taken with food. Psychological and perhaps physical dependency have been recorded but are uncommon: as in the case of other hypnotics, prolonged administration is undesirable.

▲ Usually 500 mg–1 G at night, with food or hot milk.

★ Contra-indicated in porphyria and known hypersensitivity. Caution in impaired liver or kidney function. Ethchlorvynol decreases the effects of oral anticoagulants and dosage should be reduced if antidepressants (whether tricyclic or MAO-inhibitor) are taken at the same time.

➤ Precautions are generally as for BARBITURATES (Essay III and Chart III).

◆ USA:
Ethchlorvynol Capsules USP: available as
Placidyl (Abbott): Caps 100, 200, 500 & 750 mg

ETHINAMATE

● Ethinamate is a non-barbiturate hypnotic unrelated to any of the major classes of soporific agents. Its onset of action is rapid but its short duration of effect (2–4 hours) makes the compound unsuitable for individuals who have difficulty staying asleep. It is not appropriate for daytime sedation, except perhaps to allay anxiety prior to minor dental and surgical procedures. Hangover, dizziness, and unsteady gait are not infrequent adverse effects, and confusion, paradoxical excitement and digestive disturbances occur in some cases. Rarely disorders of blood function follow repeated use of ethinamate. Prescription of the drug for prolonged periods is inadvisable because of the risk of tolerance and physical dependency. Patients who have been receiving it regularly should be withdrawn slowly, as a withdrawal syndrome similar to that of the barbiturates may otherwise be precipitated. Rashes and other skin reactions indicate hypersensitivity to the drug.

▲ 500 mg–1.5 G at night. Lower doses are advised for elderly or debilitated patients. For daytime use: a single dose of 500 mg ½-hour before surgery.

★ The compound should not be given in porphyria and only with circumspection in severe liver and kidney ailments. Contra-indicated during pregnancy and lactation. The central depressant actions of barbiturates, narcotics, tranquillizers and alcohol are enhanced by ethinamate, and the effects of oral anticoagulants decreased.

◆ USA:
Ethinamate Capsules USP: available as
Valmid (Lilly): Caps 500 mg

ETHOHEPTAZINE

● Although this drug is a chemical analogue of PETHIDINE (MEPERIDINE), it is of only moderate pain-relieving potency and is far less likely to induce tolerance and habituation. Ethoheptazine is prescribed, often in conjunction with aspirin and other simple analgesics, to alleviate chronic or intermittent pain which is not sufficiently severe to warrant the administration of narcotics. It is especially useful in inflammatory and musculo-skeletal pain states. Interestingly, it has been found that doses of ethoheptazine 100 mg by subcutaneous injection, given at four-hourly intervals, proved effective in suppressing morphine withdrawal symptoms. However, the drug is not marketed in injectable form, partly because administration by this route appears to provoke undesirable excitation of the central nervous system. In practice this type of reaction occurs only if unacceptably large numbers of tablets have been taken. Side-effects are seldom troublesome at recommended dosages, but those in excess of recommended regimens can produce itching, drowsiness, dizziness, and gastro-intestinal upsets. Protracted use has occasionally resulted in addiction.

▲ 75–150 mg four- or five-hourly. Somewhat higher doses may be required in certain cases.

★ A popular preparation of ethoheptazine also contains the tranquillizer MEPROBAMATE, so warnings, contra-indications etc. relevant to that drug should be observed. The compound is not recommended in severe kidney disorders, disturbances of blood metabolism, or during pregnancy.

➤ For further information, see Essay IV and Chart IV: Morphine and Other Potent Analgesics.

◆ UK:
Equagesic (Wyeth): Tabs ethoheptazine citrate 75 mg, meprobamate 150 mg, aspirin 250 mg, calcium carbonate 75 mg
Zactipar (Wyeth): Tabs ethoheptazine citrate 75 mg, paracetamol 400 mg
Zactirin (Wyeth): Tabs ethoheptazine citrate 75 mg, aspirin 325 mg, calcium carbonate 97 mg
   USA:
Ethoheptazine Citrate Tablets USNF 1970: available as
Zactane (Wyeth): Tabs 75 mg
Equagesic (Wyeth): as UK
Zactirin (Wyeth): as UK
Zactirin-Co (Wyeth): Tabs ethoheptazine citrate 100 mg, aspirin 222 mg, phenacetin 162 mg, caffeine 32.4 mg

ETHYLMORPHINE R

● Ethylmorphine, a drug seldom prescribed today, has a pain-relieving action midway between that of CODEINE and that of MORPHINE. As an analgesic, it is available only as a branded tablet which also contains glyceryl trinitrate, for use in angina pectoris: each has a quantity of ethylmorphine which is likely to have only marginal pain-relieving efficacy. The compound is very rarely given as eye-drops, to stimulate production of lymph in glaucoma and other optical disorders: however, direct application has an irritant action, causing the eyelids and conjunctivae to redden and swell up. In chronic catarrhal middle-ear deafness, injection of ethylmorphine through the tympanic membrane has been reported to be effective. It is as a cough-suppressant only that the drug has current therapeutic use. Chronic administration of the drug at analgesic doses (far higher than those required to control coughs) may result in habituation and addiction of the morphine type.

▲ For suppression of cough: 5–10 mg in a suitable mixture or elixir. Maximum single dose 60 mg.

➤ Warnings and contra-indications are essentially as for MORPHINE: see Essay IV and Chart IV: Morphine and Other Potent Analgesics.

◆ UK:
Ethylmorphine Hydrochloride BP Addendum 1977: bulk powder
Natirose (Lewis): Chewable SC Tabs ethylmorphine hydrochloride 3 mg, glyceryl trinitrate 0.75 mg, hyoscyamine hydrobromide 0.05 mg

ETORPHINE R

● This compound is a narcotic analgesic which, by weight, is some 200 or more times as potent as MORPHINE. It is marketed only for use in veterinary medicine, to tranquillize or anaesthetize animals of various kinds. The available solution of the drug is so powerful that even a single drop absorbed through the skin has been known to be lethal in man. See DIETHYLTHIAMBUTENE.

◆ UK:
Etorphine and Acepromazine Injection BPC, BVetC &
Etorphine and Methotrimeprazine Injection BPC, BVetC: available as
Immobilon (Reckitt & Colman): Large Animal Pack: Vials etorphine hydrochloride 24.5 mg, acepromazine maleate 100 mg/10 ml (coloured yellow); Small Animal Pack: Vials etorphine hydrochloride 1.48 mg, methotrimeprazine tartrate 360 mg/10 ml (clear solution)

FENCAMFAMIN

● Fencamfamin is a central nervous system stimulant whose potency lies midway between that of caffeine and that of AMPHETAMINE. The drug is prescribed to relieve lassitude, fatigue and somnolence in the recuperative period following surgical operations or when potent analgesics of the MORPHINE type must be taken regularly: the latter often produce drowsiness at effective dose levels. An extremely useful medicament, fencamfamin is generally well tolerated, and regular use over periods of months does not appear to lead to a significant degree of tolerance, and psychological habituation is not commonly seen. These are possible hazards, as the drug is somewhat euphoriant at doses only slightly in excess of those recommended. Dry mouth, headache, dizziness, abdominal upsets are among the unwanted reactions which have been noted. The compound is not marketed in the USA and the only preparation available in the UK also contains a number of vitamins of the B group. There seems no reason why fencamfamin should not be tried as an alternative to amphetamines in a number of clinical indications, e.g. narcolepsy. The drug has been prescribed experimentally in cases of dementia: an improvement in alertness and orientation was observed but restlessness occurred in a number of patients. The elderly are in general more susceptible than persons of other age groups to the effects of psychotropic agents.

▲ 10–20 mg twice or occasionally three times daily, the last dose taken not later than 4 p.m.: otherwise sleep may be difficult.

★ Not recommended in severe hypertension or cardiac disease, hyperthyroidism, glaucoma and states of agitation or hyperexcitability; nor for concurrent use with antidepressants of the MAO-inhibitor series.

➤ For a comparison with other stimulants, and further information on interactions, etc., see Essay I and Chart I: Amphetamines.

◆ UK:
Reactivan (E. Merck): Tabs fencamfamin hydrochloride 10 mg, thiamine 10 mg, pyridoxine 20 mg, cyanocobalamin (vit. B_{12}) 10 μg, vitamin C 100 mg

FENFLURAMINE

● This compound is unusual among AMPHETAMINE derivatives in that it produces no stimulation of the central nervous system, and indeed at therapeutic doses it may be soporific. It is prescribed to decrease appetite in obesity. Claims that the drug has a more profound influence on weight have proved extravagant: like other amphetamine analogues, its effect on appetite is short-lived and unlikely to last for more than a few weeks. It should be prescribed only as part of a complete programme including strict diet and exercise. Adverse effects are unpleasant at the higher dosage levels, and severe depression, diarrhoea, nausea, urinary frequency, anxiety and disturbances of REM or dreaming sleep have been noted. It is rather surprising that several reports of fenfluramine abuse have been published, suggesting that some patients find the drug euphoriant. This appetite-suppressant is one of three psychotropic agents currently being studied for their possible damaging effect on brain function in the foetus. The likelihood of dependency has not been established reliably, but practitioners should err on the side of caution and give the drug on a short-term basis only.

▲ 60–120 mg daily: the appearance of a delayed-release formulation may make dosage more convenient. One or two of these capsules, taken at breakfast, may be appropriate for some patients, but lower doses are effective for others.

★ Contra-indicated in pregnancy, for children, in hypertension and for persons with a history of drug abuse. Interactions with other drugs which can have serious consequences are several: particularly, fenfluramine should not be given at the same time as amphetamines or other appetite-suppressants, antidepressants (tricyclic or MAO-inhibitor), antihypertensive and oral anti-diabetic drugs. CNS depression caused by tranquillizers, alcohol etc. is enhanced.

➤ For further information, see Essay I and Chart I: Amphetamines.

◆ UK:
Fenfluramine (Hydrochloride) Tablets BPC: available as
Ponderax (Servier): Tabs 20 & 40 mg; SR Caps 60 mg
    USA:
Pondimin (Robins): Tabs 20 mg

FENTANYL R

● Although fentanyl is a narcotic analgesic whose potency is comparable to that of MORPHINE, this synthetic drug is almost exclusively used in a specialized situation. With the technique of neuroleptanalgesia, a patient is enabled to remain conscious, albeit pain-free, during a surgical operation or a diagnostic procedure (e.g. bronchoscopy). The compound's extremely short duration of action (½–1 hour after intravenous injection) lends itself to this type of application, in which fentanyl is often given with the tranquillizer DROPERIDOL. This drug is also administered in conjunction with anaesthetic agents to provide 'balanced anaesthesia', for instance in heart surgery. Fentanyl has been given for postoperative pain relief, and it has been found that intramuscular rather than intravenous injection significantly prolongs its effect. This has not been tried often, partly because the drug has significant respiratory depressant activity and additionally because duration of pain relief (2–3 hours after IM dosage) is still shorter than that afforded by MORPHINE and most analogues. Side-effects are typical of the opiates (nausea, itching, constipation, mood changes) except that fentanyl in certain cases produces muscular rigidity of the chest wall which may be hazardous. The combination with droperidol can be dangerous because the latter compound is far longer-acting and has been claimed to produce stressful reactions in patients postoperatively. Fentanyl theoretically has a high potential for habituation, and is therefore under international legal restriction; but because it is almost never prescribed outside hospitals or for other than very short periods the problem scarcely arises.

▲ Postoperative pain relief: 0.05–0.1 mg intramuscularly, two- to three-hourly.

★ Contra-indicated in severe respiratory problems, coma, convulsive disorders, and generally as for MORPHINE. Fentanyl's action is potentiated by other CNS depressants, and the drug should not be given to patients under treatment with MAO-inhibitor antidepressants. In the case of combinations with DROPERIDOL, additional interactions and precautions should be considered.

➤ For further information, see Essay IV and Chart IV: Morphine and Other Potent Analgesics.

◆ UK:
Fentanyl Citrate BPC: present in
Sublimaze (Janssen): Amps 0.1 mg/2 ml; Vials 0.5 mg/10 ml
Thalamonal (Janssen): Amps fentanyl citrate 0.1 mg, droperidol 5 mg/2 ml
Hypnorm (Crookes): Vials fentanyl citrate 3.15 mg, fluanisone 100 mg/10 ml (For veterinary use only)
  USA:
Fentanyl Citrate Injection USP: available as
Sublimaze (McNeil): Amps 0.1 mg/2 ml & 0.5 mg/5 ml
Innovar (McNeil): Amps fentanyl citrate 0.1 mg, droperidol 5 mg/2 ml & 0.25 + 12.5 mg/5 ml

FLUPENTHIXOL

● This compound is one of the more recent introductions to the antipsychotic tranquillizers (neuroleptic agents): it belongs to the thioxanthene series of compounds. Its principal applications are in the symptomatic treatment of withdrawn, confused, apathetic and delusional states as these may figure prominently in schizophrenia and other forms of psychotic illness. At dosages far lower than those required to control such symptoms, flupenthixol has been proposed to relieve non-psychotic conditions, and appears successful in anxiety, tension and depression. A very important point about the thioxanthene class of drugs is that, unlike the more conventional phenothiazine antipsychotic agents, they do not provoke mental depression and do not enhance this if it is already present. Because schizophrenics and other patients with severe mental disturbances are often unreliable about taking medication by mouth, a number of preparations have come on to the market which circumvent the problem.

Among these, flupenthixol as the decanoic acid ester (a suspension of the drug in vegetable oil) is available as a depôt injection, a single dose of which will produce effects lasting two to four weeks. With the availability of convenient formulations of this kind, there is a danger that patients may not be monitored as closely or as regularly as if they were on oral antipsychotic drugs. Adverse reactions are less frequent and often less serious with thioxanthene compounds than with other neuroleptics: drowsiness and lethargy are commonly reported, as well as anticholinergic effects (blurred vision, dry mouth) and changes in libido and sexual potency. Parkinsonian reactions, so often a problem with CHLOR-PROMAZINE and other major tranquillizers, do occur with flupenthixol but are more likely at higher doses. Somewhat confusingly, the oral tablet preparation has two brand names, Depixol and Fluanxol, the latter being only 1/6th as potent and intended for use in less severe anxious and depressed states.

▲ Orally: Non-psychotic states: 2–3 mg daily. Schizophrenia and other psychoses: 3–18 mg daily by mouth, or 20–40 mg by deep intramuscular injection 2–4 weekly; up to 200 mg may sometimes be required.

★ Principal contra-indications are severe cardiac or cardiovascular, liver and kidney ailments, Parkinson's disease, and states of agitation or hyperexcitability. Should not be given concurrently with MAO-inhibitor antidepressants.

➤ See also under CLOPENTHIXOL and Essay VI and Chart VI(B): Antipsychotic Tranquillizers.

◆ UK:
Fluanxol (Lundbeck): Tabs 0.5 mg (hydrochloride)
Depixol (Lundbeck): Tabs 3 mg (hydrochloride); Amps & Syrettes 20 mg/ 1 ml & 40 mg/2 ml; Concentrated Amps 100 mg/1 ml (decanoate)

FLUPHENAZINE

● This compound has become one of the most extensively administered chemicals in current psychiatric practice. Fluphenazine is a derivative of CHLORPROMAZINE, possessing an exceedingly potent antipsychotic activity. Like many other drugs of the phenothiazine class it is prescribed to control hallucinations, delusions, hyperagitation and other symptoms of schizophrenia and psychological complaints of comparable severity. Fluphenazine, in addition to oral preparations, is presented in the form of two depôt injections: the enanthate and the decanoate. A single deep intramuscular injection of the former acts for up to 28 days and of the more widely used decanoate for 5 to 8 weeks. The convenience of such formulations, particularly because of the problem of non-compliance with regimens of tablets by psychotic patients, is obvious. But the dangers tend to be underestimated: for example, psychiatric outpatients may not be monitored as often or as thoroughly as they ought to be if long-acting injections are given, and severe adverse effects from fluphenazine often occur between hospital appointments. A particular danger with depôt phenothiazines (and to a lesser extent of most neuroleptic agents) is that pre-existing mental depression may be intensified or provoked by them, and a number of cases of suicide following fluphenazine injections have been reported. Other common side-effects are apathy and loss of interest in the individual's surroundings, docility and loss of motivation: parkinsonian reactions are more often seen with this than with some other antipsychotic medicaments. Long-term administration, especially of large doses, may lead to tardive dyskinesia, a severe and perhaps irreversible form of Parkinson's disease. The prescription of oral fluphenazine in combination with an antidepressant such as NORTRIPTYLINE, in the treatment of non-psychotic anxiety, tension and depression, may be justified in some instances but many practitioners evidently do not understand the nature or quality of fluphenazine's effects. Fixed-dose combinations are particularly undesirable since these are unlikely to contain the optimum dose of one or other of their constituents and they are pharmacologically unsound. While fluphenazine has an undoubted role in controlling psychotic states, its increasing use to alleviate minor emotional disturbances is regrettable, since there are safer alternative drugs whose unwanted effects are negligible in comparison to those so often provoked by major tranquillizers of this type.

▲ Outpatients: 1–5 mg daily. Inpatients: up to 60 mg daily (by mouth), according to severity of symptoms and response. Enanthate and decanoate: initially 12.5 mg intramuscularly, followed by 12.5–25 mg after 7–10 days, depending on response; thereafter, 12.5–50 mg 3–4 weekly and 5–8 weekly respectively.

★ Contra-indicated in sclerosis of brain vessels, severe cardiac, liver and kidney disorders; depressive states; convulsive disorders; cases of intolerance to other antipsychotic drugs of the phenothiazine type; and phaeochromocytoma. Potentially serious interactions may occur with oral anticoagulants, some antihypertensive and antidiabetic drugs and with antidepressants of the MAO-inhibitor group.

➤ For further information, see Essay VI(B) and Chart VI: Antipsychotic Tranquillizers.

◆ UK:
Fluphenazine Hydrochloride Tablets BPC: available as
Moditen (Squibb): Tabs 1, 2.5 & 5 mg; Elix 2.5 mg/5 ml (deleted 1981)
Motipress (Squibb): Tabs fluphenazine hydrochloride 1.5 mg, nortriptyline hydrochloride 30 mg

Motival (Squibb): Tabs fluphenazine hydrochloride 0.5 mg, nortriptyline hydrochloride 10 mg
Fluphenazine Enanthate Injection BPC: available as
Moditen-Enanthate (Squibb): Amps 25 mg/1 ml; Vials 250 mg/10 ml
Fluphenazine Decanoate Injection BPC: available as
Modecate (Squibb): Amps 12.5 mg/0.5 ml; Amps & Syrettes 25 mg/1 ml; Vials 250 mg/10 ml; Concentrated Amps 100 mg/1 ml
   USA:
Fluphenazine Hydrochloride Tablets USP
Fluphenazine Hydrochloride Elixir USP
Fluphenazine Hydrochloride Injection USP &
Fluphenazine Hydrochloride Oral Solution USP: available as
Permitil (Schering): Tabs 0.25, 2.5, 5 & 10 mg; SR Tabs 1 mg; Soln 5 mg/ml
Proxilin (Squibb): Tabs 1, 2.5, 5 & 10 mg; Elix 2.5 mg/5 ml; Vials 25 mg/1 ml
Fluphenazine Enathate Injection USP: available as
Prolixin Enathate (Squibb): Syrettes & Cartridges 25 mg/1 ml; Vials 125 mg/5 ml
Fluphenazine Decanoate Injection USP: available as
Prolixin Decanoate (Squibb): Syrettes 25 mg/1 ml; Vials 125 mg/5 ml

FLURAZEPAM

● Flurazepam is a sleep-inducing drug of recent introduction. Chemically and otherwise it is a close analogue of DIAZEPAM (Valium) and belongs to the benzodiazepine class of compounds. It has become a popular alternative to the barbiturates for promoting sleep, in part because it is effective even in fairly intractable cases of insomnia but chiefly because of its low toxicity. Flurazepam exerts its soporific action more selectively than do AMYLOBARBITONE (AMOBARBITAL) and the rest of the barbiturates, damping down REM (dreaming) sleep less than these. Side-effects are seldom of sufficient severity that use of the compound has to be discontinued. However, flurazepam is longer-acting than is often believed, and so hangover and oversedation the following day may be experienced: reflexes too may be impaired after ingestion of the drug. At large doses paradoxical excitement and disinhibition occasionally occur. Protracted use of any benzodiazepine leads in many cases to psychological habituation: physical addiction is not frequent but should be considered as a possibility. Prescription of flurazepam for long periods is not advised.

▲ 15–60 mg at night.

★ Contra-indicated in cases of severe respiratory distress, myasthenia gravis, and known hypersensitivity to any of this class of compounds.

Particular caution in impaired liver or kidney function. The CNS-depressant effects of barbiturates, tranquillizers and alcohol are increased.

➤ For further information, see Essay III and Chart III: Barbiturates.

◆ UK:
Dalmane (Roche): Caps 15 & 30 mg
   USA:
Flurazepam Hydrochloride Capsules USP: available as
Dalmane (Roche): Caps 15 & 30 mg

FLUSPIRILENE

● This drug is an addition to the already extensive range of major tranquillizers or antipsychotic agents. It is presented as a micro-crystalline suspension for injection into muscle: a single dose will act for approximately 7 days. This is a shorter period of effect than that provided by other depôt antipsychotics, e.g. FLUPHENAZINE DECANOATE, but still has obvious advantages over oral preparations, which must be taken at least once daily. Fluspirilene is prescribed to control acute episodes – hallucinations, delusions, agitation – and to prevent their relapse in schizophrenia. The drug's unwanted effects compare favourably with those provoked by other neuroleptics at equivalent doses: parkinsonian reactions, mental depression, apathy, and sedation may be expected but are perhaps less severe than the adverse reactions from CHLORPROMAZINE and other phenothiazine tranquillizers. Occasionally nodules are formed in the subcutaneous tissues after injection: these have been shown to contain particles of the drug, and their presence indicates that the present formulation could be improved. The insidious form of parkinsonism known as tardive dyskinesia is probably a hazard of long-term administration of fluspirilene, as of other antischizophrenic agents.

▲ In the range of 2–12 mg weekly, by deep intramuscular injection, depending on the severity of the condition and personal idiosyncrasy.

★ Contra-indicated in convulsive disorders and for patients who cannot tolerate the related drug PIMOZIDE: not established as safe for use during pregnancy.

➤ For further information on interactions with other drugs, warnings, etc., see Essay VI(B) and Chart VI: Antipsychotic Tranquillizers.

◆ UK:
Redeptin (Smith Kline & French): Amps 2 mg/1 ml & 6 mg/3 ml; Vials 12 mg/6 ml

GLUTETHIMIDE

● This compound is prescribed mainly to aid sleep and, more rarely, for daytime sedation. Glutethimide is not a barbiturate, though it shares many of the characteristics of this type of hypnotic: regular use over weeks or months leads to a reduction in the drug's efficacy and hence tolerance develops. Physical addiction has been reported which is again similar in type, if less severe, to that which follows chronic barbiturate taking. This does not occur in every case, and some patients can be maintained at constant dosage regimens for long periods. But glutethimide should not be prescribed for long-term administration and is not advised for patients with a history of drug abuse. This is not only because of the dependency hazard but also because certain individuals find high doses of the compound euphoriant and enjoy the paradoxical excitement which can then arise. Hangover, oversedation and unsteadiness of gait may be experienced the morning after a night's sleep induced by this medicament. Allergic skin reactions occur in a few hypersensitive patients. Glutethimide is relatively less dangerous in overdosage than barbiturates, but much more so than FLURAZEPAM and other hypnotics of the benzodiazepine type, which may be preferable for the relief of insomnia.

▲ 250–750 mg at night.

★ This drug should not be prescribed for patients who suffer from convulsive disorders such as epilepsy, nor for those hypersensitive either to glutethimide or its chemical relative METHYLPRYLONE. Caution in impaired liver or kidney function, and if other central depressant agents or oral anticoagulants are given concurrently.

➜ For comparison with other hypnotics and further information, see Essay III and Chart III: Barbiturates.

◆ UK:
Glutethimide Tablets BPC: available as
Doriden (Ciba): Tabs 250 mg
   USA:
Glutethimide Tablets USP &
Glutethimide Capsules USP: available as
Doriden (USV): Tabs 250 & 500 mg; Caps 500 mg
Dorimide (Cenci): Tabs 500 mg
Rolathimide (Robinson): Tabs 500 mg

HALOPERIDOL

● While principally administered for its antipsychotic effect, haloperidol is also given, at lower doses, to control nausea and vomiting, and by injection for premedication before surgical operations. The drug is effective in alcoholic withdrawal and controls delirium tremens (DTs). Primarily this butyrophenone compound is prescribed to control mania, agitation, aggressiveness, hallucinations and other symptoms of schizophrenia and other disorders which are classified as psychotic. Use of this extremely potent neuroleptic to alleviate mild emotional or psychosomatic complaints such as anxiety and tension is inadvisable except in unusual cases. Not only does haloperidol tend to provoke a range of very disagreeable side-effects – parkinsonism, oversedation, apathy, loss of motivation – it can considerably enhance the intensity of mental depression which often coexists with anxiety states. Prolonged treatment with haloperidol, especially in long-stay psychiatric patients, often results in tardive dyskinesia, a severe form of Parkinson's disease which may not be reversible: this and other drugs of the butyrophenone class are even more apt to provoke this syndrome than other antipsychotic agents. Even small therapeutic doses of haloperidol may exacerbate depression and produce other adverse effects, so the medicament should be reserved for treatment of serious psychological disturbances.

▲ Outpatients: 2–6 mg daily. Hospital inpatients may require up to 100 mg daily for relief of symptoms.

★ Contra-indicated in spastic cerebral conditions, Parkinson's disease, and severe liver disease. Concomitant use of MAO-inhibitor antidepressants is dangerous, and potentially serious interactions occur with amphetamines and other stimulants, and some antihypertensive agents. Utmost caution if other CNS depressants are required.

➤ For further information, see Essay VI(B) and Chart VI: Antipsychotic Tranquillizers.

◆ UK:
Haloperidol Tablets BPC &
Haloperidol Injection BPC: available as
Haldol (Janssen): Tabs 500 µg, 1.5, 5, 10 & 20 mg; Oral Conc 2 mg/1 ml; Amps 5 mg/1 ml & 10 mg/2 ml
Serenace (Searle): Caps 500 µg; Tabs 1.5, 5 & 10 mg; Oral Conc 2 mg/1 ml; Amps 5 mg/1 ml
    USA:
Haloperidol Tablets USP
Haloperidol Oral Solution USP &
Haloperidol Injection USP: available as
Haldol (McNeil): Tabs 500 µg, 1, 2, 5 & 10 mg; Oral Soln 2 mg/1 ml; Amps 5 mg/1 ml; Vials 50 mg/10 ml

HARMALINE and HARMINE

● Harmine and harmaline are the principal alkaloids of a South American vine, *Banisteriopsis caapi.* Both substances are also present in the plant *Peganum harmala,* whose habitat ranges from Central and South America to the Asian steppes. Harmine, originally named telepathine, has definite psychedelic effects which qualitatively resemble those produced by LYSERGIDE (LSD). The difference between their psychological actions is hard to describe: the term 'oneirophrenic' has been coined for harmine and harmaline by Claudio Naranjo, to suggest the dream-like states provoked by these compounds. Perception is altered more subtly by harmine than by LSD, though not less profoundly. Not only may visions ('hallucinations') be seen, but a fascinating aspect of these alkaloids' activity is that two or more individuals to whom one or other has been administered may see the *same* visions. The indigenous people of Peru, who smoke or snuff *Peganum* in powdered form, believe that *yage* or *ayahuasca,* as they call the substance, inspires telepathic communication: hence the original name for harmine. Taken by mouth, harmine is virtually inactive; but smoked, snuffed, or administered by intramuscular injection, a dose of 100–300 mg is likely to promote profound psychological effects. Harmaline and harmine are not available for prescription as they are not considered medicinally useful; neither have they appeared on the illicit market. Nobody should contemplate taking these or any other psychedelics except under expert medical supervision and with additional safeguards. Harmine is a mild inhibitor of the enzyme MAO (monoamine oxidase), like certain antidepressants.

➤ For further information, see Essay V and Chart V: Psychedelics. For warnings and other data on MAO-inhibitors, see Chart II: Antidepressants.

HEPTABARBITONE (HEPTABARBITAL)

● This drug is typical of the intermediate-acting members of the barbiturate class, possessing most of the attributes of AMYLOBARBITONE (AMOBARBITAL). Heptabarbitone is almost exclusively prescribed as a remedy for insomnia. While it is effective in this indication, the drug suffers from all the disadvantages of barbituric acid derivatives: chronic use tends to habituation and frank addiction, and non-medical consumption of high doses may induce a state of paradoxical excitement and euphoria of a type favoured by many drug abusers. Although heptabarbitone is often classed as 'short-acting', hangover effects may be apparent and oversedation, with consequent slowing of reflexes, is common the morning after a nocturnal dose. Given the drug's abuse liability and its potential for suicidal use, prescription of this as of other barbiturates as hypnotics is considered inappropriate by many practitioners. With the advent of safer alternatives, such as members of the benzodiazepine group of sedative/tranquillizers (e.g. NITRAZEPAM, Mogadon), there is certainly no therapeutic necessity to prescribe barbiturates to aid sleep.

▲ 100–300 mg at night.

★ In common with other barbiturates, heptabarbitone should be avoided in porphyria, severe respiratory ailments, and hypersensitivity to any drug of this type. Concurrent administration of other central depressants, including alcohol, is not recommended.

➤ For further information, see Essay III and Chart III: Barbiturates.

◆ UK:
Medomin (Geigy): Tabs 200 mg
　USA:
Medomin (Geigy): Tabs 200 mg

HEXOBARBITONE (HEXOBARBITAL)

● The data provided in the preceding entry (HEPTABARBITONE) apply to hexobarbitone also. In the UK this compound is available only as a tablet which also contains CYCLOBARBITONE. The combination of two barbiturates is unnecessary, as all those of intermediate duration of action have practically identical effects.

▲ Between 125 and 500 mg at bedtime. Repeated use is not advised.

★ See under HEPTABARBITONE and Essay III and Chart III: Barbiturates, for warnings, contra-indications and interactions with other drugs.

◆ UK:
Evidorm (Winthrop): Tabs hexobarbitone 250 mg, cyclobarbitone calcium 100 mg
　USA:
Hexobarbital Tablets USP: available as
Sombulex (Riker): Tabs 250 mg
Ultrased (Scrip): Tabs 250 mg

HYDROCODONE (DIHYDROCODEINONE) R

● Hydrocodone is a CODEINE derivative and shares its two principal effects: relief of moderately severe pain and the control of intractable cough. This compound is more morphine- than codeine-like, however, and for this reason any preparation containing it is restricted under the UK Misuse of Drugs Act. In fact the only such product marketed in Britain is a cough syrup of which a very small dose of hydrocodone is among the ingredients. In the USA only pure formulations of the drug are so controlled. Hydrocodone has slightly better pain-relieving activity than its close analogue DIHYDROCODEINE but neither is effective in the most severe pain states. Various products are available in the USA which combine the opiate with simple analgesics such as paracetamol (acetaminophen). While these may be therapeutically useful in mitigating recurrent or chronic pain, the dependence liability of the drug is such that use over protracted periods, or by individuals predisposed to abuse narcotics, should be monitored carefully. Side-effects characteristic of the opiates – nausea, constipation, dizziness, drowsiness, and mood changes – occur if large doses are given, but are less pronounced than those provoked by MORPHINE and other narcotics of greater absolute analgesic potency. Long-term consumption of hydrocodone-containing syrups and elixirs is, unless therapeutically justified, inadvisable.

▲ Relief of severe cough. Most syrups contain between 1 and 4 mg of hydrocodone per 5 ml (teaspoonful): 1.5–4 mg 3- to 4-hourly. As an analgesic: 5–15 mg at similar intervals.

★ Contra-indications include severe respiratory, liver or kidney disorders, alcoholism, and convulsive conditions. Concurrent administration of MAO-inhibitor antidepressants may be dangerous.

➤ For further information, see Essay IV and Chart IV: Morphine and Other Potent Analgesics.

◆ UK:
Dimotane-DC (Robins): Syr hydrocodone bitartrate 1.8 mg, brompheniramine maleate 2 mg, guaiphenesin 100 mg, phenylephrine hydrochloride 5 mg, phenylpropanolamine hydrochloride 5 mg/5 ml
    USA:
Hydrocodone Bitartrate Tablets USP: available as
Dicodid (Knoll): Sol Tabs 5 mg
Codone (Lemmon): Tabs 5 mg
Anexsia-D (Beecham): Tabs hydrocodone bitartrate 7 mg, aspirin 230 mg, phenacetin 150 mg, caffeine 30 mg
Coditrate (Central): Tabs hydrocodone bitartrate 2.4 mg, potassium guaiacolsulfonate 120 mg; Syr 10 ml equiv 1 Tab
Dicodrine (O'Neal, Jones & Feldman): Syr hydrocodone bitartrate 1.67 mg, potassium guaiacolsulfonate 83.34 mg, phenylephrine hydrochloride 5 mg, thenyldiamine hydrochloride 3.34 mg/5 ml
Duradyne-DHC (O'Neal, Jones & Feldman): Tabs hydrocodone bitartrate 5 mg, aspirin 230 mg, paracetamol (acetaminophen) 150 mg, caffeine 30 mg
Hycodan (Endo): Tabs hydrocodone bitartrate 5 mg, homatropine hydrobromide 1.5 mg; Syr 5 ml equiv 1 Tab; Powder for Soln 770 + 230 mg per G
Norcet (Frye): Tabs hydrocodone bitartrate 7.5 mg, paracetamol 650 mg

Tussend (Dow): Tabs hydrocodone bitartrate 5 mg, phenylephrine hydrochloride 25 mg; Syr 5 ml equiv 1 Tab
Tussionex (Pennwalt): Tabs & Caps hydrocodone bitartrate 5 mg, phenyltoloxamine resinate 10 mg; Syr 5 ml equiv 1 Tab or Cap
Vicodin (Knoll): Tabs hydrocodone bitartrate 5 mg, paracetamol (acetaminophen) 500 mg

HYDROMORPHONE R

● Hydromorphone possesses one of the highest analgesic potencies of MORPHINE-like drugs. While no longer marketed in Britain, the medicament is prescribed in several other countries, including the USA, to relieve very severe pain states and, at appreciably lower dosages, as a cough suppressant. Whatever the clinical indication and the form in which the drug is taken, it has a capacity for inducing tolerance and dependency which is no less than that of morphine itself or DIAMORPHINE (heroin). Hydromorphone is administered in myocardial infarction (coronary thrombosis), renal colic, severe burns and fractures, for postoperative analgesia and the pain of terminal cancer. Its use except on a short-term basis should be considered only when morphine would otherwise be prescribed. It may seem astonishing that one American medical journal carries regular advertisements for hydromorphone to relieve 'the pain you [the physician] see every day'. On the illicit market for narcotics, this drug is almost as much sought after as heroin, since it is powerfully euphoriant. Side-effects closely resemble those of morphine: nausea, constipation, dizziness, sedation, mood changes and particularly respiratory depression appear to arise more often after hydromorphone administration. Like other narcotic agonists, this agent at the molecular level binds to specific sites in the brain (especially the μ-receptors which are associated with analgesia, euphoria and other effects). This activity has a strong bearing on the phenomena of tolerance and addiction. Hydromorphone may be given orally, but it is more effective by injection or as rectal suppositories. Although cough syrups contain relatively low doses of the drug, repeated use may still lead to dependency: therefore these should be avoided for all but the most intractable types of cough (e.g. in tuberculosis, severe acute bronchitis).

▲ As an antitussive, 1–2 mg 4-hourly. Pain relief: orally, 1–4 mg; by subcutaneous or intramuscular injection, up to 4 mg. A marked loss of analgesic potency has been reported following intravenous injection. Patients with very intense chronic pain may need much higher doses.

★ Contra-indicated in raised intracranial pressure. Utmost caution in respiratory depression, convulsive states, liver and kidney dysfunction.

Concomitant prescription of MAO-inhibitor antidepressants and partial or pure narcotic antagonists may be dangerous.

➤ For further information, see Essay IV and Chart IV: Morphine and Other Potent Analgesics.

◆ USA:
Hydromorphone Hydrochloride Tablets USP: 1, 2, 3 & 4 mg
Hydromorphone Hydrochloride Injection USP: 1, 2, 3, 4 mg/1 ml
Dilaudid (Knoll): Tabs 1, 2, 3 & 4 mg; Amps 1, 2, 3 & 4 mg/1 ml; Vials 15 mg/10 ml; Suppos 3 mg; Powder for Solution: Bottles 1 & 3.5 G
Dilaudid Cough Syrup (Knoll): Syr hydromorphone hydrochloride 1 mg, glyceryl guaiacolate 100 mg/5 ml
Dilocol (Bell): Syr hydromorphone hydrochloride 1 mg, sodium citrate 250 mg, antimony potassium tartrate 1 mg/5 ml

HYDROXYZINE

● This is one of a very few anxiety- and tension-relieving drugs which are not related to DIAZEPAM (Valium) and other benzodiazepines. Like these, hydroxyzine has muscle-relaxant effects: it is also useful as an antiemetic and antihistamine, and may be given by injection as well as orally. Although it has been claimed that the drug's anxiolytic action is simply due to its general sedative properties, there is no doubt that hydroxyzine is in some cases a successful alternative to the benzo-diazepines. When administered concurrently with MORPHINE or other potent analgesics, pain-relieving effectiveness is considerably increased. Some patients experience disturbances of visual accommodation, sleepi-ness, dry mouth, and itching, and if the intramuscular route is used discomfort or pain at the injection site may be felt. Because of its antispasmodic action, the medicament is prescribed for relief of asthma; and in certain gastro-intestinal complaints marked by excessive gut motility, together with EPHEDRINE and other compounds whose effec-tiveness is considered to be enhanced. Hydroxyzine appears to have little potential for abuse or habituation.

▲ 50–300 mg daily, in 2 or 3 divided doses (orally). By injection, up to 100 mg. The drug must never be administered intravenously.

★ Patients should be warned that reflexes may be affected. Hydroxyzine is contra-indicated during pregnancy and in cases of known hypersensi-tivity. The CNS-depressing effects of barbiturates, opiates, tranquillizers and alcohol may be greatly increased.

➤ For further information, see Essay VI and Chart VI(A): Tranquil-lizers.

◆ UK:
Atarax (Pfizer): Tabs 10 & 25 mg; Syr 10 mg/5 ml
  USA:
Hydroxyzine Hydrochloride Tablets USP
Hydroxyzine Hydrochloride Syrup USP &
Hydroxyzine Hydrochloride Injection USP: available as
Atarax (Roerig): Tabs 10, 25, 50 & 100 mg; Syr 10 mg/5 ml; Syrettes 100 mg/2 ml; Vials 500 mg/10 ml
Ataraxoid (Pfizer): Tabs hydroxyzine hydrochloride 10 mg, prednisolone 2.5 or 5 mg
Cartrax (Roerig): Tabs hydroxyzine hydrochloride 10 mg, penta-erythirotol tetranitrate 10 or 20 mg
Enarax (Beecham): Tabs hydroxyzine hydrochloride 25 mg, oxyphencyc-limine hydrochloride 5 or 10 mg
Marax (Roerig): Tabs hydroxyzine hydrochloride 10 mg, ephedrine sulfate 25 mg, theophylline 130 mg; Syr 20 ml equiv 1 Tab
Vistrax (Pfizer): Tabs as *Enarax*
Hydroxyzine Pamoate Capsules USP &
Hydroxyzine Pamoate Oral Suspension USP: available as
Vistaril (Pfizer): Caps 25, 50 & 100 mg; Oral Susp 25 mg/5 ml; Syrettes 25 & 50 mg/1 ml, 100 mg/2 ml; Vials 250 & 500 mg/10 ml

IBOGAINE R

● Despite the fact that this chemical is nowhere obtainable on prescription, and has never been seen on the illicit markets, ibogaine is classed as a Controlled Drug, to which the most stringent restrictions apply. Doubtless this is because, from what sketchy evidence is available, it has psychedelic or 'hallucinogenic' activity. Ibogaine has been isolated from the root of *Tabernanthe iboga,* a shrub native to Central and West Africa and principally found in Zaire. Locally, this root is chewed to combat fatigue and to aid witch-doctors in divination, and is taken at religious ceremonies in Gabon. Reports of the effects of ibogaine on Western subjects have been few and provide us with insufficient data for a detailed account. Nevertheless, it appears that this alkaloid has genuine psychedelic qualities analogous to those of LYSERGIDE (LSD) but probably more similar to HARMALINE and HARMINE. In man, doses of about 300 mg orally, and approximately one-third of this quantity by injection, induce perceptual changes, visions, and other phenomena which are associated with psychedelic or 'psychotomimetic' substances, for a period of 3–5 hours. Early accounts of the activity of *T. iboga* root have suggested that it is a stimulant or that its effects resemble those of alcohol: in the absence of a conceptual frame of reference for describing psychedelic actions such statements, while understandable, are seriously misleading. No agent of this kind should ever be taken except under expert medical supervision.

➤ For further information, including criteria for use of such drugs, see Essay V and Chart V: Psychedelics.

IMIPRAMINE

● Next to AMITRIPTYLINE, imipramine is the most frequently prescribed of the tricyclic class of antidepressants. Not surprisingly, its chief application lies in the treatment of depressive states, and the drug may mitigate anxiety and tension to some extent also. Like all tricyclics, its action is far from immediate: two to four weeks of regular use must elapse before alleviation of symptoms, if this is forthcoming, will begin. Other effects, usually of an unwanted kind, tend to occur within two or three days of the commencement of therapy, and commonly include dry mouth, blurred vision, minor gastro-intestinal disturbances, changes in libido, and sedation. Because the latter effect may be pronounced, after dosage has been stabilized, a single daily dose at bedtime is often appropriate. Imipramine has been tried, with moderate success, to treat enuresis (bed-wetting) in children, and is currently promoted as an adjunct to analgesics in chronic rheumatic conditions. Some patients find that, particularly early in imipramine treatment, their depression is intensified. A great many physicians still apparently do not realize that relatively small numbers of tablets of this and other tricyclic antidepressants may be lethal in overdosage, which is difficult to reverse. In particular the toxic effects of this class of compounds on the heart have not been sufficiently emphasized, and it is not always possible to predict which patients may be susceptible to imipramine and its alternatives in this way.

▲ For the first week, 25 mg three times daily; thereafter 50 mg at similar intervals until response is obtained. Dosage may then be reduced and the drug taken as a single nightly regimen.

★ Contra-indicated in urinary retention, glaucoma, hyperthyroidism, prostatic enlargement. Especially serious interactions may occur with amphetamines and other stimulants and MAO-inhibitor antidepressants.

➤ For more information on warnings, interactions etc., see Essay II and Chart II: Antidepressants.

◆ UK:
Imipramine (Hydrochloride) Tablets BPC: 10 & 25 mg
Berkomine (Berk): Tabs 10 & 25 mg (deleted 1981)
Tofranil (Geigy): Tabs 10 & 25 mg; Syr 25 mg/5 ml; Amps 25 mg/2 ml
    USA:
Imipramine Hydrochloride Tablets USP: 10, 25 & 50 mg
Imipramine Hydrochloride Injection USP: 12.5 mg/ml

Tofranil (Geigy): Tabs 10, 25 & 50 mg; Amps 25 mg/2 ml
Imavate (Robins): Tabs 10, 25 & 50 mg
Janimine (Abbott): Tabs 10, 25 & 50 mg
Presamine (USV): Tabs 10, 25 & 50 mg; Amps 25 mg/2 ml
SK-Pramine (Smith Kline & French): Tabs 10, 25 & 50 mg
WDD (Tutag): Tabs 25 mg
Tofranil-PM (Geigy): Caps 75, 100, 125 & 150 mg (pamoate)

IPRINDOLE

● Iprindole is an antidepressant drug of the tricyclic type, with properties similar to those of IMIPRAMINE and AMITRIPTYLINE. It has been prescribed for a whole range of depressive conditions, from mild forms associated with anxiety and tension to the manic-depressive syndrome, a severe psychotic state. At the beginning of treatment with this compound, anticholinergic reactions (disturbances in visual accommodation, dry mouth, urinary hesitancy) may be expected: the incidence and severity of unwanted effects will depend partly on dosage and also on individual idiosyncrasy. If the medicament is effective in a particular case, its antidepressive action will not be apparent for up to 4 weeks of regular dosage. As is the situation with other tricyclic agents, patients with very profound depression may find this intensified. Although lethal overdosage with iprindole has not been recorded (possibly because the drug is infrequently prescribed), this should be regarded as a potential hazard. The possibility that it may be cardio-toxic in some patients should be considered.

▲ At first, 30 mg three times daily, up to 180 mg/day. After stabilization, 15–60 mg thrice daily according to response.

★ Not advised for patients with severe liver disorders, glaucoma, urinary retention, prostatic hypertrophy or within 4 weeks of treatment with antidepressants of the MAO-inhibitor group.

➤ For further information, see Essay II and Chart II: Antidepressants.

◆ UK:
Prondol (Wyeth): Tabs 15 & 30 mg (hydrochloride)

IPRONIAZID

● This drug is chiefly of historical interest, in that it was the first specifically antidepressive agent to be made available. It belongs to a small class known as monoamine-oxidase (MAO) inhibitors, because such compounds inhibit this enzyme, high concentrations of which have been recorded in depressed patients. Iproniazid, ISOCARBOXAZID, NIALAMIDE and TRANYLCYPROMINE are currently prescribed for relief of depressive states refractory to treatment with the standard (and generally safer) tricyclic agents such as AMITRIPTYLINE. MAO-inhibitors, though still considered to have a place in the therapeutic repertory, cannot be drugs of first choice because they interact, in some instances fatally, with a large number of other drugs of different kinds and with several foods and drinks: particularly to be avoided are concentrated meat and yeast extracts (e.g. Marmite, Bovril), caviare, beers and wines (especially Chianti), hard cheeses, pickled herrings, broad bean pods, bananas, and textured vegetable proteins. Patients under treatment with iproniazid and related drugs should be given a special card by the prescriber, to warn about food reactions and, especially in emergency, to alert other physicians not to administer any of a large list of other medicines: for example, following injury, PETHIDINE (MEPERIDINE) and other strong analgesics are dangerous in combination with MAO-inhibitors. As with other antidepressants, this compound must be taken for 2–4 weeks before therapeutic benefit is likely to occur. Dry mouth, fatigue, nausea, headache, dizziness and restlessness are among the more often experienced adverse effects. Combinations of these antidepressants with other psychotropic drugs (such as antipsychotic tranquillizers) are occasionally prescribed but only in exceptional circumstances.

▲ 100–150 mg daily as a single dose, reducing over 2–4 weeks to a maintenance regimen of 25–50 mg daily, on average, depending on the severity of the condition and on response.

★ MAO-inhibitors are contra-indicated in liver disorders, severe cardiac, cardiovascular and cerebrovascular complaints, epilepsy, and phaeo-chromocytoma. The principal types of drugs with which toxic reactions may occur are: tricyclic antidepressants, opiate analgesics, amphetamines and other stimulants and appetite-suppressants (including many cough remedies), barbiturates and some other sedative and hypnotic agents, antihistamines, anti-diabetic drugs and antihypertensive medicaments.

➤ For further information, see Essay II and Chart II: Antidepressants.

◆ UK:
Marsilid (Roche): Tabs 25 & 50 mg (phosphate)

ISOCARBOXAZID

● Isocarboxazid is an antidepressant of the MAO-inhibitor type, with actions and effects very similar to those described in the preceding entry, for IPRONIAZID. The same potentially dangerous interactions with tyramine-containing foods and with the same types of other drugs occur. The therapeutic benefits of isocarboxazid and other compounds of this class are limited by the often unpleasant side-effects, and numerous toxic reactions with foods, drinks and drugs, and should not be the first choice in the chemical treatment of depression. MAO-inhibitors are spectacularly successful in a few patients, but the restrictions are difficult to follow. After-effects, following weeks or months of such therapy, have barely been touched on in the clinical literature: these resemble the drug's immediate side-effects but may set on with greater intensity, and the original depression may be increased in severity.

▲ For the first weeks 30 mg daily, reducing to 10–20 mg daily (maximum of 40 mg) according to response. Isocarboxazid should be discontinued gradually.

➤ See preceding entry, IPRONIAZID, and Essay II and Chart II: Antidepressants.

◆ UK:
Isocarboxazid Tablets BPC: available as
Marplan (Roche): Tabs 10 mg
   USA:
Isocarboxazid Tablets USP: available as
Marplan (Roche): Tabs 10 mg

KETAZOLAM

● The reader of any of the Charts or Essays in this book will hardly fail to notice numerous examples of redundancy, i.e. of drugs which possess virtually identical chemical structure and pharmacological effects but which are marketed as distinct entities. This phenomenon particularly applies to the benzodiazepine class of tranquillizers, the best-known example of which is DIAZEPAM (Valium). Ketazolam is a derivative of diazepam and, so far as the present authors can determine, offers no advantages of any importance over the original compound. The drug has this year (1980) become available in the UK as a 'new' remedy for anxiety and tension, and to relieve muscular spasticity associated with injury to the spinal cord and multiple sclerosis. As far as the latter indications are concerned, it remains unclear whether ketazolam is superior to diazepam, also a potent muscle-relaxant. At comparable doses the new compound is said to be less likely than diazepam to produce oversedation, impairment of reflexes, and similar reactions typical of the benzodiazepine class. Already ketazolam seems well on the way to commercial success in a market that has been crowded for years past. A factor which is often overlooked in UK prescribing, because of nominal prescription charges, is the real cost of drugs, particularly psychotropic agents. In the case of ketazolam, this is more than five times the actual NHS cost of diazepam tablets or capsules. Psychological dependency having occurred on a large scale with other diazepines, it is a probable effect of long-term administration of this drug, which is not advised unless compelling medical reasons exist.

▲ 15–60 mg daily: usually a single dose (average 30 mg) at bedtime.

★ Like other diazepam-type agents, ketazolam should be avoided in severe respiratory insufficiency and known hypersensitivity to any drug of this class. Effects of other CNS depressants, including alcohol, are enhanced.

➤ For further information, see Essay VI and Chart VI(A): Tranquillizers.

◆ UK:
Anxon (Beecham): Caps 15 & 30 mg

LEVALLORPHAN

● This compound is a partial narcotic antagonist which is administered to counteract the effects of MORPHINE and similar 'agonists' in overdosage, especially the respiratory depression which the latter may provoke. Levallorphan is also occasionally used for diagnostic purposes: if given to a patient who is physically dependent on an opiate of the morphine type, it will precipitate withdrawal symptoms almost immediately. In combination with PETHIDINE (MEPERIDINE) injections of the drug are given to relieve labour pains and in anaesthesia, and the presence of an ampoule formulation containing both the narcotic and the antagonist encourages its use. The principle is that concurrent administration will stop respiratory depression from occurring. Since pethidine and levallorphan cross the placental barrier, it is assumed that breathing difficulties in the newborn baby (neonatal apnoea) will be prevented by the antagonist. In practice this may not be the case, because levallorphan has a far shorter duration of action than pethidine, and by the time delivery has occurred its effects may have worn off while those of the analgesic continue to act on the child (and the mother). In the treatment of overdosage from a narcotic, the compound has been superseded by the pure opiate antagonist NALOXONE, which seldom provokes the adverse reactions of levallorphan, such as drowsiness, fatigue, and sweating.

▲ To restore normal respiration to patients who have received excessive doses of opiates: 0.3–1.2 mg intravenously (0.3–0.5 mg for each 15 mg of morphine) and 1–1.5 mg for each 100 mg of pethidine. Infants: 0.05–0.25 mg intravenously.

★ Not indicated in the treatment of barbiturate poisoning. The drug may be dangerous if given to patients on long-term therapy with morphine-like drugs, including PENTAZOCINE and other partial antagonists which are prescribed for pain relief.

➤ For further information, see Essay IV and Chart IV: Morphine and Other Potent Analgesics.

◆ UK:
Levallorphan (Tartrate) Injection BPC: available as
Lorfan (Roche): Amps 1 mg/1 ml
Pethilorfan (Roche): Amps pethidine hydrochloride 50 mg, levallorphan
tartrate 0.625 mg/1 ml
   USA:
Levallorphan Tartrate Injection USP: available as
Lorfan (Roche): Amps 1 mg/1 ml; Vials 10 mg/10 ml

LEVONANTRADOL (CP 50,556)

● To include more than a small number of compounds which are still
experimental would bulk out the present work considerably. However,
since it appears to possess some remarkable properties and because it will
probably become available to prescribers relatively soon, levonantradol is
considered briefly here. The substance was developed from Δ^9-tetrahydro-
cannabinol (THC), one of the active alkaloids of CANNABIS. There is
evidence that cannabis derivatives have pain-relieving activity and a
recent trial has clearly indicated that THC is a strong anti-emetic: but
these also produce mood changes (euphoria or dysphoria) and what some
clinicians are pleased to call 'psychotomimetic' (psychosis-mimicking)
reactions, such as hallucinations. The THC molecule has been very
greatly modified to achieve levonantradol: experiments with laboratory
animals, backed now by some clinical experience, indicate that the new
compound is much more effective as an anti-emetic than PRO-
METHAZINE, PROCHLORPERAZINE and other phenothiazine
derivatives which are routinely given in this indication. In particular, the
nausea and vomiting which several drugs used in cancer chemotherapy
promote are evidently counteracted more successfully with levonantradol.
It has also been found that the compound provides a level of analgesia
comparable to that yielded by MORPHINE and its analogues and is
approximately five times as active as morphine on a weight basis. Yet it
does not bind to the opiate receptors, is not antagonized by NALOX-
ONE, and apparently has little dependence potential. Side-effects
reported to date include somnolence, dry mouth, dizziness, postural
hypotension and occasionally mood changes of either a positive or
negative kind: it is too early to be able properly to assess the incidence of
such unwanted reactions, but in terms of frequency and intensity these
compare favourably with the side-effects of both phenothiazine anti-
emetics and narcotic analgesics. Evidently 'psychotomimetic' reactions
are uncommon with levonantradol. If further research confirms these
results, then the drug will be a valuable addition to the therapeutic
armamentarium. Studies of levonantradol soon to be published indicate,
interestingly, that the compound binds to the receptor site(s) specific for

tranquillizers of the diazepam (Valium) type. A further finding from the Salk Institute in California may widen the spectrum of potential clinical applications still further. In experimental animals, levonantradol enhances the effectiveness of sodium valproate (Epilim, UK; Depakene, USA), one of the most useful modern anti-epileptic agents: earlier research had demonstrated a significant anticonvulsant effect for TET-RAHYDROCANNABINOL (THC), but adverse effects limited the latter's therapeutic use.

▲ To relieve nausea/vomiting: 0.5–1 mg. Pain relief: 1–3 mg, every 4–6 hours. Most of the research relates to an injectable formulation of the drug: this is dissolved in the rather viscous propylene glycol, and must be given by deep intramuscular injection.

★ At present use of the compound is not advised during pregnancy, in cases of known hypersensitivity to cannabis or its derivatives, for patients who are psychotic or emotionally unstable, and in brain tumours. Caution is required when the brain or spinal column is being irradiated, for concurrent administration with other psychotropic agents, and in myocardial infarction. The manufacturer's suggestion that dysphoric reactions to levonantradol be treated with phenothiazine tranquillizers is inappropriate, as these agents are likely to intensify mental depression.

➤ Under investigation: Pfizer Ltd, Groton, Connecticut and Sandwich, Kent.

LEVORPHANOL R

● Levorphanol is one of the most effective synthetic morphine analogues for relief of intractable pain. It is prescribed for premedication before surgery, to alleviate postoperative pain and other forms of very severe acute and chronic pain states. A particular advantage which this medicament shares with few other analgesics of comparable potency (PHENAZOCINE is one such) is that the unwanted reactions which typically follow morphine administration – drowsiness, dizziness, nausea, vomiting, mood changes (euphoria/dysphoria) – are considerably less severe with levorphanol at equivalent dosage. The assertion that, weight for weight, the compound is almost as effective by mouth as by injection is not supported by clinical experience: commonly, potent analgesics are less (and sometimes much less) than half as active for pain relief when taken orally. In the case of levorphanol, analgesic action following oral administration appears to be one-half to one-third of that afforded by injection (intramuscular). Because the drug is an opiate agonist it is necessarily under legal restriction along with morphine, pethidine etc. However, very few cases of physical addiction to it have been reported. The reason for this is almost certainly that levorphanol is much less likely to promote euphoria than most other highly potent analgesics. Tolerance to its effects develops slowly in comparison to morphine and the majority of its analogues. On a weight basis, it has been estimated that orally 1.5 mg of levorphanol approximates to 5 mg of diamorphine (heroin).

▲ The drug's duration of action (4–6 hours) has been overestimated. Orally, 1.5–3 mg and by any of the injectable routes 2–4 mg 4-hourly. Patients with terminal cancer and analogous pain states, who have been taking opiates regularly, may require considerably in excess of these doses.

★ Contra-indicated in raised intracranial pressure. Utmost caution in severe liver disorders, respiratory insufficiency. Combination with MAO-inhibitor antidepressants may be dangerous.

▶ For further information, see Essay IV and Chart IV: Morphine and Other Potent Analgesics.

◆ UK:
Levorphanol (Tartrate) Tablets BPC &
Levorphanol (Tartrate) Injection BPC: available as
Dromoran (Roche): Tabs 1.5 mg; Amps 2 mg/1 ml
   USA:
Levorphanol Tartrate Tablets USP &
Levorphanol Tartrate Injection USP: available as
Levo-Dromoran (Roche): Tabs 2 mg; Amps 2 mg/1 ml; Vials 20 mg/10 ml

LITHIUM CARBONATE

● This salt of an element, lithium, a compound of almost absurd simplicity, would not be expected to have psychotropic properties. It has, however, and is one of the most potent and toxic of the drugs employed in contemporary psychiatry. Lithium's value in controlling symptoms associated with the manic phase of manic-depressive psychosis, first proposed almost two decades ago, has now been established. Exactly how it exerts this effect is completely unknown. The drug's indications have been extended to include the prevention of recurrent mania, and in chronic and recurrent severe depression; but so far from being universally beneficial in mitigating these conditions, it may exacerbate them. This is particularly true of certain forms of chronic and intermittent depression, and some practitioners still claim that lithium has no real advantages over standard antipsychotic drugs (such as CHLORPROMAZINE, Largactil, Thorazine) in the treatment of mania. Lithium carbonate is one of the most toxic agents in current therapeutic use: this may be illustrated by the fact that doses of 0.8–1.5 mEq (milli-equivalent) per litre of blood produce effects regarded as beneficial, while 2.0 mEq/L and over are likely to provoke toxic reactions. Dosage is expressed in this way because blood lithium levels must be regularly monitored during treatment and individual response to the same milligramme dose may be different. Early adverse reactions are numerous: even at therapeutic dose levels nausea, vomiting, fine tremor, diarrhoea, thirst, fatigue, and muscular weakness may be experienced. In some patients two or more of these unwanted effects occur at the beginning of therapy. Other reactions, which may arise at any time, such as unsteadiness of gait, double vision, severe tremor, incoherent speech and difficulty in concentrating, and epileptiform fits, show that dangerous (toxic) levels of the drug are circulating in the system. If any of the above reactions are noted, lithium should be stopped, and large doses of sodium chloride (salt: 12 grammes per 24 hours, orally, in four or more doses) administered. Because lithium tends to cause fluid retention, kidney dialysis may be needed, but conventional diuretics are contra-indicated. Long-term administration of the drug may impair renal function and cause hypothyroidism. It should be obvious from these observations that prescription of the compound should be restricted to severely psychotic illnesses, and even then only under close supervision. Not all persons suffering from manic-depression benefit from lithium; but some respond well provided that the necessary precautions are taken. During the first week of treatment, blood samples should be taken at least twice, in order to establish an effective dose and to ensure that toxicity does not occur, and weekly thereafter. There is at present a disturbing trend: an increasing number of general practitioners are prescribing lithium for non-psychotic depression, which may conceivably be justified in rare cases, but without performing the mandatory blood-tests or observing the proper precautions.

▲ 1.2–1.6 G in two or three divided doses (severely psychotic patients): the elderly and debilitated may require less. In any event, as already stated, the object is to achieve plasma levels of about 1.0–1.5 mEq/L: higher concentrations will often lead to the toxic reactions described.

★ Contra-indicated in impaired kidney function, cardiac failure, and for patients on low-salt diets. Not advised in pregnancy, lactation, hypothyroidism. Lithium should not be given concurrently with diuretics, barbiturates, and combinations with antipsychotic tranquillizers or tricyclic antidepressants may exacerbate adverse effects.

➤ For further information, see Essay VI and Chart VI(B): Tranquillizers.

◆ UK:
Lithium Carbonate Tablets BPC: 250 & 400 mg
Slow Lithium Carbonate Tablets BPC: 300 & 400 mg
Camcolit (Camden): Tabs 250 & 400 mg
Phasal (Pharmax): SR Tabs 300 mg
Priadel (Delandale): SR Tabs 400 mg

Liskonum (Smith Kline & French): SR Tabs 450 mg
    USA:
Lithium Carbonate Tablets USP &
Lithium Carbonate Capsules USP: available as
Eskalith (Smith Kline & French): Caps 300 mg
Lithane (Roerig): Tabs 300 mg
Lithobid (Rowell): Tabs 300 mg (+ sodium chloride 40 mg)
Lithonate (Rowell): Caps 300 mg
Lithonate-S (Rowell): Liq 0.8 mEq/5 ml (citrate)
Lithotabs (Rowell): Tabs 300 mg
Pfi-Lithium (Pfi-Pharmecs): Tabs 300 mg

LORAZEPAM

● This tranquillizer, prescribed to alleviate anxiety and tension states, closely resembles DIAZEPAM (Valium) in its pharmacological profile. Both drugs belong to the benzodiazepine class of sedative and anxiolytic drugs, and lorazepam is becoming popular in general practice. The latter has a somewhat shorter duration of action than diazepam, but a single daily or nightly dose is adequate for many patients. Repeated use leads to tolerance and some form of dependency, so unless the psychological state being treated is chronic and other modes of therapy are inappropriate prescription of the compound on an open-ended basis is not recommended. Physical addiction, indicated by the appearance of a definite withdrawal syndrome on abrupt discontinuation of other benzodiazepines, may occur with this drug of the class: the incidence of such dependency has probably been underestimated. Dosages in excess of those indicated produce oversedation, hangover (if lorazepam is taken at night), and paradoxical excitement. Headache, nausea, dizziness and blurred vision are less regularly observed unwanted effects. Benzodiazepine tranquillizers are often prescribed together with other sedative agents to promote sleep. This is quite unnecessary in the great majority of cases, since if lorazepam is taken on retiring it is likely to be just as effective in combating insomnia as other soporifics. According to one study, 2–4 mg of this drug are equivalent to 30 mg of FLURAZEPAM, the latter marketed as a hypnotic.

▲ Between 1 and 6 mg daily, according to requirements and individual response. As an injection, lorazepam (4–8 mg intramuscularly) may be effective for premedication before surgery and to control convulsive disorders.

★ Not to be given in severe respiratory insufficiency and known hypersensitivity to any benzodiazepine drug. Central depressant actions of opiates, other tranquillizers and alcohol are increased.

➤ For further information, see Essay VI and Chart VI(A): Tranquillizers.

◆ UK:
Ativan (Wyeth): Tabs 1 & 2.5 mg: Amps 4 mg/2 ml (half-filled)
    USA:
Ativan (Wyeth): Tabs 500 µg, 1 & 2 mg

LOXAPINE

● As if the repertory of antipsychotic drugs were not already sufficiently large, loxapine has recently been added to the list for prescription in the USA. The drug is proposed to relieve the symptoms of schizophrenia. Although it does not belong to any of the principal chemical classes of major tranquillizers (neuroleptics), loxapine seems to provoke similar types of unwanted effects: among the commoner of these dizziness, sedation, fatigue and parkinsonian episodes have been noticed. Again, like antipsychotics of the CHLORPROMAZINE (Largactil, Thorazine) type, protracted administration of high doses to psychiatric inpatients may result in the insidious form of Parkinson's disease known as tardive dyskinesia: this may be irreversible. It is far from clear whether loxapine offers any substantial advantages over conventional antischizophrenic drugs.

▲ Outpatients: 15–40 mg daily, and psychiatric inpatients up to a maximum of 160 mg/day, usually in divided doses, depending on severity of symptoms and individual response.

★ Contra-indicated in pregnancy, cardiac disease, severe respiratory and liver disorders, convulsive states, and urinary retention.

➤ Precautions and interactions are likely to be similar to those for phenothiazine tranquillizers: see Essay VI and Chart VI(B): Antipsychotic Tranquillizers.

◆ USA:
Loxitane (Lederle): Caps 10, 25 & 50 mg (succinate); Oral Conc 25 mg/1 ml (hydrochloride)
Daxolin (Dome): Caps 10, 25 & 50 mg (succinate)

L-TRYPTOPHAN

● L-tryptophan is an amino acid which occurs naturally in the body and is a precursor of 5-hydroxytryptamine (serotonin): inhibition of the latter is believed to alleviate mental depression. There is still some argument among psychiatrists about this chemical's presumed antidepressant activity. Some studies indicate that l-tryptophan may be as effective as standard tricyclic antidepressants such as IMIPRAMINE, while others suggest that its effects are merely sedative. According to one source, the drug may provoke hypersexuality in schizophrenics. Dry mouth, over-sedation, or nausea are experienced by some patients.

▲ 2–4 G daily, in two or three doses. Because l-tryptophan may inhibit production of the B vitamin pyridoxine, the latter has been added to one formulation.

★ Not recommended in severe depression, nor for use during pregnancy or by children. If the anticonvulsant levodopa is being taken, the preparation without pyridoxine should be given. L-tryptophan enhances the effects of allopurinol (Zyloric), a medicament prescribed to relieve gout.

➤ For further information, see Essay II and Chart II: Antidepressants

◆ UK:
Pacitron (Berk): Tabs 500 mg
Optimax (E. Merck): Tabs l-tryptophan 500 mg, pyridoxine 5 mg, ascorbic acid (vitamin C) 10 mg; Powder 1 G + 10 mg + 20 mg per 10 G (also without pyridoxine)

LYSERGAMIDE (ERGINE) R

● Lysergamide, or *d*-lysergic acid amide, is an alkaloid found in the Mexican plant *Rivea corymbosa* (locally named ololiuqui) and in some species of Morning Glory, e.g. *Ipomoea violacea*. Ololiuqui was employed ceremonially by the Aztecs and still plays a part in the rituals of indigenous Central and South American peoples. Lysergamide is one of several active ingredients of *Rivea* and of *Ipomoea* and some other Convolvulaceae, being present in the seeds of these plants. The compound has some psychedelic or hallucinogenic effect, but this has not been fully investigated by pharmacologists. Intoxication with Morning Glory seeds has been reported, chiefly from the USA: a number of these cases were serious enough to warrant hospitalization because of unpleasant perceptual alterations and nausea, vomiting, flushed skin, widely dilated pupils, fast heart-rate (tachycardia) and abrupt fall in blood-pressure following ingestion of 150 or more such seeds. Whether lysergamide provokes psychological effects which are genuinely psychedelic (i.e. similar to those promoted by the closely related synthetic drug LYSER-GIDE or LSD) remains unclear. Doses of between 1 and 5 mg orally may produce alterations in perception, but the drug has a narrow margin of safety. If available, it should be taken only under expert medical supervision and with several additional safeguards.

➤ For additional warnings and other data, see Essay V and Chart V: Psychedelics.

LYSERGIDE (LSD) **R**

● Lysergic acid diethylamide, or lysergide, is a semisynthetic derivative
of ergot, a fungus which grows on rye. Its extraordinary effects on
perception, discovered accidentally in 1938, are now well documented.
Lysergide is among the most stringently restricted of Controlled Drugs,
and illegal use has become so widespread in the Western world as to be for
practical purposes ineradicable. Young and inexperienced individuals,
who may try LSD for 'kicks', find that they experience more than they
bargained for and frightening reactions may ensue. The drug so profoundly alters perception, and induces synaesthesia (all the senses becoming apparently jumbled) and depersonalization, that it has been termed
'psychotomimetic', i.e. mimicking a spontaneous psychotic state. Its use
in psychiatry, for many years apparently discredited, has lately begun
again in a tentative fashion, despite the fact that reputable researchers
have considerable bureaucratic difficulties in obtaining supplies of the
compound. Among a number of potential medical applications for LSD
experimentation with terminally ill patients is proving of particular
interest: their sensation of pain appears to be altered such that this does
not worry them, and, if lysergide is given very soon before death, the
passing seems more peaceful and dignified than when conventional
medication is administered. A detailed description of the psychological
effects of lysergide will be found in Essay V. Unwanted physical reactions
may include in some cases nausea, trembling, dilatation of pupils, and
fatigue. The sensationalistic accounts of dangerous delusions arising from
non-medical use of lysergide have seldom been substantiated. Nevertheless, extreme caution is required if the taking of so potent a psychotropic
agent is contemplated: not only should this be under expert medical
supervision, but other precautions detailed in Essay V must be observed.
Doses of pure drug in the region of 150–300 µg exert definite psychedelic
activity. Among the antidotes which have been suggested, nicotinic acid
(niacin), a B vitamin, at doses of 1–2 G two or three times daily may be
helpful in mitigating after-effects. Antipsychotic drugs such as
HALOPERIDOL are likely to do more harm than good. See also under
MESCALINE.

➤ For further information, see Essay V and Chart V: Psychedelics.

MAPROTILINE

● Maprotiline has a chemical structure containing four rings, rather than
the usual three, for an antidepressant of the tricyclic type. This medicament is among a few recent additions to the range of drugs which
counteract depression, and not unnaturally is referred to as a tetracyclic.
The addition of this further ring to the basic skeleton of configurations

required for a substance to exert such an effect does not necessarily imply a therapeutic advantage. According to objective experiments in which maprotiline has been compared to standard antidepressants (e.g. AMITRIPTYLINE and IMIPRAMINE), it appears that onset of depression-relieving action occurs rather more rapidly with the new drug than with alternatives: within 7–10 days vs 2–4 weeks for amitriptyline and other tricyclics. Adverse effects depend partly on the dosage administered, and it is not obvious whether maprotiline really provokes fewer of these than imipramine. Certainly drowsiness, ataxia, fine tremor, dizziness, and anticholinergic reactions (blurred vision, dry mouth) do occur in a proportion of cases, particularly during the early phase of treatment. A potentially important point is that this compound appears to have a lower convulsive threshold (i.e. it may provoke fits) than comparable antidepressants, and these do sometimes arise even at therapeutic dosages. Maprotiline is probably as dangerous in overdosage as the tricyclic antidepressants, to which their cardio-toxicity may contribute. This is significant because some forms of severe depression are enhanced by compounds of this type.

▲ Usually in the range of 25–150 mg daily, dosage being determined empirically over a period of 2–3 weeks, as for other antidepressants.

★ Contra-indicated in severe heart disease, convulsive conditions, glaucoma, urinary retention and enlargement of the prostate; and for concurrent use with MAO-inhibitors or amphetamines and other stimulants and appetite-suppressants, and certain antihypertensives.

➤ For further information, see Essay II and Chart II: Antidepressants.

◆ UK:
Ludiomil (Ciba): Tabs 10, 25, 50, 75 & 100 mg (hydrochloride)

MAZINDOL

● Mazindol is the most recently introduced appetite-suppressant agent, which is now available in the USA as well as the UK. Although the compound is not chemically related to AMPHETAMINE, it is probable that its anorexiant activity is at least partly due to the fact that it has stimulant properties. In any event mazindol, like the amphetamines and their other analogues, should be prescribed in reduction of obesity on a short-term basis only (not longer than a few weeks), and then only in conjunction with exercise and diet. According to experimental evidence the drug may be less effective than PHENMETRAZINE, a powerful amphetamine-like stimulant, in promoting weight loss. Adverse reactions from mazindol include nausea, vertigo, chills, agitation, fast heart-beat and other effects reminiscent of amphetamine. Some patients have reported amphetamine-like euphoria after taking the compound. Its potential for abuse and dependency have not yet been established, but in the circumstances described the practitioner would be wise to err on the safe side and prescribe mazindol on a shut-ended basis, and not for individuals with a history of drug abuse. Claims have been made by laypeople that mazindol has aphrodisiacal properties: one of the present writers has commented on this in detail elsewhere, observing in particular that the compound is if anything more likely to reduce libido and sexual potency than to enhance them. This drug is under investigation for possible use as an antidepressant, but as yet this application has not been adequately tested.

▲ Usually, a single dose of between 1 and 3 mg on rising; a second dose at lunchtime may be required by some patients. The drug is intrinsically long-acting.

★ Principal contra-indications are glaucoma, peptic ulcer, cardiac disease, hypothyroidism, and agitated states. Caution in hypertension. Possibly serious interactions may occur with some antihypertensive drugs, amphetamines, and antidepressants, especially MAO-inhibitors.

➤ For further information, see Essay I and Chart I: Amphetamines.

◆ UK:
Teronac (Wander): Tabs 2 mg
    USA:
Sanorex (Wander): Tabs 1 & 2 mg

MECLOFENOXATE

● Meclofenoxate is a mild central nervous system stimulant which is prescribed to aid recovery from strokes and reverse intellectual impairment associated with ageing. Historically, the drug has also been given to control delirium tremens in alcoholic withdrawal, to elevate respiratory function in carbon monoxide poisoning, and in breathing difficulties of newborn babies (neonatal apnoea). Paediatric tablets are marketed which are intended to help in treatment of motor retardation in children. The evidence for meclofenoxate's usefulness in any of the above indications is meagre. A small-scale clinical trial found that the stimulant could be beneficial in some cases of dementia in the elderly. In the absence of objective, well-controlled studies, and given that alternative medication known to be effective is available for some of the proposed indications, the routine prescription of meclofenoxate is not justified. Side-effects are purported to be mild and transient, with a few patients experiencing agitation or insomnia. Abuse liability appears to be negligible.

▲ Adults: 300 mg three times daily (maximum 1.5 G).

★ Caution in severe cardiac and kidney disorders.

> For further information, see Essay I and Chart I: Amphetamines.

◆ UK:

Lucidril (Reckitt & Colman): Tabs 300 mg; Paediatric Tabs 100 mg (hydrochloride: latter deleted 1981)

MEDAZEPAM

● Medazepam is a close analogue of DIAZEPAM (Valium), prescribed to relieve tension and anxiety and states of hyperagitation. The drug is a benzodiazepine: one of a large and increasing number of tranquillizers with a virtually identical spectrum of activities. Medazepam was introduced as a 'new entity' and its manufacturers asserted that it was even more effective than diazepam, with fewer unwanted reactions. A familiar claim, but one which is not backed up by objective evidence. Therapeutic doses of medazepam may provoke drowsiness, oversedation, impairment of reflexes and other side-effects typical of this class of drugs. Consumption of large doses can result in paradoxical excitement and a stripping away of inhibitions (disinhibition), a phenomenon similar to that produced by alcoholic excess. Prolonged administration of this and related compounds is inadvisable because tolerance develops quickly and psychological dependence is then likely.

▲ 10–40 mg daily: a single night-time dose is often sufficient.

★ Should not be prescribed in cases of severe respiratory distress or known sensitivity to benzodiazepine tranquillizers. The actions of other drugs which depress the central nervous system, such as other tranquillizers, barbiturates, narcotic analgesics and alcohol, are likely to be intensified.

> For further information, see Essay VI and Chart VI(A): Tranquillizers.

◆ UK:

Nobrium (Roche): Caps 5 & 10 mg

MEPHENESIN

● This compound is an obscure, old-fashioned muscle-relaxant with mild analgesic and sedative properties. It is sometimes prescribed to enhance the effectiveness of aspirin and other simple pain-killers in the treatment of inflammatory conditions (e.g. arthritis) and other chronic or intermittently painful states. Large doses may induce drowsiness, nausea, and less frequently double vision, lethargy and muscular disco-ordination. The US Food and Drug Administration has ruled that mephenesin is ineffective for the indications claimed by the manufacturers.

▲ 500 mg–1 G up to 6 times daily. The drug should be taken with food or milk; otherwise gastro-intestinal upsets may arise.

★ Contra-indicated in severe liver or kidney disease.

◆ UK:
Myanesin (Duncan, Flockhart): Tabs 500 mg (deleted 1981)
   USA:
Mervaldin (Lannett): Tabs 500 mg

MEPHENTERMINE R

● Mephentermine, an amphetamine derivative, is an obsolescent drug administered by injection as a respiratory stimulant in anaesthetics. For reasons which are obscure, the drug appears on the UK schedules of restricted substances although it is many years since mephentermine was discontinued. The compound is still listed as being available in the USA but is seldom prescribed. Even high doses do not often provoke the euphoriant effects characteristic of amphetamines: anxiety, restlessness, rapid rise in blood-pressure and heart-rate (tachycardia) are more likely.

▲ 30–45 mg intravenously or intramuscularly, depending on the specific indication (e.g. hypotension following spinal anaesthesia in Caesarian section).

★ More specific and reliable respiratory stimulants are marketed for all the indications in which mephentermine was once appropriate. Contra-indicated in hypotension induced by CHLORPROMAZINE and other antipsychotic agents; for patients under treatment with MAO-inhibitor antidepressants; and in cases of hypersensitivity to amphetamine-like compounds.

➤ For further information, see Essay I and Chart I: Amphetamines.

◆ USA:
Mephentermine Sulfate Injection USP: available as
Wyamine (Wyeth): Amps & Syrettes 15 & 30 mg/1 ml, 30 mg/2 ml; Vials 150 & 300 mg/10 ml

MEPROBAMATE

● Until the advent of DIAZEPAM (Valium) and other tranquillizers of the benzodiazepine category, meprobamate was for several years the most popular remedy for anxiety and tension taken in the USA: it is perhaps better known under its first trade-name Miltown. Meprobamate was originally believed to exert a more selective action on the central nervous system than the barbiturates, which up to the time of its introduction in

1951 had been prescribed for their calming and sedative effects. Unfortunately, though this is not as widely appreciated as it should be, apart from its shorter duration of action (3–5 hours) the substance suffers from practically all the disadvantages of barbiturate therapy. Tolerance sets on rapidly with repeated administration, and both psychological and physical dependency are considerable hazards: the withdrawal syndrome which occurs on abrupt discontinuation of meprobamate, like that associated with barbiturates, may be so severe as to be life-threatening if left untreated. Not every patient who takes the medicament becomes dependent with regular use, but many do. Meprobamate was once prescribed as an anti-epileptic and anti-allergic agent but has been superseded. Side-effects at higher dose levels include oversedation, loss of appetite, allergic skin rashes, and sometimes jaundice, convulsions, and disorders of blood function. Meprobamate is marketed both alone and in preparations containing other drugs, such as analgesics, diuretics, and hormones, for the relief of pain states accompanied by anxiety (e.g. premenstrual distress, psychological changes associated with the menopause). Fixed-dose combinations of this type are pharmacologically unsound. For the chemical treatment of anxiety, tension and similar states, diazepam and other, less toxic modern alternatives are available.

▲ 200–800 mg daily for relief of moderate anxiety. Dosage should not exceed 1.6 G daily, in 3 or 4 divided doses.

★ Contra-indicated in porphyria, known hypersensitivity, epilepsy, alcoholism. Caution in impaired liver or kidney function.

➤ For further information, see Essay VI and Chart VI (A): Tranquillizers; and for interactions with other drugs, see Chart III: Barbiturates.

◆ UK:
Meprobamate Tablets BPC: 200 & 400 mg
Equanil (Wyeth): Tabs 200 & 400 mg
Milonorm (Wallace): Tabs 400 mg
Miltown (Carter-Wallace): Tabs & SR Caps 400 mg
Tenavoid (Burgess): Tabs meprobamate 200 mg, bendrofluazide 3 mg
  USA:
Meprobamate Tablets USP: 200 & 400 mg
Meprobamate Oral Suspension USP: 200 mg/5 ml
Meprobamate Injection USP: 400 mg/5 ml
Amosene (Ferndale): Tabs 400 mg
Arcoban (Arcum): Tabs 400 mg
Bamate (Century): Tabs 400 mg
Bamo (Misemer): Tabs 400 mg
Equanil (Wyeth): Tabs 200 & 400 mg; SR Caps 400 mg; Susp 200 mg/5 ml
Kalmm (Scrip): Tabs 200 & 400 mg
Maso-Bamate (Mason): Tabs 400 mg

Meprocon (CMC): Tabs 200 & 400 mg
Meprospan (Wallace): SR Caps 200 & 400 mg
Pax-400 (Kenyon): Tabs 400 mg
Saronil (Saron): Tabs 400 mg
Miltown (Wallace): Tabs 200, 400 & 600 mg; Amps 400 mg/5 ml
SK-Bamate (Smith Kline & French): Tabs 200 & 400 mg
Tranmep (Reid-Provident): Tabs 400 mg
Milpath (Wallace): Tabs meprobamate 200 mg, benzhexol (trihexi-
phenidyl) 25 mg
Milprem (Wallace): Tabs meprobamate 200 or 400 mg, conjugated
oestrogens 0.25 mg (NB Observe precautions for oestrogens)
Miltrate (Wallace): Tabs meprobamate 200 mg, pentaerythritol tetra-
nitrate 10 or 20 mg
Pathibamate (Lederle): Tabs as *Milpath*
PMB (Ayerst): Tabs as *Milprem*
See also under BENACTYZINE, DEXAMPHETAMINE, ETHOHEP-
TAZINE

MESCALINE R

● Mescaline has been called by Brimblecombe and Pinder, in their book
on psychedelics, 'the paradigm of a hallucinogenic drug'. This substance
was the first of its kind to be investigated scientifically. It is an alkaloid of
the cactus *Lophophora williamsii* and is known by the people of Mexico
and Peru, where this grows, as *peyotl* (peyote). Structurally mescaline is
not dissimilar to AMPHETAMINE, but its psychological activity puts it
into an entirely different class. At doses of 200–750 mg orally, physical
effects from the alkaloid begin in 20–40 minutes and may be felt as
unpleasant: nausea, perspiration, an increase in heart-rate, and trembling
are often experienced immediately prior to the onset of profound
alterations in consciousness. Perception is so radically altered that the
phenomenon virtually defies description: an apparent merging of the
faculties (synaesthesia) makes the taker see the music issuing from the
record player, smell the picture on the wall. Colours are vastly intensified,
and visions may appear before one's eyes. The term 'hallucinations'
suggests that what is perceived does not exist, but there are many who
would dispute this. Perhaps the most remarkable reaction triggered by
mescaline, as by other psychedelic drugs, is depersonalization, a deep
feeling that one is no longer there as an individual entity, with the paradox
that sensations are still flooding in. This state, among others provoked by
the 'hallucinogens', may be extremely frightening to a subject who either
has not experienced it before or does not anticipate it. It is chiefly when
depersonalization occurs that, if a psychiatrist of conventional views is
brought in, the individual undergoing the 'trip' is regarded as suffering

from a drug-induced psychosis, and 'treatment' is likely to be the same as if an acute spontaneous psychotic state had developed: usually this involves administration of a powerful neuroleptic such as HALO-PERIDOL. Such steps are very seldom necessary and may do more harm than good. To obviate this type of situation, and for other sound reasons, mescaline should not be taken unless expert medical supervision is available. A number of additional criteria for the use of psychedelic agents are set down elsewhere. Aldous Huxley's book *The Doors of Perception* offers an intelligent and literate introduction to the subject of the psychological effects of hallucinogens.

➤ For further information, see Essay V and Chart V: Psychedelics.

MESORIDAZINE

● The above-named compound is one of a plethora of major tranquilliz-ers related to, and with effects like, CHLORPROMAZINE (Largactil, Thorazine). Mesoridazine, in common with certain other potent antipsy-chotic drugs, has been irresponsibly advertised in the USA for use in 'common adjustment problems in our society', and we have been told that it 'benefits personality disorders in general'. In 1970 the American Food and Drug Authority compelled the manufacturer to cancel an extensive campaign in the medical press promoting its use in chronic alcoholism. The only legitimate application for mesoridazine is the control of acute and chronic schizophrenic, and perhaps other severely psychotic, condi-tions. A number of controlled trials have indicated that this compound possesses no real advantages over chlorpromazine, though some prac-titioners may disagree. Certainly the adverse effects which it is likely to provoke – sedation, rapid fall in blood-pressure, apathy, fatigue, anti-cholinergic reactions (blurred vision, dry mouth) are common – should contra-indicate its administration for all but the most severe psychic disturbances, and particularly in minor emotional problems. Like other phenothiazine antipsychotics, this agent often produces parkinsonian effects and, if given at high doses for prolonged periods, a chronic form of Parkinson's disease which may be irreversible. Another frequent ill-effect is the enhancement of mental depression, which can become of great intensity.

▲ Outpatients: 25–200 mg daily. Psychiatric inpatients: up to a maximum of 400 mg daily, usually in divided doses.

★ Should be avoided in severe liver, kidney or cardiac disorders, convulsive states, alcoholism, and pre-existing mental depression.

➤ For further information, see Essay VI and Chart VI(B): Antipsychotic Tranquillizers.

◆ USA:
Mesoridazine Besylate Tablets USP
Mesoridazine Besylate Oral Solution USP &
Mesoridazine Besylate Injection USP: available as
Serentil (Boehringer Ingelheim): Tabs 10, 25, 50 & 100 mg; Oral Soln
25 mg/1 ml; Amps 25 mg/1 ml

METHADONE R

● The lack of availability of opium, from which to obtain MORPHINE, during the early part of the Second World War in Germany, provided a particular stimulus in the search for alternatives. Methadone and PETHIDINE were the most important synthetic pain-killers of comparable potency to morphine to emerge during this time. Subsequently both compounds became established as standard drugs for relief of severe pain. Methadone is prescribed to control postoperative pain and in other conditions when a narcotic is indicated: it is not, however, administered during labour, because its respiratory depressant action is much greater than that of pethidine. Its duration of action (4–7 hours) exceeds that of morphine and is considerably longer than that afforded by pethidine. Methadone is also given, at relatively small doses, to suppress chronic cough. Dizziness, drowsiness, nausea, vomiting, constipation and mood changes are side-effects characteristic of the opiate agonists: these are more pronounced with methadone than with other drugs of comparable analgesic activity. Tolerance develops readily with repeated use, and the compound has an abuse and addiction liability equivalent to that of morphine. Mood changes, experienced by some individuals as euphoria, are similar to those provoked by morphine or DIAMORPHINE (heroin). For the past 12 years, since Drug Dependency Clinics were set up in the UK, and for almost as long in the USA, methadone (usually in a non-injectable form, such as a syrup) has increasingly been prescribed for opiate addicts. The 'methadone maintenance' idea, whereby patients who were unable to forsake narcotic use were given a single dose of the drug daily, has become accepted practice in a number of countries. The theory is that addicted persons, prescribed conservative doses which are dispensed by pharmacies on a daily basis, will have their need for opiates satisfied to the point where they will not resort to injectable heroin. It has been asserted that, when previously habitués led unstable and socially 'undesirable' lives, using methadone syrup they can be rehabilitated, take jobs, and be useful to society. There is much controversy about the matter, but it is at least arguable that the administration of methadone merely replaces one addiction with another. Indeed, the withdrawal syndrome on abrupt discontinuation of the drug is more prolonged than are heroin abstinence reactions (4–7 days vs 2–3 for the acute phase), and is at least as severe. The argument that addicts are better off with an oral than an injectable drug has some substance; but in a recent survey, which compared patients who received oral methadone and injectable heroin respectively, no significant differences were seen in terms of life-style, criminal activity and other parameters. The proponents of the methadone maintenance policy have consistently underestimated the dependence liability and other undesirable effects of the drug. Partly because of the British Clinics' practice of prescribing only the substitute drug, and that in small doses, many opiate-dependent individuals buy their supplies of heroin, generally in impure, adulterated form, on the illicit market. For relief of severe pain states, a number of alternative medicaments are available which are equally effective and have less potential for abuse.

▲ Pain relief: initially 5–10 mg orally or by intramuscular injection, repeated 4–6 hourly. In intractable cough: 2–4 mg in an appropriate syrup or linctus at similar intervals.

★ Contra-indicated in respiratory insufficiency, severe head injury, hypersensitivity to the compound. There is danger of drug accumulating in the body with repeated use. Methadone should not be given concurrently with antidepressants of the MAO-inhibitor type, nor with partial narcotic antagonists (e.g. PENTAZOCINE) for use in analgesia. Respiratory and CNS depressant effects of barbiturates, tranquillizers, and alcohol are increased.

➤ For further information, see Essay IV and Chart IV: Morphine and Other Potent Analgesics.

◆ UK:
Methadone (Hydrochloride) Tablets BPC: 5 mg
Methadone (Hydrochloride) Linctus BPC: normally 2 mg/5 ml; also 5 mg/5 ml (for use in Drug Dependency Units)
Methadone (Hydrochloride) Injection BPC: Amps 10 mg/1 ml
Physeptone (Burroughs Wellcome): Tabs 5 mg; Linct 2 mg/5 ml; Amps 10 mg/1 ml
    USA:
Methadone Hydrochloride Tablets USP: 5 & 10 mg
Methadone Hydrochloride Oral Solution USP: 10 mg/1 ml
Methadone Hydrochloride Dispersible Tablets USP: 40 mg
Methadone Hydrochloride Injection USP: 10 mg/1 ml
Dolophine (Lilly): Tabs 5 & 10 mg; Amps 10 mg/l ml; Vials 200 mg/20 ml
Methadone Diskets (Lilly): Dispersible Tabs 40 mg
Westadone (Vitarine): Effervescent Tabs 2.5, 5, 10 & 40 mg
Nodalin (Table Rock): Tabs methadone hydrochloride 2.5 mg, aspirin 200 mg, phenacetin 120 mg, caffeine 20 mg
Methenex (Bristol): Effervescent Tabs methadone hydrochloride 40 mg,

naloxone hydrochloride 2 mg; Powder for Oral Susp 10 + 500 µg/10.5 G (temporarily deleted)

METHAQUALONE R

● This drug has the dubious distinction of being the only hypnotic restricted under the UK Misuse of Drugs Act: even the barbiturates are not at present so controlled. When methaqualone was first marketed in Britain, as a tablet also containing the sedative antihistamine DIPHENHYDRAMINE, a familiar type of claim was put forth by the manufacturers: that the compound was a safe and effective alternative to the barbiturates in promoting sound sleep; that it had low toxicity and presumably low dependence potential. The preparation in question was called Mandrax. Within a very short time after its introduction this became popular among drug abusers and was preferred by some to AMYLOBARBITONE (AMOBARBITAL) and similar barbiturates. The particular reason for the phenomenon was that, at doses only slightly greater than those required as a hypnotic, methaqualone exerts a peculiar type of euphoria, with paradoxical excitement. One of the most insidious effects of the drug is that memory of what took place following its ingestion may be lost: a patient of one of the present authors found, some days following a dose of Mandrax, that under its influence he had typed, and posted, several letters, which were found to contain gibberish. The patient had no recollection whatever of what he had done. Psychological habituation to methaqualone occurs readily and rapidly, and genuine physical addiction, with a withdrawal syndrome comparable to that which obtains for barbiturates, is a special hazard. Methaqualone has no therapeutic applications except as a soporific, and there are numerous alternatives. In the USA misuse of the drug happens on a large scale, notably with the tablet trade-named Quaalude, and the expression 'luding out' (meaning to get 'stoned' on the drug) has become part of the subculture's vocabulary. There is absolutely no legitimate indication for prescribing the compound. So far from having a low toxicity, in addition to its other adverse effects methaqualone is highly dangerous in over-dosage, especially in combination with alcohol.

▲ 125–250 mg at night.

★ Contra-indicated in severe liver disorders, alcohol or other drug dependence, convulsive disorders, during pregnancy and lactation. Repeated use cannot be justified. Effects of other CNS depressants are enhanced.

➤ For further information, see Essay III and Chart III: Barbiturates.

◆ UK:
Mandrax (Roussel): Tabs & Caps methaqualone 250 mg, diphenhydramine
hydrochloride 25 mg (to be deleted December 1980)
    USA:
Methaqualone Tablets USP &
Methaqualone Hydrochloride Capsules USP: available as
Mequin (Lemmon): Tabs 300 mg
Parest (Parke Davis): Caps 200 & 400 mg
Quaalude (Lemmon): Tabs 150 & 300 mg
Sopor (Arnar-Stone): Tabs 150 & 300 mg

METHARBITONE (METHARBITAL)

● Not to be confused with METHYLPHENOBARBITONE (MEPHOBARBITAL), also a very long-acting compound, metharbitone is a barbiturate prescribed almost exclusively to prevent convulsions from occurring in epilepsy. This drug is far less popular than PHENOBARBITONE, which has essentially the same sedative and anticonvulsant activity, but may be helpful for epileptic patients who cannot tolerate any of the newer and less toxic alternatives such as ethosuximide and sodium valproate (Epilim). The risk with this as with other long-acting barbiturates is that accumulation in the body of dangerous quantities of drug may follow regular use. Psychological and physical dependency are less likely with phenobarbitone and metharbitone than with short-acting compounds of the same class, such as AMYLOBARBITONE (AMOBARBITAL) or PENTOBARBITONE; but the potential should be borne in mind. Adverse effects are typical of the barbiturates, and may include oversedation (with reflex impairment), confusion, hangover, unsteadiness of gait and, at high doses, some euphoria.

▲ 50–100 mg once or twice daily. Larger doses may be needed by patients on long-term anticonvulsant therapy.

★ Principal contra-indications are porphyria, hypersensitivity to any barbiturate, and severe respiratory and liver disorders. Drugs of this class antagonize the effects of analgesics and potentiate the effects of other central depressants, including tranquillizers and alcohol. Caution if concurrent prescription of oral anticoagulants, antipsychotic agents, or the contraceptive Pill is needed.

➤ For further information, see Essay III and Chart III: Barbiturates.

◆ USA:
Metharbital Tablets USP: available as
Gemonil (Abbott): Tabs 100 mg

METHOTRIMEPRAZINE (LEVOMEPROMAZINE)

● Chemically, methotrimeprazine is closely related to CHLOR-PROMAZINE (Largactil, Thorazine) and other antipsychotic tranquilliz-ers; but this drug is given chiefly as premedication before surgery, in obstetrics together with opiate analgesics, and postoperatively to aid pain relief. It has recently been deleted in the UK and is available only as an injection in the USA. Side-effects are characteristic of the phenothiazine class of medicaments: dizziness, drowsiness, rapid fall in blood-pressure, fatigue, mental depression, and nausea are not uncommon.

▲ 10–20 mg every 4–6 hours, by deep intramuscular injection. The ampoule formulation is compatible only with atropine and scopolamine, and nothing else should be mixed in the same syringe. Particular caution must be exercised if either drug is combined to avoid the risk of tachycardia (fast heart-rate) and other undesirable effects.

★ Contra-indicated in severe cardiac, liver and kidney dysfunction; cases of known hypersensitivity to any phenothiazine derivative; concurrent administration of antihypertensive drugs or MAO-inhibitor antidepress-ants.

➤ For further information, see Essay VI(B) and Chart VI: Antipsychotic Tranquillizers.

◆ USA:
Methotrimeprazine Injection USP: available as
Levoprome (Lederle): Amps 20 mg/1 ml; Vials 200 mg/10 ml

★ Contra-indicated in severe cardiac, liver and kidney dysfunction; cases of known hypersensitivity to any phenothiazine derivative; concurrent administration of antihypertensive drugs or MAO-inhibitor antidepress-ants.

➤ For further information, see Essay VI(B) and Chart VI: Antipsychotic Tranquillizers.

◆ USA:
Methotrimeprazine Injection USP: available as
Levoprome (Lederle): Amps 20 mg/1 ml; Vials 200 mg/10 ml

METHYLAMPHETAMINE (METHAMPHETAMINE) R

● Methylamphetamine, known as methamphetamine in the USA, is the most powerful central nervous system stimulant of the amphetamine class of compounds, even more potent in this respect than DEXAM-PHETAMINE. Because of the intense, energetic euphoria which even small doses of the drug often provoke, methylamphetamine is always at a premium on the illicit market. Orally, it has been prescribed to reduce appetite in obesity, to relieve the hyperkinetic syndrome in children, and to control the sleeping disorder narcolepsy. By injection, the medicament is sometimes given to reverse the effects of barbiturates and other sedatives in overdosage, and in psychiatry to induce talkativeness in otherwise taciturn patients. For all these indications alternative treatments are available; only perhaps in narcolepsy is the prescription of methylamphetamine justified. Regular use in any other condition is contra-indicated: even patients not normally considered likely to abuse drugs, such as overweight housewives, may find themselves craving further and further doses. Whether physical addiction to amphetamines occurs is disputed, but there is no doubt that psychological habituation is almost inevitable with repeated administration. Non-medical use of this type of compound, particularly when stimulants are taken by injection, often leads to 'amphetamine psychosis', a condition characterized by delusions, bizarre stereotyped behaviour, formication (a sensation that insects are crawling on one), and other reactions which may be indistinguishable from spontaneously occurring psychoses. Even at therapeutic doses, agitation, restlessness, tachycardia, gatro-intestinal disturbances and mental depression (the latter as the drug's action wears off) are often experienced. The formidable misuse and dependence potential of methylamphetamine has resulted in its restriction in the UK for hospital use only.

▲ 2.5–15 mg daily is the average range. For patients suffering from narcolepsy, who may need to take the drug on a regular basis, much higher dosages may be required.

★ Contra-indicated in hypertension, glaucoma, cardiac and cardiovascular disease, hyperthyroidism, urinary retention, and in cases of anxiety or hyperagitation. The drug should not be prescribed concomitantly with MAO-inhibitor or other antidepressants, antipsychotic tranquillizers, antihypertensive agents, inter alia.

➤ For further information, see Essay I and Chart I: Amphetamines.

◆ UK:
Methylamphetamine (Hydrochloride) Tablets BP 1973 &
Methylamphetamine (Hydrochloride) Injection BP 1973: available as
Methedrine (Burroughs Wellcome): Tabs 5 mg; Amps 30 mg/1.5 ml (hospitals only)
    USA
Methamphetamine Hydrochloride Tablets USP 1970: 2.5, 5, 7.5, 8 & 10 mg
Dee-10 (Scrip): Tabs 10 mg
Desoxyn (Abbott): SR Tabs 5, 10 & 15 mg
Methampex (Lemmon): Tabs 10 mg

Obedrin (Beecham-Massengill): SR Tabs 10 mg
Aridol (MPC): Tabs methylamphetamine hydrochloride 1.5 mg, pama-brom 52 mg, pyrilamine maleate 30 mg, homatropine methylbromide 1.2 mg, hyoscine sulfate 0.1 mg, scopolamine hydrobromide 0.02 mg
Obe-Slim (Jenkins): Tabs methylamphetamine hydrochloride 10 mg, amylobarbitone (amobarbital) sodium 50 mg, homatropine methyl-bromide 7.5 mg
Span-RD (Metro): Tabs methylamphetamine hydrochloride 12 mg, dl-methylamphetamine hydrochloride 6 mg, secbutobarbitone (butabarbital) 30 mg
Mediatric (Ayerst): Tabs & Caps methylamphetamine hydrochloride 1 mg, conjugated oestrogens 0.25 mg, methyltestosterone 2.5 mg, vitamins; Liq: 15 ml equivalent to 1 Tab or Cap

METHYLPHENIDATE R

● Methylphenidate is an analogue of the AMPHETAMINES and is considered by many, incorrectly, to have much less potential for abuse and dependency. The restless, energetic 'high' which the drug provokes is very similar to amphetamine-engendered euphoria and only slightly less intense. For this reason illicit trafficking in methylphenidate, which may be somewhat easier to obtain than amphetamines, occurs and is increas-ing. The drug is prescribed in narcolepsy, for relief of the hyperactive or hyperkinetic syndrome in children, and, with scant justification, to reverse fatigue and lethargy (e.g. during convalescence). It is regularly advertised in US medical journals to counteract apathy and loss of motivation in the elderly: convincing evidence that the compound exerts such an effect, without patients becoming tolerant to its action and psychologically dependent, is lacking. Chronic abuse of methylphenidate often results in 'amphetamine psychosis' and is similar in this respect to METHYL-AMPHETAMINE and DEXAMPHETAMINE. Nervousness, agitation, insomnia, dizziness and other unwanted reactions are similar to, if not so pronounced as, those produced by amphetamines. Long-term administra-tion of the substance should be avoided unless absolutely necessary, e.g. in narcolepsy.

▲ 5–30 mg daily, usually in two doses: at breakfast and lunchtime. The last dose should be taken not later than 4 p.m., otherwise insomnia is likely.

★ The principal contra-indications and warnings are as for the amphetamines, the former including hypertension, hyperthyroidism, heart disease, and agitated states. Methylphenidate is not advised for concurrent treatment with antidepressants, antipsychotic tranquillizers, and certain drugs prescribed in hypertension.

➤ For further information, see Essay I and Chart I: Amphetamines.

◆ UK:
Ritalin (Ciba): Tabs 10 mg; Amps 20 mg/2 ml + solvent (Amps restricted to hospital use only)
　　USA:
Methylphenidate Hydrochloride Tablets USP &
Methylphenidate Hydrochloride for Injection USNF 1970: available as
Ritalin (Ciba): Tabs 5, 10 & 20 mg; Amps 20 mg/2 ml + solvent

METHYLPHENOBARBITONE (MEPHOBARBITAL)

● This compound is a long-acting barbiturate with actions and uses like those of BARBITONE and PHENOBARBITONE. It is occasionally prescribed for daytime sedation, though there exist many more modern drugs which may be given for this purpose. Methylphenobarbitone is now almost exclusively employed for its anticonvulsant properties: to prevent the occurrence of fits in individuals suffering from epilepsy. Psychological habituation and, to a lesser extent, physical dependency can occur with this compound as with all barbiturates. However, since some epileptics are unable to tolerate other, less toxic and non-habituating anti-epileptic agents, long-acting barbiturates may be needed on a long-term basis. Tolerance to the principal adverse effects may develop quickly, but for patients who are not accustomed to barbiturates hangover, oversedation, unsteadiness, lethargy and, at substantial doses, paradoxical excitement may be a problem. Reflexes may be affected to a greater extent than is subjectively believed. Methylphenobarbitone and related drugs are unsuitable for concurrent use with analgesics, although such combinations were once traditional remedies for chronic or intermittent ailments: barbiturates antagonize the effects of pain-killers except insofar as general sedation may be increased.

▲ As a sedative: 30–100 mg daily in two divided doses. The administration of longer-acting barbiturates to promote sleep at night is not recommended. In epilepsy: average 200–400 mg/day in divided doses, but dosage must be tailored to meet individual requirements.

★ Contra-indicated in porphyria, severe respiratory and liver disorders, and known hypersensitivity to any barbiturate. Should not be prescribed together with oral anticoagulants, antipsychotic tranquillizers or other CNS depressants unless reasons are compelling.

➤ For further information, see Essay III and Chart III: Barbiturates.

◆ UK:
Prominal (Winthrop): Tabs 30, 60 & 200 mg

USA:
Mephobarbital Tablets USP: available as
Mebaral (Winthrop): Tabs 32, 50, 100 & 200 mg
Menta-Bal (Walker): Tabs 30 mg
Mephoral (Campbell): Tabs 30 & 100 mg

METHYLPRYLON(E)

● Methylprylon is a member of a small chemical class of non-barbiturate sedative and hypnotic drugs. It possesses all the important attributes of its close analogue GLUTETHIMIDE, the only other compound in the piperidinedione category. It is effective in promoting sleep, particularly in cases where early waking is a problem, and has sometimes been pre-scribed for daytime sedation: for the latter indication other medicaments are more appropriate (e.g. tranquillizers of the DIAZEPAM [Valium] type). Concomitant use of methylprylon with simple analgesics such as aspirin, for relief of chronic or intermittent pain states, is not recom-mended because the soporific may antagonize the action of pain-relieving agents. Unwanted side- and after-affects of the drug are generally mild at therapeutic doses, but even so hangover, oversedation and slowing of reflexes may follow a nocturnal dosage. Paradoxical excitement and euphoria may occur if excessive quantities are taken. Regular administra-tion of methylprylon to relieve insomnia is not generally advisable because tolerance and psychological (and rarely physical) habituation may result. However, for short courses of treatment for intractable sleeping difficulty this medicament is often very effective. The assumption that methylprylon has an abuse and dependence liability equal to that of the barbiturates is unfounded. Nevertheless, due care is always required in prescription of strong hypnotics.

▲ In the range of 200–600 mg at night. Elderly and debilitated patients will usually require smaller doses than other groups of patients.

★ Known hypersensitivity to methylprylon or to GLUTETHIMIDE and epilepsy are the chief contra-indications. Caution in severe liver and kidney disease. The drug should not be given with antipsychotic tranquillizers or, ideally, with other centrally depressant drugs or oral anticoagulants.

➤ For further information, see Essay III and Chart III: Barbiturates.

◆ UK:
Methylprylone Tablets BPC: available as
Noludar (Roche): Tabs 200 mg
     USA:
Methylprylon Tablets USP &
Methylprylon Capsules USP: available as
Noludar (Roche): Tabs 50 & 200 mg; Caps 300 mg

MIANSERIN

● A recent addition to the armamentarium of antidepressants, mianserin has been shown to possess both antidepressive and anti-anxiety activity: it may offer some advantages over conventional tricyclic compounds such as AMITRIPTYLINE and IMIPRAMINE in alleviating mixed states of agitation, tension and depression. As is the case with all antidepressants, mianserin does not exert its psychotropic effect immediately but appears to do so more rapidly than the tricyclics: i.e. within 7–10 days vs up to 4 weeks for amitriptyline and comparable drugs. Adverse effects, which are dose-related and tend to occur early after commencement of therapy, include dry mouth, disturbances of visual accommodation, dizziness, drowsiness, constipation, nausea, and fine tremor. It is uncommon for a patient to experience more than one or two of these reactions at appropriate doses; but the optimal dose must be worked out empirically by the prescriber. Generally both early and regular unwanted effects are less common and less severe than those resulting from treatment with tricyclics. The distinct sedative actions of mianserin should be taken into account: the corollaries of this can be overcome by giving the drug as a single night-time dose. This compound lacks the cardio-toxicity of amitriptyline and other similar antidepressants, which may be a great boon when severely depressed patients are being treated: fatal over-dosage with antidepressants is increasing rapidly, chiefly due to cardiac effects. Overall mianserin seems to be less toxic than analogous drugs. So far as its therapeutic effectiveness is concerned, one particular clinical trial found it no more beneficial than imipramine in depressed patients. Other studies, however, suggest that it may be of greater benefit in some cases.

▲ Initially, 20–30 mg at night, gradually increasing over 7–10 days to a maximum of 200 mg, depending on response.

★ Caution in patients with suicidal tendencies, as these may be enhanced. Likewise in patients with cardiac, liver or kidney disorders or epilepsy. Should not be given concurrently with MAO-inhibitors, the anti-hypertensive clonidine (Catapres), or alcohol. Serious interactions appear less likely to arise with drugs used to control blood-pressure and other compounds which affect the activity of most antidepressants.

➤ For further information, see Essay II and Chart II: Antidepressants.

◆ UK:
Bolvidon (Organon): Tabs 10, 20 & 30 mg
Norval (Bencard): Tabs 10, 20 & 30 mg (hydrochloride)

MOLINDONE

● As if there were not already more than enough medicaments available to control the symptoms of schizophrenia (cf Chart VIB), molindone has now been introduced for prescription in the USA. It is chemically unrelated to the phenothiazines and other classes of antipsychotic tranquillizers, but its activity is similar. Adverse effects following molindone administration include drowsiness, restlessness, insomnia, mental depression, heavy or absent menstruation in women, gastro-intestinal upsets, changes in libido, and extra-pyramidal (parkinsonian) reactions. It is noteworthy that all these effects may follow treatment with CHLOR-PROMAZINE (Largactil, Thorazine) and other conventional antipsychotic agents. As yet it is still too early to tell the incidence of unwanted reactions and how intractable any of these might be. On the face of it, this drug does not appear to offer any special advantages over other major tranquillizers or neuroleptics, even though it may be effective in diminishing hyperagitation, aggressiveness, and delusions in individuals suffering from schizoid disorders. Molindone may exacerbate mental depression if this is already present, and the risk of attempted suicide should then be borne in mind or, better, the drug not prescribed at all. Since the compound is sedative at therapeutic doses, patients should be warned about possible impairment of reflexes when driving or operating machinery. It is too soon to tell whether molindone is as likely as other neuroleptics to provoke tardive dyskinesia, a severe form of Parkinson's disease, if administered over a prolonged period. Certainly, given the pharmacological profile of the drug, molindone should only be prescribed in psychotic conditions, and not for relief of minor psychological or emotional complaints.

▲ 15–60 mg daily (outpatients): dosage must be adjusted according to individual response.

★ Molindone increases the toxicity of ORPHENADRINE (Disipal) and may antagonize the effects of tetrabenazine (Nitoman) and other anti-parkinsonian drugs. This is very unfortunate because parkinsonian reactions occur so often with antipsychotic drugs. Contra-indicated in CNS depression due to alcohol, barbiturates and other central depressants. Absorption of the anticonvulsant phenyoin (Epanutin) and the tetracycline antibiotics may be affected. Molindone's anti-emetic effect may obscure signs and symptoms of acute abdominal illness and brain tumours.

➤ For further information, see Essay VI(B) and Chart VI: Antipsychotic Tranquillizers.

◆ USA:
Lidone (Abbott): Caps 5, 10 & 25 mg
Moban (Endo): Tabs 5, 10 & 25 mg (hydrochloride)

MORPHINE R

● Morphine, the principal alkaloid of the OPIUM poppy, *Papaver somniferum*, was first isolated by Sertürner early in the last century; and it remains the yardstick by which other potent analgesics are judged. It is one of the few old-generation drugs of vegetable origin which not only are still used but considered an essential part of the pharmacopoeia. Morphine is even today the drug of choice for many practitioners to relieve severe pain, whether traumatic and acute or spontaneous and chronic: in renal and biliary colic, myocardial infarction (coronary thrombosis), pre- and postoperatively and in terminal pain states, some consider morphine superior to all the more recently introduced alternatives, of which there are many. In pain of visceral origin the drug is often given with atropine to prevent nausea and other cholinergic (e.g. nauseant) effects of the opiate. Administration of morphine may be oral, rectal, or by the different routes of injection: weight for weight, and perhaps absolutely too, it is much less effective when given by mouth, and oral preparations of morphine are seldom used in the USA. Frequently encountered side-effects are drowsiness, dizziness, nausea, vomiting, constipation, respiratory depression (though this is less of a problem than is usually suggested), and mood changes, which some patients experience as euphoria and some as dysphoria. In other words, while certain individuals enjoy the dreamy, 'floating' psychological state induced by the drug, probably as many again do not find this sensation agreeable. Those who do, of course, are far more likely to become psychologically or physically dependent on morphine, and the same applies for other opiates. In the treatment of terminal pain states, such as those in advanced cancer, the phenomena of tolerance and addiction are of no consequence, and the possibility of either should not prevent the responsible practitioner from prescribing as appropriate: that many physicians withhold opiates from patients in very severe pain, while overprescribing almost anything else, is shocking. Now, so far as non-medical use of morphine is concerned, there exist many misapprehensions. First, true addiction occurs only after regular administration for months, rather than days or weeks, as attested by the onset of withdrawal symptoms if the drug is discontinued. And, as with DIAMORPHINE (heroin), even when this does develop, any deterioration in physical or psychological health (unless enormous doses are taken) is much more likely to result from indirect than from direct effects of the compound. There is no evidence that even prolonged use of morphine or diamorphine *per se* produces mental or physical ill-effects: it is the circumstances in which the drug may be used to which one must look for a proper explanation of the unfortunate state of many street addicts. Morphine and similar potent opiate 'agonists' lock into special receptor sites in the brain which are specific for such drugs (μ receptors). At these sites chains of proteins, known as endorphins and enkephalins, are bound, mimicking the action of morphine-like agents and themselves provide naturally-occurring pain relief. It has been hypothesized that opiate addicts, or persons predisposed to take such drugs, suffer from a deficiency of these 'natural opiates', which only use of morphine or one of its analogues can bring up to appropriate levels. This could explain the fact that, whereas some patients who have been receiving medically prescribed morphine for months can be withdrawn easily and with very slight or absent withdrawal symptoms, others require to increase the dose after a short time and can be weaned off the drug only with difficulty. The recent finding that ordinary milk contains morphine, and that the compound is present in plants other than the poppy, may give further insights into such problems.

▲ In the range of 5–20 mg, orally or by injection. There is considerable variation in individual response, so dosage must be determined to meet the individual patient's requirements. If morphine is injected, the intramuscular route is preferable to the intravenous, for duration of effect will be noticeably longer: 3–5 hours vs 2–4. In very severe chronic and terminal pain states, single doses of up to 100 mg may be needed in certain cases.

★ The risk of physical dependency should be borne in mind if morphine is prescribed other than in terminal patients. It is contra-indicated in respiratory depression, bronchial asthma, and hypersensitivity to the drug. Caution in convulsive states, and impaired liver or kidney function. Morphine should not be given at the same time as antidepressants of the MAO-inhibitor group, nor, except in overdosage, with analgesics which are partial opiate antagonists (e.g. PENTAZOCINE [Fortral, Talwin]).

➤ For further information, see Essay IV and Chart IV: Morphine and Other Potent Analgesics.

◆ UK:
Morphine Hydrochloride Solution BPC: 10 mg per ml
Morphine Hydrochloride Suppositories BPC: 15 & 30 mg
Morphine Sulphate Tablets BP 1973: 15 & 30 mg
Morphine Sulphate Suppositories BPC: 15 & 30 mg
Morphine Sulphate Injection BPC: Amps 10, 15, 20 & 30 mg/1 ml, 30 mg/2ml
Morphine and Atropine (Sulphates) Injection BPC: Amps 10 + 0.6 mg/1 ml
Morphine and Cocaine (Hydrochlorides) Elixir BPC: each 5 mg/5 ml

Duromorph (Laboratories for Applied Biology): Amps micro-crystalline morphine 70.4 mg/1 ml
MST-1 (Napp): SR Tabs morphine sulphate 10 mg
Nepenthe (Evans): Amps anhydrous morphine equiv. 4.2 mg/0.5 ml; Oral Soln 8.4 mg/1 ml (extracted from papaveretum and opium tincture)
Cyclimorph (Calmic): Amps morphine tartrate 10 or 15 mg, cyclizine tartrate 50 mg/1 ml
   USA:
Morphine Sulfate Tablets USP 1970: Hypo Tabs 8, 10, 15 & 30 mg
Morphine Sulfate Injection USP: Amps & Syrettes 8, 10 & 15 mg/1 ml or 2 ml
Morphine and Atropine Sulfates Tablets USNF 1970: Hypo Tabs 15 + 0.4 mg
   Unbranded Amps morphine sulfate 15 mg, atropine sulfate 0.4 mg/ 2 ml; Vials 20 ml
see also under OPIUM and PAPAVERETUM

NABILONE (LILLY 109514)

● This is an experimental compound derived from TETRAHYDRO-CANNABINOL (THC), one of the active constituents of CANNABIS. Nabilone was first proposed as a drug to alleviate anxiety: in normal volunteers doses in the range of 2.5–5 mg orally provoked euphoria and dry mouth as well as making the subjects less tense. These and smaller doses had muscle-relaxant effects but did not significantly affect heart-rate or blood-pressure. Other studies indicated that dosages in excess of 2.5 mg produced marijuana-like 'high' states, to which tolerance quickly developed, as well as drowsiness, dizziness and transient fall in blood-pressure. The purpose of synthesizing drugs such as nabilone, which requires considerable technical expertise, is hopefully to dissociate the euphoriant action of cannabis from properties which are therapeutically useful: THC itself has been clearly shown to possess such attributes but does tend to promote psychological effects which investigators consider undesirable. According to some published studies, nabilone appears to show promise as an anti-emetic, particularly in the control of intractable nausea provoked by anti-cancer drugs. In this respect it is certainly superior to standard phenothiazine derivatives such as PRO-CHLORPERAZINE (cf Essay VIB). For the time being, studies with nabilone have been suspended because of unexpected toxic reactions in laboratory animals: one hears, however, that this situation is likely to be temporary. So far as the drug's anti-nauseant action is concerned, this appears on the basis of research so far unpublished to be inferior to that of another THC derivative, LEVONANTRADOL, which though still experimental seems to have a number of other important potential applications.

◆ under study: Lilly Research Laboratories, Indianapolis, Indiana, USA

NALBUPHINE

● Nalbuphine is a potent analgesic which was introduced for prescription in the USA in 1978. Although it is structurally related to the conventional opiates, such as MORPHINE and particularly OXYCODONE, this new compound is different from these in an important respect: it is a partial antagonist of morphine-like drugs while retaining their pain-relieving efficacy. Research in the field of strong analgesics has for some years centred on compounds which partially reverse the actions of 'agonist' opiates and which are believed to possess a much lower potential for abuse and dependency. The problem with many of these antagonists, such as NALORPHINE, was that at analgesic doses they tended to provoke such serious adverse effects as to make them unacceptable for clinical use in pain relief. Nalbuphine has been extensively tested for various types of pain and is recommended by its manufacturers for administration in postoperative pain, during labour, as a supplement to surgical anaesthetic agents, as well as in other conditions for which an opiate would normally be prescribed. Comparative studies appear to show that the new drug is superior to BUTORPHANOL, PENTAZOCINE and other partial antagonists, and as effective for pain control as morphine or pethidine (meperidine). The most frequently reported side-effects in a large series of patients were sedation, sweating, nausea/vomiting, dizziness or vertigo, headache and dry mouth: generally adverse reactions seemed to be less troublesome than those provoked by morphine and other analgesics of comparable potency. Nalbuphine does not depress respiration as much as standard opiates, and unlike buprenorphine its action can be reversed by the pure antagonist NALOXONE. Euphoria evidently does not occur often, and when it does mood changes are slight, and psychotomimetic reactions (e.g. hallucinations) which may be experienced after taking pentazocine have seldom been noted. Whether the claim that this compound is virtually devoid of abuse and addiction liability, only time will tell.

▲ 10–20 mg by intramuscular or subcutaneous injection, 3–6 hourly: maximum 160 mg per 24 hours.

★ Caution in impaired respiratory or liver function, head injury, myocardial infarction, sensitivity to the drug. Nalbuphine should not be given concurrently with MAO-inhibitor antidepressants or with opiate agonists such as morphine: in the latter cases, patients undergoing long-term treatment with narcotics may be dependent and any antagonist may provoke the appearance of withdrawal symptoms.

➤ For further information, see Essay IV and Chart IV: Morphine and Other Potent Analgesics.

◆ USA:
Nubain (Endo): Amps 10 mg/1ml, 20 mg/2 ml; Vials 100 mg/10 ml (hydrochloride)

NALORPHINE

● This compound, a partial opiate antagonist, has been administered to reverse the effects of overdosage from MORPHINE, PETHIDINE (MEPERIDINE) and similar narcotic analgesics. In particular it was used to restore normal respiration, a function which can be much depressed by morphine-like drugs, in poisoning with these compounds; and to relieve breathing difficulties in the newborn (neonatal apnoea). Additionally nalorphine has been given to diagnose the presence or absence of opiate dependency: patients addicted to heroin or one of its analogues will, if injected with the antagonist, almost immediately begin to experience withdrawal symptoms. While nalorphine and its analogue LEVALLOR-PHAN remain available in many countries, the former is not now marketed in the UK and only a veterinary preparation is obtainable in the USA. This is entirely because both these partial opiate antagonists have been superseded by the much safer and more effective pure antagonist NALOXONE, for which see the following Alphabetical Entry. Nalor-phine has analgesic properties and has been tried for pain relief: unfortunately very unpleasant, indeed unacceptably severe, side-effects occur at the required doses, including bizarre psychological states such as delusions and depersonalization.

▲ Adults: 5–10 mg intravenously, repeated as required.

★ Contra-indicated in overdosage from barbiturates and other sedative and hypnotic agents. Obviously, concurrent administration of morphine or a similar narcotic 'agonist' is undesirable except in the situations mentioned above.

➤ See also Essay IV: Morphine & Other Potent Analgesics.

◆ UK:
Nalorphine (Hydrochloride) Injection BPC: 10 mg/1 ml (not available)
    USA:
Nalorphine Hydrochloride Injection USP: available only as
Nalline (Merck Animal Health): Amps 5 mg/1 ml (veterinary use only)

NALOXONE

● Naloxone is one of the most important drugs to be introduced during the past decade. It is administered to reverse the effects of accidental or deliberate poisoning with morphine and other narcotic 'agonists' as well as some partial antagonists prescribed for pain relief (e.g. PENTAZOCINE, Fortral, Talwin). In very much smaller doses naloxone has proved of remarkable benefit in restoring normal breathing in newborn babies suffering from apnoea, e.g. respiratory distress which may be produced if the mother has been given PETHIDINE (MEPERIDINE) during labour: this and other drugs used in obstetrics cross the placental barrier and provoke the condition in neonates. Naloxone is a derivative of OXY-MORPHONE and was – a rare phenomenon – first prepared in a private laboratory. It is completely superseding the older partial narcotic antagonists such as NALORPHINE and LEVALLORPHAN for the indications described: the new drug is a pure antagonist, it is highly effective, and side-effects are uncommon. In addition it has a much wider margin of safety than previously available opiate antidotes, which themselves could be unreliable and sometimes dangerous. An interesting application for the compound is in treatment of opiate addicts, and a formulation containing naloxone in combination with the heroin substitute METHADONE has been prescribed in the USA. One of the problems which arose with this preparation, Methenex, was that naloxone is only about 1/100th as effective orally as by injection and its duration of action is far shorter than that of methadone (up to 5 hours vs 24+ hours for methadone). It has been found that an intravenous injection of naloxone 1 mg can block completely the euphoriant effects of DIAMOR-PHINE (heroin) 25 mg, a moderately high dose, and larger quantities of naloxone will have this effect for longer periods. Further research in this area is progressing: the potential benefits for opiate habitués with a tendency to recidivism seem clear. Naloxone has been given experimentally with some success to patients suffering from anorexia nervosa, the drug being administered by intravenous infusion. For reasons that are not yet clear, the compound seems to produce weight gain in such patients, who are notoriously difficult to treat.

▲ In opiate overdose, 0.4–1.2 mg intravenously, repeated once or twice at intervals of 5–10 minutes, until normal respiration is restored.

★ Contra-indicated during pregnancy (except in labour) and, ordinarily, for administration to persons known to be, or suspected of being, addicted to morphine or similar opiate analgesics.

➤ For further information, see Essay IV and Chart IV: Morphine and Other Potent Analgesics.

◆ UK:
Naloxone (Hydrochloride) Injection BPC: available as
Narcan (Winthrop): Amps 0.4 mg/1 ml & 0.04 mg/2 ml (neonatal)
   USA:
Naloxone Hydrochloride Injection USP: available as
Narcan (Endo): Amps 0.4 mg/1 ml; 0.04 mg/2 ml (neonatal) see also
under METHADONE (Methenex)

NIALAMIDE

● This antidepressant of the monoamine-oxidase (MAO) inhibitor type
has essentially the same actions, uses, adverse effects, contra-indications
and, importantly, interactions with other drugs, as IPRONIAZID and
ISOCARBOXAZID. It has been deleted recently in both the UK and the
USA: the drug is, however, still marketed in some Western European
countries, though its use is declining. The principal reason for nialamide's
lack of popularity is that, like other MAO-inhibitors, it is incompatible
with a considerable number of other drugs (including some very commonly prescribed) and with several types of foods and drinks.

➤ For further information, see Essay II and Chart II: Antidepressants.

◆ *Nialamide Tablets* BPC: formerly available as
Niamid (Pfizer): Tabs 25 & 100 mg

NITRAZEPAM

● A close analogue of DIAZEPAM (Valium), nitrazepam has over the
past decade become the most widely prescribed remedy for insomnia in
the UK, having to a considerable extent supplanted the barbiturates as
sedative/hypnotic medication. The rationale of this is clear: compounds of
the benzodiazepine class, some of which are given as anxiety-relieving
tranquillizers and others (like nitrazepam) to promote sleep, are much
less toxic than AMYLOBARBITONE (AMOBARBITAL, Amytal) and
its analogues among the old-generation soporific agents. Psychological
and physical dependency are probably less likely to occur. Side-effects of
nitrazepam are characteristic of diazepam-type drugs: hangover, oversedation, confusion, and similar reactions, while usually mild and transient, may follow a nightly dose of the compound. It is not commonly
realized that central depressant actions may persist well into the day
subsequent to administration, with some risk that reflexes may be
impaired. Certain patients complain of moderate retrosternal pain
('heartburn') shortly after taking a dose of nitrazepam, and a few
experience numbness of the extremities, effects which are not characteristic of the diazepine class of drugs: but these generally last only a very short

time. Large doses of the substance may cause paradoxical excitement occasionally. The Committee on Review of Medicines, which studied nitrazepam and its chemical relatives in detail in 1980, recommend that these drugs should not be prescribed for prolonged periods, because tolerance develops quickly to their sedative and other effects and psychological habituation to them is likely to arise with repeated use. These hazards are relatively minor in comparison with those associated with barbiturates, but the tendency among practitioners, even so, has been to underestimate them.

▲ The standard dosage unit is a 5 mg tablet or capsule. Many patients, however, require more than this to send them to sleep: 20 mg is not an excessive quantity for some. Individual response to nitrazepam and its analogues is very variable, and so dosage should be adjusted according to the patient's response.

◆ Contra-indicated in severe respiratory distress, during pregnancy, and in cases of known hypersensitivity to any benzodiazepine, including those prescribed as daytime tranquillizers. Caution in impaired liver or kidney function. The CNS-depressant actions of other drugs, such as barbiturates, tranquillizers, strong analgesics, and alcohol are likely to be enhanced.

➤ For further information, see Essay III and Chart III: Barbiturates. For diazepam-type compounds in general, see Essay VI(A): Tranquillizers.

◆ UK:
Nitrazepam Tablets BPC: 5 mg
Mogadon (Roche): Tabs & Caps 5 mg
Nitrados (Berk): Tabs 5 mg
Remnos (DDSA): Tabs 5 & 10 mg
Somnased (Duncan, Flockhart): Tabs 5 mg (deleted 1981)
Somnite (Norgine): Tabs 5 mg
Surem (Galen): Caps 5 mg
Unisomnia (Unigreg): Tabs 5 mg

NOMIFENSINE

● Nomifensine is a new antidepressant unrelated to either the tricyclic compounds such as AMITRIPTYLINE and IMIPRAMINE, which are standard drugs, or to the MAO-inhibitors. On the available evidence it appears that this agent is effective in depressive states of various types and degrees of severity, and may be superior to the conventional tricyclics. Nomifensine has been in clinical use on the continent of Europe for several years and its actions extensively studied. There is little question but what it is at least as beneficial for certain conditions as imipramine, the drug with which it has most often been compared. Adverse effects are dose-related and seldom serious: palpitations, nausea, headache, dry mouth, and dizziness have occasionally been reported but such reactions tend to be transient. The toxic action on the heart which is such a potentially dangerous attribute of all the tricyclic antidepressants seems to be absent with nomifensine: nevertheless the practitioner should be cautious in prescribing large quantities of the drug to severely depressed patients, whose condition may possibly be intensified before symptoms are relieved and therefore may become suicide-prone. An advantage claimed for all antidepressants of recent introduction – e.g. MAP-ROTILINE, VILOXAZINE – is that they begin to demonstrate mood-elevating effects more quickly than amitriptyline and standard drugs: in the case of nomifensine most of the patients who are going to respond to treatment with the compound will do so within 7–10 days, vs up to 4 weeks for tricyclics. Administered in conjunction with CHLORPROMAZINE and other major tranquillizers to control schizophrenic symptoms, this drug appears to be better tolerated than other antidepressants.

▲ In the range of 50-200 mg daily, taken as two or three doses. The makers recommend 25 mg twice or thrice daily at first, increased according to response over one to two weeks.

★ Caution in cardiac disease and concurrent administration of MAO-inhibitor antidepressants. Nomifensine may antagonize the effects of certain anti-hypersensitive drugs and enhance those of levodopa and other compounds prescribed in Parkinson's disease.

➤ For further information, see Essay II and Chart II: Antidepressants.

◆ UK:
Merital (Hoechst): Caps 25 & 50 mg (hydrogen maleate)

NORTRIPTYLINE

● This medicament is closely related and similar in function to AMI-TRIPTYLINE, the prototype of the tricyclic class of antidepressants. It may help to alleviate obsessional neuroses and phobias, as well as depression of various types and grades of severity. If nortriptyline is going to elevate mood, this will occur only after regular administration for 2–4 weeks. Other reactions, most of them unwanted, tend to begin within a few days of the beginning of therapy, and some may persist: dry mouth, disturbances of visual accommodation, stomach upsets, and changes in libido are not uncommon. Like its parent drug, nortriptyline has been given to control nocturnal enuresis in children. In common with other tricyclic antidepressants, this compound may enhance states of very severe depression. Similarly, it is dangerous in overdosage, chiefly because of cardio-toxicity.

▲ Up to 200 mg/day, depending on the condition being treated and on individual response. Initially, 25 mg 2 or 3 times daily, the dosage being adjusted upwards or downwards after 2–4 weeks.

★ Contra-indicated in glaucoma, urinary retention, enlargement of the prostate, and hypothyroidism; utmost caution in cardiac, liver and kidney disorders, and in epilepsy and diabetes mellitus. Potentially serious interactions may occur with amphetamines, certain anti-hypertensive agents, barbiturates, MAO-inhibitor antidepressants, and other drugs.

➤ For further information, see Essay II and Chart II: Antidepressants.

◆ UK:
Nortriptyline (Hydrochloride) Tablets BPC &
Nortriptyline (Hydrochloride) Capsules BPC: available as
Allegron (Dista): Tabs 10 & 25 mg
Aventyl (Lilly): Caps 10 & 25 mg; Oral Conc 10 mg/5 ml
    USA:
Nortriptyline Hydrochloride Capsules USP &
Nortriptyline Hydrochloride Oral Solution USP: available as
Aventyl (Lilly): Caps 10 & 25 mg; Oral Soln 10 mg/5 ml
Pamelor (Sandoz): Caps 10 & 25 mg
see also under FLUPHENAZINE

OPIPRAMOL

● Opipramol is yet another of the class of antidepressive agents referred to, because of their three-ring chemical structure, as tricyclics. This drug may be helpful in some cases of mixed anxiety, tension, and depression, and some physicians believe it to be useful in relieving symptoms associated with the menopause. Opipramol is not effective in all types of depressive illness and may indeed exacerbate some such conditions. It appears to be better tolerated than comparable antidepressants, in that side-effects typical of this class of compounds – dizziness, drowsiness, dry mouth are perhaps the most common – are milder than those provoked by AMITRIPTYLINE and standard drugs. These occur chiefly at the beginning of therapy. Alleviation of symptoms will not begin until the drug has been taken regularly for 2–4 weeks. The cardio-toxicity of opipramol may be less than that of other tricyclics, but due care should be taken nevertheless, and its potential suicidal use borne in mind.

▲ 50–150 mg daily. A regimen recommended by the drug's manufacturers is 50 mg at midday, followed by 100 mg on retiring. Dosage must be tailored to meet individual requirements.

★ Contra-indications etc.: as for NORTRIPTYLINE (preceding entry).

➤ For further information, see Essay II and Chart II: Antidepressants.

◆ UK:

Insidon (Geigy): Tabs 50 mg (dihydrochloride: deleted 1981)

OPIUM R

● Opium is the latex, or gum, which is harvested from the unripe seed-pods of the opium poppy, *Papaver somniferum*. This is brown, sometimes almost black in colour, and may be in the form of dry blocks or slightly sticky material. For medicinal purposes powdered opium is standardized to contain 10% morphine, while 'raw' extract may contain between 5% and 20%, depending upon its quality and where the poppy is cultivated. While morphine is by far the most important alkaloid of the plant, its exudate contains a number of other ingredients, of which CODEINE, present as only 1% or less, and papaverine are therapeutically useful: the former chiefly as a cough-suppressant and antidote in diarrhoea and the latter as a muscle-relaxant. Most modern authorities assert that the therapeutic action of opium in relieving pain is entirely due to the presence in it of MORPHINE, possibly also to a slight extent of codeine (chemically methylmorphine). However, others believe that the dozen or so other alkaloids complement morphine's effects and produce a more balanced form of analgesia. Hence the fact that purified total alkaloids of opium, or PAPAVERETUM, prepared in the form of tablets or an injection, remain popular for premedication, in terminal pain states and for various other indications. The rationale of these products is that the unwanted effects characteristic of morphine, such as nausea/vomiting, are to some extent negated by the presence of papaverine, which reduces the motility of the gut. Opium as such is principally prescribed in the form of papaveretum, and also as Opium Tincture (which is seldom dispensed except in diluted, flavoured form), Camphorated Opium Tincture (Paregoric) and Dover's Powder. The last is a preparation containing equal parts of opium and the emetic ipecacuanha. While these formulations are occasionally given for pain relief, more commonly they are administered to relieve severe cough and diarrhoea. Even at the rather low doses recommended in these indications, practitioners are not fond of prescribing opium, certainly not for more than very limited periods. The abuse and addiction liability of opium, due chiefly to its morphine content, are well known but often overstated. Non-medical use of opium has occurred for thousands of years, and in the West many notable writers and artists have become habitués: among these Thomas De Quincey, Samuel Taylor Coleridge and J. M. W. Turner may be mentioned. Today the substance is still smuggled into Western countries in its raw form, though supplies are generally too erratic for more than a few people to be able to take it regularly (unlike its derivative DIAMORPHINE or heroin). The resin is more likely to be smoked than eaten, for effect is more rapid. The euphoria provoked by opium has often been described poetically: this is different from the morphine or heroin 'high'. One of the present authors, as an Oxford postgraduate, undertook a personal experiment with high-quality opium from Pakistan. The object of the exercise, which was monitored by impartial observers, was to establish whether at least once-daily consumption for a period of two weeks would be sufficient to elicit withdrawal symptoms on abrupt cessation of the drug at the end of the pre-determined time. The author, having planned the trial well in advance, smoked a quantity of opium (a sufficiently large quantity to provoke distinct, dreamy euphoria) each evening for fourteen days. For four days thereafter he was observed closely: absolutely no abstinence signs or symptoms, objectively recorded or subjectively experienced, developed. In addition, no craving for further quantities of drug was evinced. It might have been supposed that the undertaking of such an experiment would preclude other normal activities on the part of the participant during the trial: this proved not to be the case, and normal working was continued throughout except during the evenings. Having noted this phenomenon, one does not wish to claim that other individuals, who may be predisposed to opiate dependency, would necessarily emerge from a comparable study in the same way. Opium is certainly a drug of addiction, whether taken as extract or in the form of morphine, and by whatever route of administration. For details, see under MORPHINE and below.

▲ To control chronic, severe cough: 5 ml of Camphorated Tincture of Opium (Paregoric: see below). Pain relief: 1–2 ml of Opium Tincture.

➤ For further information, see Essay IV and Chart IV: Morphine and Other Potent Analgesics.

◆ UK:
Powdered Opium BPC: bulk powder to contain anhydrous morphine 10%
Camphorated Opium Tincture BPC: opium tincture 5 ml, benzoic acid 5 G, camphor 300 mg, anise oil 0.3 ml, alcohol (60%) to 100 ml (contains anhydrous morphine 0.05% w/v)
Opium Tincture BPC: powdered opium in alcoholic (90%) solution (contains anhydrous morphine 10 mg per ml or 1.0% w/v)
Concentrated Camphorated Opium Tincture BPC: opium tincture 40 ml, benzoic acid 40 G, camphor 2.4 G, anise oil 2.4 ml, alcohol (60%) 40 ml, water to 100 ml (to contain anhydrous morphine 0.4% w/v)
Ipecacuanha and Opium (Dover's Powder) Tablets BPC 1973: powdered opium 30 mg, powdered ipecacuanha 30 mg (or to contain equal parts)
USA:
Powdered Opium USP: to contain between 10.0% and 10.5% anhydrous morphine

Opium USP: to contain not less than 9.5% anhydrous morphine
Opium Tincture USP: to contain 1 G/100 ml (1.0% w/v: as BPC)
Paregoric USP: essentially the same concentration and ingredients as Camphorated Opium Tincture BPC
B & O Supprettes (Webcon): Suppos powdered opium 30 or 60 mg, extract of belladonna 15 mg
see also under MORPHINE and PAPAVERETUM

ORPHENADRINE

● Orphenadrine is chiefly prescribed as a remedy for parkinsonism, the disorder characterized by motor and muscular disco-ordination, whether this is of spontaneous occurrence or (as frequently happens) it is induced by treatment with major tranquillizers or antipsychotics: all the phenothiazines, the butyrophenones, and to a lesser extent members of other classes of drugs administered in the treatment of psychotic states, tend to provoke parkinsonian reactions. Some practitioners give orphenadrine or a similar anti-tremor agent concurrently with CHLOR-PROMAZINE, HALOPERIDOL and other antipsychotic medicaments, to prevent these distressing side-effects from occurring. Others believe that such prophylactic treatment is inappropriate, and prefer to wait for the onset of extra-pyramidal reactions, as these are known, before instituting orphenadrine. Whatever the clinician's judgement this compound is among the most effective for mitigating parkinsonian effects: the recently-established drug levodopa, often dramatically successful in controlling tremors, involuntary movements and other phenomena of Parkinson's disease, may interact seriously with major tranquillizers and so alternative medication is required. Orphenadrine is also clinically useful, in conjunction with paracetamol and sometimes on its own, for alleviating painful muscular conditions (including some rheumatic states), tension headache and dysmenorrhoea (painful periods). Dry mouth, sensitivity to light, and palpitations may be experienced, and at high doses, particularly following injection of orphenadrine, a light euphoria is felt by some patients.

▲ To control parkinsonism: up to 200 mg daily orally or by intramuscular injection, in two or three divided doses. Pain relief: 50–150 mg three or four times daily.

★ Contra-indicated in glaucoma, urinary retention, prostatic enlargement, myasthenia gravis; and caution in impaired cardiac, liver and kidney function. Orphenadrine must not be given concurrently with DEXTROPROPOXYPHENE (PROPOXYPHENE) or with amphetamines or other central nervous system stimulants.

◆ UK:
Orphenadrine Citrate Tablets BP 1973: 100 mg
Slow Orphenadrine Citrate Tablets BPC: 100 mg
Norflex (Riker): Tabs 100 mg; Amps 60 mg/2 ml
Norgesic (Riker): Tabs orphenadrine citrate 35 mg, paracetamol 450 mg
Orphenadrine Hydrochloride Tablets BPC: available as
Disipal (Brocades): Tabs 50 mg; Amps 40 mg/2 ml
   USA:
Orphenadrine Citrate Injection USP: available as
Flexon (Keene): Vials 300 mg/10 ml
Myotran (Hyrex): Vials 300 mg/10 ml
Myotrol (Legere): Amps 60 mg/2 ml
Norflex (Riker): Tabs 100 mg; Amps 60 mg/2 ml
Norgesic (Riker): Tabs orphenadrine citrate 25 mg, aspirin 225 mg,
phenacetin 160 mg, caffeine 30 mg (NB formulation different from UK)
Disipal (Riker): Tabs orphenadrine hydrochloride 50 mg

OXAZEPAM

● One of the close analogues of DIAZEPAM (Valium), oxazepam
similarly is prescribed to alleviate anxiety and tension states. For this
purpose it possesses few if any advantages over diazepam or CHLOR-
DIAZEPOXIDE (Librium). The assertion that the drug is 'short-acting'
in comparison with diazepam, made in more than one reference text, is
misleading: a single dose may exert noticeable effects for between 12 and
24 hours. Thus a single daily dose regimen, with the compound taken at
night, may be satisfactory for some patients who ordinarily would be
asked to take one tablet (or however many) three times during the day.
Because oversedation, confusion, and impairment of reflexes are frequently encountered side-effects from this as from other benzodiazepine
tranquillizers, nightly dosage has obvious advantages. Oxazepam should
not be prescribed on an open-ended basis unless there is clear clinical
justification: tolerance and psychological dependency are real hazards of
prolonged use of any drugs of this class. High doses can induce states of
paradoxical excitement and breakdown of the faculty which 'builds in'
social inhibitions, with bizarre and sometimes violent behaviour. For
patients who do require more than one daily dose, the minimum should be
given which adequately controls symptoms.

▲ Up to 120 mg daily, in divided doses, in severe anxiety. More usually,
15–30 mg twice or three times daily (but see above).

★ Contra-indicated in severe respiratory distress, known hypersensitivity
to any benzodiazepine (including NITRAZEPAM and others of this
chemical class used as hypnotics), myasthenia gravis. Caution in severe

liver or kidney disorders, and for concurrent administration of other drugs which depress the CNS, including barbiturates, other tranquillizers, potent analgesics and alcohol.

→ For further information, see Essay VI and Chart VI(A): Tranquillizers.

◆ UK:
Serenid-D (Wyeth): Tabs 10 & 15 mg
Serenid-Forte (Wyeth): Caps 30 mg
   USA:
Oxazepam Tablets USP &
Oxazepam Capsules USP: available as
Serax (Wyeth): Tabs 15 mg; Caps 10, 15 & 30 mg

OXILORPHAN (BC–2605)

● This experimental drug is one of a very few pure narcotic antagonists, whose closest analogue among compounds currently marketed is NALOXONE. Such agents are so called because they completely reverse the effects of MORPHINE and similar opiate 'agonists', and if administered to narcotic habitués will precipitate withdrawal symptoms. Among their clinical applications are in treatment of opiate overdosage and diagnosis of heroin addiction. Oxilorphan, which despite several years' experimental and clinical study is not yet available for prescription, provokes a moderate degree of euphoria, but evidently not the 'psychotomimetic' effects (e.g. hallucinations) characteristic of some antagonists (e.g. NALORPHINE, PENTAZOCINE). Duration of action at doses of between 1 and 4 mg appears to be about 24 hours, as against one hour or less for naloxone. Physical dependence liability seems to be minimal. The principal potential therapeutic indication for oxilorphan will probably be in the maintenance treatment of opiate addicts. A number of approaches have been tried to wean people off heroin: maintenance of the habitué with oral METHADONE, a synthetic narcotic with the same abuse potential as the original drug, is the standard technique in several countries (see Essay IV); but this has many disadvantages, some obvious, some less so. The pharmaceutical company which patented oxilorphan has experimented with a tablet containing methadone together with naloxone, for the patient to take daily, the latter compound hopefully blocking the effects of any heroin taken subsequently. Among the problems encountered with this product, Methenex, was the short duration of action of the antagonist, the very high oral dose required, and the considerable cost of naloxone. Treatment with oxilorphan may circumvent the first two of these difficulties, and the fact that it yields some euphoria may make it more acceptable to patients than other medication which might be offered.

◆ Under study: Bristol Laboratories Inc, Syracuse, NY.

OXYCODONE R

● This compound is a valuable alternative to MORPHINE for the relief of severe pain states. Currently oxycodone is available to prescribers in the UK only in the form of suppositories, which may be obtained solely through one chain of pharmacies. Drugs for rectal administration are not popular in Britain, unlike France and some other continental countries, but oxycodone suppositories (which are small and easily inserted) may be very useful for patients suffering from terminal illness: particularly at night, sleep may have to be disturbed for the regular tablet or injection of opiate. This can be obviated by administration of oxycodone rectal tablets: these are quickly absorbed. The drug has a significantly longer duration of action than morphine and almost all analgesics of comparable potency, i.e. 6 hours or more, vs 3–5 for morphine and less for DIAMORPHINE, particularly in patients who have acquired some tolerance to narcotics. In the USA no pure preparations of the drug are marketed: only tablets and capsules which also contain simple analgesics (the APC mixture) or paracetamol, and one product which incorporates a moderately high dose of the barbiturate HEXOBARBITONE (HEXOBARBITAL). The addition of barbiturates to formulations of analgesics, particularly strong ones, is highly undesirable for two reasons: firstly, hexobarbitone and its congeners antagonize the pain-relieving effects of oxycodone and other analgesics, and secondly, repeated administration of such combination products may result in a dual physical (as well as psychological) dependency. In any case, being a potent opiate, oxycodone has a high potential for abuse and habituation, and thus should not be prescribed for other than short courses of treatment except in the most severe pain states, when the question of addiction becomes irrelevant. Side-effects from the drug are typical of the narcotics, and commonly include drowsiness, nausea/vomiting, dizziness, constipation, and mood changes (which some experience as euphoria).

▲ In the range 5–60 mg, depending on the severity of pain and individual susceptibility. Terminal patients may require doses much in excess of this.

★ Contra-indicated for use in obstetrics, because oxycodone tends to cause as much respiratory depression as MORPHINE, and, for this reason, in bronchial asthma and other disorders of breathing function. Precautions and interactions with other drugs: essentially as for morphine. Concomitant use of antidepressants of the MAO-inhibitor type is particularly to be avoided.

➤ For further information, see Essay IV and Chart IV: Morphine and Other Potent Analgesics.

◆ UK:

Proladone (Boots): Suppos 30 mg (pectinate: limited availability)
   USA:
Percobarb (Endo): Caps oxycodone hydrochloride 4.5 mg, oxycodone terephthalate 0.38 mg, hexobarbital 100 mg, aspirin 224 mg, phenacetin 160 mg, caffeine 32mg, homatropine 0.3 mg (also half-strength)
Percocet (Endo): Tabs oxycodone hydrochloride 5 mg, acetaminophen (paracetamol) 325 mg
Percodan (Endo): Tabs oxycodone hydrochloride 4.5 mg, oxycodone terephthalate 0.38 mg, aspirin 224 mg, phenacetin 160 mg, caffeine 32 mg, homatropine hydrobromide 0.38 mg (also half-strength)
Tylox (McNeil): Caps oxycodone hydrochloride 4.5 mg, oxycodone terephthalate 0.38 mg, acetaminophen (paracetamol) 500 mg

OXYMORPHONE R

● Like the compound described in the preceding Entry, oxymorphone is a semisynthetic derivative of MORPHINE. In milligramme potency, 1.0–1.5 mg of it is equivalent to morphine 10 mg for relief of very severe pain. The drug, now available in the USA only in injectable and suppository form, is given for premedication prior to surgery, and for very intense pain states (e.g. terminal cancer) when morphine or a medicament of comparable analgesic strength is indicated. In 1955, an expert committee of the World Health Organization found that oxymorphone had 'particularly dangerous addiction-producing properties' and recommended the abolition of its manufacture. The same committee modified its position in 1959, deciding that in some circumstances it had medicinal advantages over morphine. However, there is no doubt that oxymorphone has a dependence liability at least equal to, and possibly surpasssing, that of morphine, and one study in particular showed that some degree of habituation could occur in cancer patients within four weeks of regular administration. This, if true, would make the drug exceptional: when morphine and similar analgesics are given regularly, addiction by no means always supervenes even after months of treatment, and it is generally the case that, so far as non-medical use is concerned, repeated administration of a narcotic for 2–3 months is required before severe withdrawal symptoms are elicited when the drug is abruptly discontinued. In terms of side-effects, oxymorphone provokes similar reactions to morphine but these tend to be more pronounced: nausea/vomiting, drowsiness, dizziness, constipation, and mood changes (euphoria or dysphoria) are common, and respiratory depression, which all morphine analogues produce, is often more severe.

It is hard to see the clinical justification for the continued availability of the drug.

▲ 1–2 mg initially, 4–6 hourly: patients being treated regularly with the drug may require much higher doses as tolerance develops.

➤ As for OXYCODONE. For further information, see Essay IV and Chart IV: Morphine and Other Potent Analgesics.

◆ USA:
Oxymorphone Hydrochloride Injection USP &
Oxymorphone Hydrochloride Suppositories USP: available as
Numorphan (Endo): Amps 1 & 1.5 mg/1 ml; Vials 10 & 15 mg/10 ml; Suppos 2 & 5 mg

OXYPERTINE

● Oxypertine is one of the least often prescribed of psychotropic agents. It possesses antidepressant and anti-anxiety effects and is given in the treatment of anxiety neuroses, severe depression, and schizophrenic states. This drug does not belong to any of the major classes of antidepressant or tranquillizing agents. Adverse effects include dry mouth, dizziness, drowsiness, nausea and other gastro-intestinal disturbances, and parkinsonian reactions. Severe depressions may be enhanced by oxypertine, so due caution in prescribing is required.

▲ Anxiety neuroses: 10 mg three or four times daily. In schizophrenic and other psychotic conditions, up to a maximum of 300 mg daily, in two or three doses.

★ Contra-indicated during pregnancy and for concomitant use with MAO-inhibitor antidepressants. Oxypertine enhances the central depressant effects of barbiturates, other sedatives, opiates, and alcohol.

➤ For further information, see Essay II and Chart II: Antidepressants.

◆ UK:
Integrin (Sterling Research): Caps 10 mg; Tabs 40 mg

PAPAVERETUM **R**

● Papaveretum is the name given to purified extracts of the alkaloids of OPIUM: such preparations contain 50% MORPHINE and 50% other substances found in the poppy, such as CODEINE, papaverine, and noscapine. Products of this type have been in clinical use for many years, and papaveretum injections were frequently given during the Second World War to relieve the pain of wounded military personnel. They are still liked by some practitioners for premedication before surgery, alone or in combination with hyoscine (which prevents nausea), to control severe pain postoperatively and in terminally ill patients. It has been argued that papaveretum provides a more balanced type of analgesia than morphine alone, e.g. that the presence in it of papaverine, a muscle relaxant, prevents the retching so often produced by opiate analgesics. This assertion has been challenged by other specialists, who say that the clinical effects of papaveretum are entirely due to the morphine as an ingredient in the mixture. For pain relief an injection of total opium alkaloids 20 mg is commonly regarded as being equivalent to morphine 13 mg. Side-effects are typical of opiates, and may include drowsiness, dizziness, vertigo, mood changes (euphoria or dysphoria) and a similar degree of respiratory depression to that provoked by morphine. Abuse and dependence potential are essentially the same as for that drug.

▲ Between 10 and 40 mg orally or by injection. A starting dose of 10 mg is appropriate except for patients already habituated to narcotics.

★ Contra-indications: as for MORPHINE. Utmost caution in severe respiratory distress and impaired liver function. Should not be used in alcoholic delirium or concurrently with MAO-inhibitor antidepressants.

➤ See also under OPIUM and Essay IV and Chart IV: Morphine and Other Potent Analgesics.

◆ UK:
Papaveretum Tablets BPC: 10 mg
Papaveretum Injection BPC: Amps 10 & 20 mg/1 ml
unbranded Amps papaveretum 20 mg, hyoscine hydrobromide 0.4 mg/1 ml
Omnopon (Roche): Tabs 10 mg; Amps 20 mg/1 ml
Omnopon Scopolamine (Roche): as unbranded Amps (+ hyoscine)
unbranded Aspirin & Papaveretum Tablets: Sol Tabs papaveretum 10 mg, aspirin 500 mg
   USA:
Pantopon (Roche): Amps 20 mg/1 ml

PARALDEHYDE

● This is a clear or yellowish volatile liquid with a characteristic pungent, indeed almost indescribably unpleasant, odour. Paraldehyde was prescribed for many decades as a sedative, hypnotic and anticonvulsant, being particularly effective in controlling the repeated fits of status epilepticus, and in tetanus, and alcoholic delirium tremens (DTs). For virtually all these purposes the compound has been superseded by less disagreeable modern drugs which are as efficacious or more so: nonetheless paraldehyde is still useful for some convulsive conditions refractory to other methods of treatment. The advantage of the drug's low toxicity is outweighed by the fact that injection of it is painful, with large volumes being required. Also, it is excreted chiefly via the respiratory system and may be smelt on the breath for hours after administration: the lingering odour is literally nauseating. Paraldehyde indeed may induce nausea or vomiting, dizziness and headache, and large doses may render the patient unconscious. When given by injection, a steel and glass syringe must be used, rather than modern disposable ones made of polypropylene or plastic, which the drug will dissolve before the practitioner's very eyes.

▲ 15–30 ml by deep intramuscular injection, delivered to at least two different sites. Paraldehyde may be taken orally but is then much less effective.

★ Paraldehyde should be administered ice-cold and oral doses accompanied by a cold drink. The compound is contra-indicated in bronchial and liver disease, and in gastro-intestinal complaints such as colitis, peptic ulcer etc. If taken repeatedly it may be habituating, but this phenomenon is very rare.

➤ For further information, see Essay III and Chart III: Barbiturates.

◆ UK:
Paraldehyde Draught BPC 1973: 6 ml/45 ml
Paraldehyde Injection BPC: Amps 2, 5 & 10 ml
Paraldehyde Enema BPC 1973: paraldehyde 10 ml, sodium chloride (0.9%) solution to 100 ml
  USA:
Paraldehyde USP: 30 ml
Sterile Paraldehyde USP: 2, 5 & 10 ml
Paral (O'Neal, Jones & Feldman): Caps 1 G; Oral Soln 30 ml; Amps 2, 5 & 10 ml

PEMOLINE

● Pemoline is a highly useful drug which is surprisingly underutilized. Its principal indications are for the control of somnolence occasioned by MORPHINE and similar potent analgesics, and to elevate patients from the fatigue and lethargy which occur during recuperation, following surgery or other treatments for severe illnesses. Pemoline may be more appropriate than AMPHETAMINE for administration to children with the hyperkinetic syndrome, because the former is a less potent stimulant than amphetamine and its analogues and its capacity for abuse and psychological dependency much smaller. As is the case with all such stimulants, physical growth in children may be slowed but to a lesser extent. One formulation (Cylert) combines pemoline with magnesium, which apparently enhances its effects: in one study Cylert was found, at a dose of 100 mg, to be equivalent to METHYLAMPHETAMINE (METHAMPHETAMINE) 20 mg for improving sustained performance by fatigued subjects. Writers and musicians, and others who may have to work intermittently very hard to meet deadlines – people who may take amphetamines occasionally – are likely to find that pemoline meets their need for increased concentration just as well as these far more dangerous compounds. In terms of stimulant action, pemoline lies midway between caffeine and methylamphetamine. While the drug produces moderate central stimulation and somewhat improved mood, the latter effect is not such that craving for further doses is common. High doses may provoke excitability, agitation, palpitations and other reactions characteristic of amphetamines, but these will be less intense. Pemoline is a particularly suitable drug for concomitant use with opiate analgesics by individuals with severe chronic or terminal pain: often the sleepiness caused by morphine and its analogues can be completely overcome. Still, recent reports (1981) of pemoline abuse should be taken seriously.

▲ 40–70 mg daily. A regimen appropriate for many patients is 10–20 mg at breakfast, and a further 10 mg at lunchtime. The last daily dose should not be taken later than 4–5 p.m., otherwise sleep may be affected.

★ Caution in glaucoma, urinary retention, prostatic hypertrophy, and the other conditions listed as contra-indications to use of amphetamines. Pemoline should not be prescribed with MAO-inhibitor antidepressants unless the patient can be closely monitored.

➤ For further information, see Essay I and Chart I: Amphetamines.

◆ UK:
Kethamed (Medo-Chemicals): Tabs 20 mg (deleted 1981)
Ronyl (Rona): Tabs 20 mg
Volital (Laboratories for Applied Biology): Tabs 20 mg
 USA:
Cylert (Abbott): Tabs 18.75, 37.5 & 75 mg; Chewable Tabs 37.5 mg (magnesium pemoline)

PENTAZOCINE

● When pentazocine was introduced for prescription 16 years ago, great claims were (and still are) made by its manufacturers: that the new compound, a partial narcotic antagonist, possessed the pain-relieving effectiveness of PETHIDINE (MEPERIDINE) or MORPHINE, that it was not habituating, and that side-effects were minimal. In the light of clinical experience it is clear that pentazocine was oversold. While it may be beneficial in alleviating mild to moderate pain, the compound is only seldom of use in the control of very severe pain states, such as those experienced postoperatively, after serious injury, or in inoperable cancer. The popularity of pentazocine with prescribers doubtless stems in part from the fact that the drug is not legally restricted as are morphine, pethidine and other potent analgesics: when any alternative is available, practitioners avoid drugs scheduled under the Misuse of Drugs Act and comparable legislation elsewhere. It was for a long time believed that because this was a partial narcotic antagonist (i.e. if given to morphine-dependent patients it would provoke withdrawal symptoms) the substance would have a low abuse and dependence liability. In the event, a number of reputable published accounts describe both illicit use of pentazocine and definite physical addiction. How common these phenomena are is difficult to determine, but there is reason to believe that they have been consistently underestimated. Not only does the drug not compare favourably with morphine and other 'agonists' for analgesic potency, its adverse effects – notably nausea/vomiting, dizziness, headache, mood changes (euphoria or dysphoria), mental depression, and bizarre psychological states such as delusions and depersonalization – may in some instances be more troublesome than those produced by standard strong analgesics. In short, a compound with limited medical applications. It is worth observing that legal restriction of pentazocine, which has been proposed in the UK, now applies in France.

▲ Orally, 25–100 mg daily, in 2 or 3 doses. By injection, usually 20–40 mg.

★ Contra-indicated in severe respiratory problems, liver and kidney disease, head injury, hypertension. Concomitant use of opiate agonists such as morphine is inadvisable and of MAO-inhibitor antidepressants contra-indicated.

➤ For further information, see Essay IV and Chart IV: Morphine and Other Potent Analgesics.

◆ UK:
Pentazocine (Hydrochloride) Tablets BPC
Pentazocine Lacate Injection BPC &
Pentazocine Lactate Suppositories BNF: available as
Fortral (Winthrop): Tabs 25 mg; Caps 50 mg; Amps 30 mg/1 ml & 60 mg/2 ml; Suppos 50 mg
Fortagesic (Winthrop): Tabs pentazocine hydrochloride 15 mg, paracetamol 500 mg
    USA:
Pentazocine Hydrochloride Tablets USP &
Pentazocine Lactate Injection USP: available as
Talwin (Winthrop): Tabs 50 mg; Amps & Syrettes 30 mg/1 ml, 45 mg/1.5 ml & 60 mg/2 ml; Vials 300 mg/10 ml
Talwin-Co (Winthrop): Caps pentazocine hydrochloride 12.5 mg, aspirin 325 mg
Talwin-Co 50 (Winthrop): Tabs pentazocine hydrochloride 50 mg, aspirin 300 mg, caffeine 32 mg

PENTOBARBITONE (PENTOBARBITAL) and PENTOBARBITONE SODIUM

● Pentobarbitone is perhaps more familiar to some readers as the branded product Nembutal, yellow capsules which have been marketed in many countries for a considerable time. The compound, and its more rapidly absorbed and metabolized sodium salt, is a sedative and hypnotic agent of the barbiturate family: it is practically identical to AMYLO-BARBITONE in its effects. It is not considered suitable in the maintenance treatment of epilepsy, unlike PHENOBARBITONE for example, because of its relatively short duration of action, and is prescribed almost always to promote sleep. This the drug does, without question, effectively. But REM or dreaming sleep is suppressed by it, as by other barbiturates, and hangover, oversedation, unsteadiness, and confusion may follow ingestion of quite small doses. Larger quantities provoke a form of paradoxical excitement which is enjoyed by many drug abusers. Repeated use is likely (though, for reasons as yet obscure, not in all cases) to lead to tolerance and psychological and/or physical habituation. Barbiturate addiction, **not** infrequent on either side of the Atlantic, may be even more devastating than narcotic dependency: withdrawal symptoms may be life-threatening and are not easy to treat. Short courses only of pentobarbitone should be prescribed for insomniacs, if indeed a barbiturate is justified for the purpose: many physicians believe this is never the case. Newer hypnotic drugs such as NITRAZEPAM and TRIAZOLAM, analogues of DIAZEPAM (Valium), are much less toxic in overdosage: dependency on these may also occur, but it is unlikely to approach that induced by protracted use of barbiturates.

▲ 50–300 mg at night (100 mg is adequate in most cases).

★ Among the principal contra-indications are porphyria and severe respiratory and liver ailments; also known hypersensitivity to any barbiturate.

➤ For additional data on precautions, interactions etc, see under AMYLOBARBITONE (AMOBARBITAL) and Essay III and Chart III: Barbiturates.

◆ UK:
Pentobarbitone Sodium Capsules BPC: 100 mg
Nembutal (Abbott): Caps 100 mg
　USA:
Pentobarbital Elixir USP: 20 mg/5 ml
Pentobarbital Sodium Capsules USP
Pentobarbital Sodium Elixir USP &
Pentobarbital Sodium Injection USP: available as
Nembutal (Abbott): Caps 30, 50 & 100 mg; SR Tabs 100 mg; Amps

100 mg/2 ml, 250 mg/5 ml, 2 G/20 ml; Vials 2.5 G/50 ml; Suppos 30, 60, 120 & 200 mg (sodium); Elix 20 mg/5 ml

Emesert (Arnar-Stone): Suppos pentobarbital 30 mg, pyrilamine maleate 25 mg; also 45 + 50 & 100 + 50 mg

Matropinal (Comatic): Tabs pentobarbital 8 mg, pyrilamine maleate 12 mg, homatropine methylbromide 10 mg; also 90 + 12.5 + 10 mg; Suppos 15 + 8 + 10 & 90 + 8 + 10 mg

Penital (Kay): Caps 90 mg (sodium)

WANS (Webcon): Suppos pentobarbital sodium 30 mg, pyrilamine maleate 30 mg; also 100 + 50 mg

Maso-Pent (Mason): Tabs 100 mg (sodium)

Night-Caps (Bowman): Caps 100 mg (sodium)

see also under CARBROMAL

PERICYAZINE (PROPERICIAZINE)

● This compound is one of the very numerous analogues of CHLORPROMAZINE (Largactil, Thorazine). It belongs to the phenothiazine class of major or antipsychotic tranquillizers. Pericyazine has been recommended not only to control hyperagitation, delusions and other severe symptoms of schizophrenias and other psychotic states, but (admittedly at far lower dosage) for alleviation of severe anxious, tense or agitated states which are not classed as psychoses. Undoubtedly pericyazine has pronounced calmative effects: it also tends to induce lethargy, apathy, indifference to surroundings, loss of motivation and often enhances mental depression. Therefore its prescription in minor emotional or psychological disturbances is not justified unless the circumstances are exceptional. Adverse effects are typical of chlorpromazinetype tranquillizers: this compound is more sedative than others of the same chemical group, and anticholinergic effects (disturbances in visual accommodation, dry mouth, gastro-intestinal upsets) are frequent. The peculiar form of Parkinson's disease which may be caused by treatment with virtually all antipsychotic agents appears less often with pericyazine than with other phenothiazines, but the risk of tardive dyskinesia – an insidious, perhaps irreversible form of parkinsonism – is probably no less with this compound than with its alternatives. This dyskinesia occurs chiefly in patients who have been receiving major tranquillizers at high doses over long periods.

▲ Outpatients: 5–25 mg daily, and inpatients up to a maximum of 90 mg daily, depending on the severity of the condition being treated and on individual response.

★ Contra-indicated in convulsive disorders, severe liver, kidney and cardiac or cardiovascular ailments. Concurrent use of anticoagulants, amphetamines and similar CNS stimulants and MAO-inhibitor anti-depressants is not advised. The effects of other drugs which are centrally depressant, i.e. other tranquillizers, barbiturates, opiate analgesics and alcohol, are increased.

➤ For further information, see Essay VI(B) and Chart VI: Antipsychotic Tranquillizers.

◆ UK:
Neulactil (May & Baker): Tabs 2.5, 10 & 25 mg; Syr 2.5 & 10 mg/5 ml

PERPHENAZINE

● Like PERICYAZINE, the subject of the preceding Entry, per-phenazine is a major tranquillizer or antipsychotic agent of the phenothiazine group whose prototype is CHLORPROMAZINE. This compound, however, is less potent in its antischizophrenic activity, while producing similar qualitative effects on the patient. Perphenazine is administered by injection to control severe nausea and vomiting, and as an adjunct to MORPHINE and other potent analgesics, whose pain-killing action it enhances. Because of its anxiety- and tension-relieving properties, the drug is often prescribed in general practice as an alterna-tive to 'minor' tranquillizers of the DIAZEPAM (Valium) type. Unfortu-nately, like almost all phenothiazine derivatives it may precipitate mental depression or intensify this if it is already present. So preparations have been devised which incorporate an antidepressant, such as AMITRIPTY-LINE, to control the triad of anxiety, tension and depression. Although such fixed-dose combination products are popular among prescribers, they are medically unsound: this is chiefly because they limit flexibility in dosage. A particular tablet may or may not contain the correct dose of each ingredient to suit an individual patient's needs. Also, side-effects, some of which are common to both tranquillizer and antidepressant, may be a problem. Dry mouth, gastro-intestinal disturbances and blurred vision are adverse effects often encountered. Parkinsonian reactions, too, may occur in susceptible individuals even at low doses. In general, perphenazine should not be the drug of first choice for the alleviation of non-psychotic anxiety or agitation: compounds of the benzodiazepine series, such as DIAZEPAM (Valium), may be more appropriate.

▲ Outpatients: 8–24 mg daily. Psychiatric inpatients: up to 64 mg daily for severely psychotic states.

★ Contra-indications are as for the preceding Entry, pericyazine, and in the case of perphenazine/amitriptyline combinations, as for AMITRIP-TYLINE and other tricyclic antidepressants.

➤ For further information, see Essay VI(B) and Chart VI: Antipsychotic Tranquillizers, and Chart II: Antidepressants.

◆ UK:
Perphenazine Tablets BPC &
Perphenazine Injection BPC: available as
Fentazin (Allen & Hanburys): Tabs 2, 4 & 8 mg; Amps 5 mg/1 ml (NB:
these are extremely sensitive to light); Syr 3 mg/5 ml
   USA:
Perphenazine Tablets USP
Perphenazine Syrup USP
Perphenazine Oral Solution USP; &
Perphenazine Injection USP: available as
Trilafon (Schering): Tabs 2, 4, 8 & 15 mg; SR Tabs 8 mg; Syr 2 mg/5 ml;
Oral Soln 16 mg/5 ml; Amps 5 mg/1 ml
see also under AMITRIPTYLINE

PETHIDINE (MEPERIDINE) R

● Since its synthesis in the 1940s pethidine, known in the USA as
meperidine, has become a standard drug. Its indications are several: in
obstetrics to relieve labour pains; postoperative analgesia; spasmodic pain
states such as renal colic; for premedication; and to control intense pain of
many kinds. In terms of absolute potency, its effectiveness does not
compare favourably with MORPHINE for control of very severe chronic
conditions and in terminal illness. Pethidine may be adequate in some
such instances, but it should be regarded as an analgesic of intermediate
strength. Its short duration of action (2–4 hours) following injection
constitutes an advantage in obstetrical analgesia, but not in cases where
regular administration of opiates is necessary: even this duration of effect
is attenuated if the drug is given regularly. Tolerance to the pain-relieving
action of pethidine is apt to develop quickly and, while addiction to the
compound is infrequent numerically, once habituation occurs the habit is
difficult to stop. For reasons which are unclear, physician addicts choose
pethidine more often than morphine: this may necessitate very frequent
injections of the drug. Withdrawal symptoms are similar to those of
MORPHINE but may be less intense. Their onset is more rapid than is
the case with morphine or METHADONE – within 12 hours or less of the
last dose – but the abstinence syndrome is also correspondingly shorter.
Euphoria occasioned by pethidine is milder than that associated with
morphine or heroin (DIAMORPHINE), and other side-effects, such as
drowsiness, dizziness, nausea, constipation, and respiratory depression,
are usually less troublesome. It is because the compound impairs respiratory function less than many of its analogues that for most obstetricians it is
the drug of choice for analgesia during labour. Even so, since some of the
drug passes via the placenta into the circulation of the foetus, breathing
difficulties in the newborn may arise: fortunately this neonatal apnoea can

be reversed by the pure narcotic antagonist NALOXONE. The combination product Pethilorfan, which contains pethidine with the partial antagonist LEVALLORPHAN, is widely used in hospitals: this is undesirable because the latter's duration of effect is considerably shorter than that of the narcotic (see under levallorphan). Pethidine is occasionally seen on the illicit market: it is acceptable if heroin is unavailable, for warding off withdrawal symptoms, but it is not as strongly euphoriant as morphine or heroin and thus less sought after. Combination products are marketed which contain pethidine and/or the anti-emetic agents scopolamine (hyoscine) and PROMETHAZINE: the latter enhances the medicament's analgesic activity. These are seldom prescribed outside hospitals.

▲ Orally, 25–100 mg and by injection 50–200 mg, depending on the clinical situation and the patient's response. Pethidine is considerably less effective orally than by injection, if a little longer-acting.

★ Pethidine should be administered with utmost caution, if at all, to patients with head injuries and impaired liver function. Elderly and debilitated persons should be monitored closely. The most important serious interaction occurs if the drug is administered to someone under treatment with antidepressants of the MAO-inhibitor type. The central depressant effects of tranquillizers, barbiturates, and alcohol may be considerably increased.

➤ For further information, see Essay IV and Chart IV: Morphine and Other Potent Analgesics.

◆ UK:
Pethidine (Hydrochloride) Tablets BPC: 25 & 50 mg
Pethidine (Hydrochloride) Injection BPC: Amps 50 mg/1 ml, 100 mg/2 ml
Pamergan P100 (May & Baker): Amps pethidine hydrochloride 100 mg, promethazine hydrochloride 50 mg/2 ml
Pamergan AP (May & Baker): Amps pethidine hydrochloride 100 mg, promethazine hydrochloride 25 mg, atropine sulphate 0.6 mg/1 ml
also see under LEVALLORPHAN (Pethilorfan)
   USA:
Meperidine Hydrochloride Tablets USP: 50 & 100 mg
Meperidine Hydrochloride Syrup USP: 50 mg/5 ml
Meperidine Hydrochloride Injection USP: as *Demerol* Amps etc
Demerol (Winthrop): Tabs 50 & 100 mg; Syr 50 mg/5 ml; Amps 25 mg/0.5 ml, Amps & Syrettes 50 mg/1 ml, 75 mg/1.5 ml, 100 mg/1 ml & 100 mg/2 ml (filled or half-filled); Vials 500 mg/10 ml, 1.5 G/30 ml, 2 G/20 ml
Demerol-APAP (Breon): Tabs meperidine hydrochloride 50 mg, acetaminophen (paracetamol) 300 mg
APC + Meperidine (Wyeth): Tabs meperidine hydrochloride 30 mg, aspirin 200 mg, phenacetin 130 mg, caffeine 30 mg

Mepergan (Wyeth): Syrettes meperidine hydrochloride 50 mg, promethazine hydrochloride 50 mg/2 ml; Vials 250 + 250 mg/10 ml
Mepergan-Fortis (Wyeth): Caps meperidine hydrochloride 50 mg, promethazine hydrochloride 25 mg

PHENAZOCINE R

● Most of the very potent analgesics, such as MORPHINE, provoke
some disagreeable side-effects, and tolerance and psychological or physical habituation occur readily with regular administration. Phenazocine,
which is now marketed only in the UK, is a useful alternative to morphine
for relief of severe acute or chronic pain, and may be equally beneficial in
controlling symptoms in terminal cancer patients. Despite the fact that the
drug falls under the same legal restriction as morphine, pethidine and the
other opiate analgesics, its abuse potential is lower than that of some
pain-relieving agents which are not so controlled (e.g. DIHYDRO-
CODEINE). Indeed, since its introduction in 1960, only two or three
cases of dependency have been notified annually to the UK Home Office.
This is no doubt because, in spite of phenazocine's excellent capacity for
mitigating severe pain, if euphoria is experienced it is likely to be mild and
transient. Other side-effects, though characteristic of the opiates, such as
nausea, drowsiness, dizziness, and oversedation, are milder following
phenazocine than after morphine administration. One disadvantage of
this compound is that, on a weight basis, it is considerably less effective
when taken by mouth than by injection: 2×5 mg tablets are approximately equivalent for analgesic potency to an injected dose of 2–3 mg.
The discontinuation of an ampoule formulation of phenazocine, which
had proved useful for premedication, analgesia for surgical procedures
(e.g. bronchoscopy) and for the most intense pain states, is regrettable.
This compound, unlike most potent analgesics (e.g. MORPHINE,
PETHIDINE), does not cause spasm of the sphincter of Oddi, and hence
may be useful to control visceral pain. Injectable phenazocine is now
marketed exclusively in Finland.

▲ Orally: 5–10 mg 4–6 hourly. Patients who have been receiving the drug
regularly may require 50 mg or more daily. Weight for weight,
phenazocine is about 5 times more potent than morphine.

★ This compound shares the contra-indications of other potent opiates.
Caution in severe respiratory depression and impaired liver function.
Concomitant administration of MAO-inhibitor antidepressants may be
hazardous.

➤ For further information, see Essay IV and Chart IV: Morphine and
Other Potent Analgesics.

◆ UK:
Phenazocine (Hydrobromide) Tablets BPC: available as
Narphen (Smith & Nephew): Tabs 5 mg

PHENBUTRAZATE

● This drug is a mild central stimulant which is incorporated into a proprietary appetite-suppressant tablet, known as Filon in the UK and Cafilon on the European continent. The principal ingredient of this formulation is PHENMETRAZINE, a very potent analogue of AMPHETAMINE. Phenbutrazate is not marketed alone in any country. It is said to balance some of the unwanted effects of phenmetrazine, but the evidence for this is anecdotal.

➤ For further information, see Essay I and Chart I: Amphetamines, and under PHENMETRAZINE.

PHENCYCLIDINE **R**

● This compound was formerly employed as an anaesthetic in veterinary medicine under the trade name Sernylan. It is not now available for prescription for any purpose. Better known as 'angel dust', phencyclidine has increasingly been seen on the illicit market. The compound has been described as a psychedelic, but this is not strictly accurate: it may provoke strange psychological states, including some which closely resemble spontaneously occurring psychotic conditions. In the USA powders which purport to contain MESCALINE or LYSERGIDE (LSD) have been shown on analysis to consist of phencyclidine. Unlike genuine psychedelics, or 'mind-revealing' agents such as lysergide, this drug has a low margin of safety between doses which provoke psychological effects and those which may be life-threatening. Under no circumstances can the present authors justify the use of phencyclidine: indeed, we absolutely contra-indicate this. Manufacturing the substance is extremely dangerous, partly because this involves highly flammable materials.

➤ For further information, see Essay V and Chart V: Psychedelics.

PHENDIMETRAZINE **R**

● Phendimetrazine is an appetite-suppressant derived from AMPHET-AMINE, although it is much less potent in its central stimulant activity. The drug (as indicated by the above legend) is restricted in the UK, where it is not available, but not in the USA, where a considerable number of branded preparations of it are marketed. Like other amphetamine analogues, phendimetrazine should be prescribed for limited periods only (not more than 4–8 weeks) because tolerance to its appetite-depressing effect develops within this time. Its abuse potential is slight because it does not, except perhaps at very high doses, produce the 'speedy' euphoria characteristic of the amphetamine class of drugs. Adverse reactions, such as restlessness, tremor, agitation and hyper-excitability depend to an extent on individual idiosyncrasy but in general they are much less pronounced than those elicited by amphetamine itself or its potent analogues METHYLPHENIDATE and PHENMETRA-ZINE, with which the compound under discussion should not be confused.

▲ 35–70 mg daily, usually as a single morning dose.

★ Caution in hypertension, glaucoma, hyperthyroidism, severe cardiac disease, and in cases of known hypersensitivity to amphetamine-type stimulants and anorexiants. Contra-indicated for use at the same time as antidepressants, whether tricyclic or MAO-inhibitor, antihypertensives, antipsychotic tranquillizers and alcohol.

➤ For further information, see Essay I and Chart I: Amphetamines.

◆ USA:
Plegine (Ayerst): Tabs 35 mg (tartrate)
Bacarate (Tutag), *Bontril-PDM* (Carnrick), *Ex-Obese* (Kay), *Minus* (Federal), *Obalan* (Lannett), *Phenzine* (Mallard), *Slim-Tabs* (Wesley), *SPRX* (Tutag), *Trimstat* (Laser) & *Trimtabs* (Mayrand): Tabs 35 mg
Adphen (Ferndale), *Melfiat* (Reid-Provident) & *Obezine* (Western Research): Tabs 35 & 70 mg
Statobex (Lemmon): Tabs 35 mg; SR Tabs & Caps 70 mg

PHENELZINE

● Phenelzine belongs to a small and diminishing group of antidepressants, the monoamine-oxidase (MAO) inhibitors. The drug is occasionally prescribed to alleviate depression in various forms as well as phobic states. Compounds of this type are not of first choice in the treatment of depressive disorders, having not quite been superseded by AMITRIP-TYLINE, IMIPRAMINE and other tricyclic agents. The difficulty about therapy with MAO-inhibitors is that they interact with several foods and drinks and with a whole host of other drugs and drug types. Among the comestibles which must be avoided are cheese, pickled herrings, concentrated meat, vegetable and vegetable protein extracts (including Marmite and Bovril), caviare, bananas; certain forms of alcohol, such as Chianti wine, are known to be dangerous in conjunction with phenelzine, but for safety no type of liquor should be taken. Among the most serious, and potentially life-threatening, interactions with other drugs can occur with

PETHIDINE (MEPERIDINE) and other opiate analgesics; with amphetamines and analogous central stimulants and appetite-suppressants; and with tricyclic antidepressants. Barbiturates, antihistamines, antihypertensives and antidiabetic medicaments may also be hazardous for concurrent administration. As if this were not enough, common side-effects of these antidepressants are nausea, dry mouth, dizziness, restlessness, fatigue and drowsiness. Onset of therapeutic effect, as in the case of most antidepressants, will not begin for 2–4 weeks following the beginning of treatment. Phenelzine may be helpful for some patients who do not respond to AMITRIPTYLINE or other members of the tricyclic class; but because of the obvious difficulties it should be tried only when alternative medication has not relieved symptoms.

▲ 10-40 mg daily, in two or three doses. Regimens must be established empirically for individual patients.

★ Contra-indicated in severe liver disorders, cardiac and cerebrovascular complaints, epilepsy, and phaeochromocytoma.

➤ For further information, see Essay II and Chart II: Antidepressants.

◆ UK:
Phenelzine (Sulphate) Tablets BPC: available as
Nardil (Warner): Tabs 15 mg
   USA:
Phenelzine Sulfate Tablets USP: available as
Nardil (Warner-Chilcott): Tabs 15 mg

PHENMETRAZINE (OXAFLUMEDRINE) ℞

● Phenmetrazine, more familiar as the branded preparation Preludin, is an analogue of AMPHETAMINE and is prescribed to suppress appetite in obesity: this should be for a strictly limited period (3–4 weeks) and only as part of a total programme including dieting and exercise. Regular use leads to tolerance and psychological dependency of the amphetamine type. The intense, energetic euphoria provoked by phenmetrazine makes it much sought after on the illicit market, particularly in the USA where extremely potent formulations are available. If the compound is taken at high doses for prolonged periods, a phenomenon called 'amphetamine psychosis' may ensue: this is almost indistinguishable from naturally-occurring psychotic states, and is characterized by delusions, auditory hallucinations, formication (a sensation that insects are crawling under the skin) and other severe symptoms. Some practitioners in the USA appear to regard phenmetrazine as less dangerous than amphetamine or DEXAMPHETAMINE: this is not so. Side-effects are likely to be very similar to these drugs', and include agitation, restlessness, stereotyped behaviour, insomnia, sweating, gastro-intestinal disturbances and changes in libido and sexual potency. In the UK Preludin has been deleted, but phenmetrazine is the principal ingredient of the Filon tablet (the other constituent, phenbutrazate, having little or no therapeutic effect) which, inexplicably, some physicians continue to prescribe for long periods. Fortunately, most practitioners now realize the potentially devastating effects of amphetamines and their surrogates and in the UK have ceased to give them.

▲ 25–75 mg daily. A single dose of a sustained-released tablet, taken at breakfast, will continue acting throughout the day.

★ Contra-indicated in hypertension, cardiac disease, hyperthyroidism, glaucoma, urinary retention, and for administration to patients considered prone to abuse drugs. Concurrent use of antidepressants, antipsychotic tranquillizers, antihypertensive agents and alcohol should be avoided.

➔ For further information, see Essay I and Chart I: Amphetamines.

◆ UK:
Filon (Berk): Tabs phenmetrazine theoclate 30 mg, phenbutrazate hydrochloride 20 mg
   USA:
Phenmetrazine Hydrochloride Tablets USP: available as
Preludin (Boehringer Ingelheim): Tabs 25 mg; SR Tabs 50 & 75 mg

PHENOBARBITONE (PHENOBARBITAL) AND PHENOBARBITONE SODIUM

● This long-acting and old-established barbiturate is today chiefly prescribed to prevent the occurrence of fits in epilepsy: for this purpose it must be taken regularly, perhaps over a period of many years. Despite the availability of more modern anticonvulsants of lower toxicity and without the dependence potential of phenobarbitone, such as ethosuximide (Zarontin) and sodium valproate (Epilim), not all sufferers from epilepsy respond to these and thus have to take a barbiturate, often in conjunction with the related compound, phenytoin sodium. The prescription of phenobarbitone (and other analogues: BARBITONE, METHARBITONE and METHYLPHENOBARBITONE) for daytime sedation and to promote sleep is seldom if ever appropriate. First, a single dose will remain in the system for 3 days or longer, and if repeated doses are taken there is a risk that toxic quantities of drug will accumulate. Then the hazards of psychological or physical habituation should be considered: these are less than for shorter-acting barbiturates such as AMYLOBARBITONE (AMOBARBITAL) and PENTOBARBITONE, but not very much. Side-effects and after-effects are typical of the chemical class to which the drug belongs, and hangover, oversedation, confusion, and reflex impairment may be expected at dosage levels likely to promote sleep. Phenobarbitone is a constituent of numerous proprietary tablets and capsules which contain aspirin and/or other simple analgesics: use of these is never therapeutically justified, in part because barbiturates antagonize the latters' pain-relieving effectiveness. The problem of 'masked barbiturates' is discussed elsewhere in this book.

▲ For maintenance treatment in epilepsy: 50–200 mg daily. Higher doses may be needed by patients who have been treated with barbiturates for long periods. As a hypnotic: 100–200 mg.

★ Contra-indicated in porphyria, and severe liver disorders, as well as known hypersensitivity to any barbiturate. Utmost caution in cardiac, kidney and respiratory ailments. Phenobarbitone potentiates the effects of other central depressants, e.g. tranquillizers, opiates, and alcohol. The drug may alter metabolism of oral anticoagulants, antipsychotic agents and the contraceptive Pill.

➔ For further information, see Essay III and Chart III: Barbiturates (NB particularly Table 4).

UK:
Phenobarbitone Tablets BPC: 7.5, 15, 30, 50, 60, 100 & 125 mg
Phenobarbitone Elixir BPC: 15 mg/5 ml
Luminal (Winthrop): Tabs 15, 30 & 60 mg
Phenobarbitone Spansules (Smith Kline & French): SR Caps 60 & 100 mg
Parabal (Sinclair): Tabs 10 mg
Epanutin with Phenobarbitone (Parke Davis): Caps phenobarbitone 50 mg, phenytoin sodium 100 mg
Phenobarbitone Sodium Tablets BPC: 30 & 60 mg
Phenobarbitone (Sodium) Injection BPC: Dry Amps 15, 30, 60 & 200 mg
For other preparations, see Table 4
  USA:
Phenobarbital Tablets USP: 8, 15, 25, 30, 60 & 100 mg
Phenobarbital Elixir USP: 7.5 & 20 mg/5 ml
Bar-8, Bar-15 etc (Scrip): Tabs 8, 15, 25, 30 & 100 mg; Elix 20 mg/5 ml
Barbipil (North American Pharmacal): Pills 32 mg
Barbita (North American Pharmacal): Pills 15 mg
Eskabarb (Smith Kline & French): SR Caps 65 & 97 mg
Henomint (Bowman): Elix 20 mg/5 ml
Hypnette (Fleming): Chewable Tabs 15 mg; Suppos 7.5 & 15 mg
Infadorm (Reid-Provident): Drops 16 mg/1 ml
Luminal (Winthrop): Tabs 15 & 30 mg
Pheno-Squar (Mallard): Tabs 16 mg
Sedadrops (Merrell-National): Drops 16 mg/1 ml
SK-Phenobarbital (Smith Kline & French): Tabs 15 & 30 mg

Solu-Barb (Fellows-Testagar): Sol Tabs 15 mg
Stental (Robins): SR Tabs 50 mg
Phenobarbital Sodium Tablets USP: 35 mg
Phenobarbital Sodium Injection USP: Amps 130 mg/1 ml
Sterile Phenobarbital Sodium USP: Powder for injection
Luminal Sodium (Winthrop): Amps 130 mg/1 ml

NB The number of compound proprietary preparations containing small doses of phenobarbitone, which are marketed in the USA, is so great that to list these would occupy excessive space in this book. For the type of products concerned, cf Essay III (Table 4)

PHENOPERIDINE R

● Phenoperidine is one of two synthetic opiates (the other being FENTANYL) which are notable for their milligramme potency and for their ultra-short duration of action (½–1 hour) following intravenous injection. Although the drug has been given to alleviate severe pain, for example postoperatively, it and fentanyl are almost exclusively administered to maintain anaesthesia when assisted ventilation is necessary during major surgery, and in the technique of neuroleptanalgesia: here the opiate is injected, alone or with an enhancing agent such as DROPERIDOL, before and during surgical procedures which require that the patient be conscious, albeit free of pain and apprehension. Phenoperidine, which is partially metabolized to PETHIDINE, has been claimed to have a lower toxicity than MORPHINE and certain analgesics of comparable potency, and that it may be more readily given to children and the elderly. Technically, the drug's capacity for abuse and addiction is similar to that of morphine; but in practical terms the question hardly, if ever, arises, since phenoperidine is used almost solely in the hospital context, only a few doses are likely to be administered, and its extremely short duration of effect would make it an unsuitable candidate for addiction. Nevertheless, because of its powerful narcotic agonist action, the medicament is restricted under the Misuse of Drugs Act.

▲ Analgesia: 1–2 mg intravenously, repeated every 30–60 minutes. For induction of anaesthesia and in neuroleptanalgesia: initially 1 mg, then 0.5 mg half-hourly, repeated as required.

★ Respiratory depression is perhaps the principal hazard associated with phenoperidine as of other drugs (e.g. FENTANYL) used in anaesthetics. Contra-indications are essentially the same as for fentanyl and other opiates.

➤ See also under FENTANYL and Essay IV and Chart IV: Morphine and Other Potent Analgesics.

◆ UK:
Operidine (Janssen): Amps 2 mg/2 ml (hydrochloride)

PHENTERMINE

● Of all the AMPHETAMINE-type appetite-suppressants, phentermine has the least stimulant activity and its use produces few if any adverse effects at therapeutic doses. The drug is generally presented in the form of a bonded resin, contained in a tablet or capsule, for prolonged release. A recent controlled experiment showed that, in overweight diabetic subjects, phentermine proved effective in promoting weight reduction without causing hypertension, agitation or other adverse reactions typical of the amphetamine class of drugs. However, tolerance to its appetite-depressing action sets in within a few weeks, and so intermittent rather than continuous prescription is advised. Even so, the compound should be given only as part of a total programme including exercise and dieting. The risk of abuse is negligible because even at extremely high doses amphetamine-like euphoria seldom occurs.

▲ 15–30 mg at breakfast (as a sustained-release tablet or capsule).

★ Caution in hypertension, hyperthyroidism, and cardiac and cardiovascular disorders. Phentermine should be avoided for patients under treatment with antidepressants of the MAO-inhibitor type.

➤ For further information, see Essay I and Chart I: Amphetamines.

◆ UK:
Duromine (Carnegie): SR Caps 15 & 30 mg (resinate)
Ionamin (Lipha): SR Caps 15 & 30 mg (resinate)
  USA:
Adipex-P (Lemmon): SR Tabs 30 mg (resinate)
Fastin (Beecham-Massengill): SR Caps 30 mg (resinate)
Ionamin (Pennwalt): SR Caps 15 & 30 mg (resinate)
Parmine (Parmed): SR Caps 30 mg (resinate)
Phentrol (North American Pharmacal): Tabs 8 & 15 mg (hydrochloride)
Rolaphent (Robinson): Tabs 8 mg (hydrochloride)
Terámine (Legere): SR Caps 30 mg (resinate)
Tora (Tutag): Tabs 8 mg (hydrochloride)
Wilpo (Dorsey): Tabs 8 mg (hydrochloride)
Wilpowr (Foy): SR Caps 30 mg (resinate)

PIMOZIDE

● Pimozide belongs to the small diphenylbutylpiperidine class of antipsychotic agents, the only other example being the depôt injectable preparation FLUSPIRILENE. In the relevant Chart, the compound is considered under the same heading as HALOPERIDOL (Haldol, Serenace), because its actions and uses are similar to those of the chemical group of which that drug is the prototype. As usual with major tranquillizers (neuroleptics) of recent introduction, pimozide has been claimed to be greatly superior to haloperidol, CHLORPROMAZINE (Largactil, Thorazine) and conventional antipsychotic medicaments in controlling the symptoms of schizophrenia. On the available evidence pimozide has been found, according to some studies, to be indistinguishable in effect from standard drugs. Other trials appear to indicate some advantage for the new agent over chlorpromazine and long-acting injectable preparations of FLUPHENAZINE. Because pimozide possesses less sedative activity than its alternatives, one authoritative review states that it has no place in the hyperactive or agitated or aggressive type of schizophrenic patient. On the other hand, pimozide is less likely than most other neuroleptics to provoke parkinsonism, mental depression, lethargy and oversedation, though such reactions have been observed in some cases. In the treatment of severe anxiety and tension states, for alleviation of which the drug has been proposed, it does not seem to be superior to DIAZEPAM (Valium) and other 'minor' tranquillizers. It is too early to tell whether pimozide precipitates tardive dyskinesia, an insidious form of Parkinson's disease, if administered at high doses for prolonged periods. Mental depression may be enhanced. Given the drug's known adverse effects and various imponderables, it is unsuitable for treatment of minor emotional or psychological disturbances. In schizophrenia real benefits compared with those yielded by standard drugs such as chlorpromazine have yet to be established.

▲ Outpatients: 2–10 mg. Psychiatric inpatients: up to 40 mg daily.

★ Particularly contra-indicated in epilepsy, for use during pregnancy, and for non-psychotic depression. Pimozide blocks the stimulant effects of AMPHETAMINES and comparable stimulants. Caution with MAO-inhibitor antidepressants.

➤ For further information, see Essay VI(B) and Chart VI: Antipsychotic Tranquillizers.

◆ UK:
Orap (Janssen): Tabs 2, 4 & 10 mg
   USA:
Orap (Janssen): Tabs 2 & 4 mg

PIPERACETAZINE

● This is one of the older antipsychotic or major tranquillizing agents. It is an analogue of and has attributes similar to CHLORPROMAZINE (Largactil, Thorazine). Piperacetazine is one of the most potent drugs of its type, often provoking apathy, mental depression, parkinsonism and other reactions characteristic of antipsychotic medications, in pronounced form, its administration should be confined to chronic cases of schizophrenia. The compound is totally unsuitable for the treatment of non-psychotic psychological disturbances. Prolonged use may cause tardive dyskinesia (cf under CHLORPROMAZINE).

▲ Outpatients: 10–40 mg daily. Hospital inpatients may require up to a maximum of 160 mg/day.

★ Contra-indicated in mental depression, severe cardiac, liver or kidney ailments, and epilepsy. The centrally depressant effects of other drugs, e.g. barbiturates, other tranquillizers and alcohol, are increased.

➤ For further information, see Essay VI and Chart VI(B): Antipsychotic Tranquillizers.

◆ USA:
Piperacetazine Tablets USP: available as
Quide (Dow): Tabs 10 & 25 mg

PIRITRAMIDE R

● Piritramide is the most recent synthetic opiate of the agonist (rather than the partial antagonist) type to be made available for prescription. The justification for the addition of still another alternative to MORPHINE and standard analgesics appears to be that the newer drug is at least as effective as others and has comparable potency. Its duration of action (more than 6 hours after intramuscular injection) is greater than that of other opiates (e.g. 4–5 hours or less for morphine and 2–4 for PETHIDINE). The manufacturers at present recommend piritramide only for administration to control postoperative pain, and not for other acute or chronic pain states. On the face of it there seems little reason to confine its use in this way. True, it produces as much respiratory depression as morphine, but the clinical importance of this is often exaggerated. Theoretically the analgesic has a moderate abuse and addiction liability, but in practice no instances of dependency have been reported (at least in the UK). Piritramide elicits morphine-like sedative and in some cases euphoric effects; and other side-effects (nausea, constipation, dizziness, confusion) are qualitatively similar. Caution should be exercised if the drug is given for other than limited periods.

▲ 15–30 mg by intramuscular injection, 5–6 hourly.

★ Piritramide should be avoided in severe respiratory, liver and biliary disorders; during pregnancy and for children. Concurrent use of MAO-inhibiting antidepressants may be dangerous, and so may administration of partial antagonist analgesics such as PENTAZOCINE. The drug increases the central depressant action of barbiturates, tranquillizers and alcohol.

➤ See also Essay IV and Chart IV: Morphine and Other Potent Analgesics.

◆ UK:
Dipidolor (Janssen): Amps 20 mg/2 ml

POTASSIUM BROMIDE

● This compound is included as an example of the now obsolete bromide type of sedatives: sodium and strontium bromide have the same effects. In spite of the risks associated with these old-fashioned remedies for insomnia and daytime sedatives, a few preparations containing one or more of them (sometimes in conjunction with barbiturates) continue to be marketed on the continent of Europe, and one in particular in the USA. Repeated administration of bromides may easily lead to psychological and physical dependency and, because of these drugs' instrinsically long duration of action, toxic quantities may accumulate in the system: this is known as bromism, a state characterized by confusion, delirium, and in severe cases convulsions and coma. Even the barbiturates, such as AMYLOBARBITONE (AMOBARBITAL), which are dangerous enough, hardly compare with the bromides in terms of undesirable short- and long-term effects.

▲ 300–600 mg at night.

➤ Contra-indications are as for BARBITURATES. See Essay III and Chart III: Barbiturates.

◆ USA:
Lanabrom (Lannett): Elix combined potassium, sodium, strontium and ammonium bromides 600 mg/5 ml

PRAZEPAM

● This is another addition to an already overcrowded market, namely the benzodiazepine class of compounds, whose most familiar exemplars are DIAZEPAM (Valium) and CHLORDIAZEPOXIDE (Librium). Prazepam is like these in all significant respects, being effective in relieving anxiety, tension, and (at the higher end of the dosage range) for promoting sleep. Oversedation, unsteadiness of gait, drowsiness, and consequent impairment of reflexes may occur and should be anticipated. At large doses all diazepam analogues can induce paradoxical excitement, and with repeated use tolerance and psychological dependency – in some cases also physical addiction – will arise. Therefore, unless the therapeutic reasons are compelling, prazepam should not be prescribed for extended periods.

▲ In the range 10–60 mg daily. Because the drug (and its active metabolites) have a duration of effect exceeding 24 hours, a single daily dose, taken at night, may serve the dual function of assisting sleep and of obviating side-effects which tend to arise during the earlier phase of the drug's activity.

★ Contra-indicated in severe respiratory distress, and in cases of known hypersensitivity to any benzodiazepine tranquillizer. Prazepam increases the CNS-depressing actions of barbiturates, other tranquillizers, strong analgesics and alcohol.

➤ For further information, see Essay VI and Chart VI(A): Tranquillizers.

◆ USA:
Verstran (Warner-Chilcott): Tabs 10 mg

PROCHLORPERAZINE

● Prochlorperazine is a member of the phenothiazine class of tranquillizers and an analogue of CHLORPROMAZINE. Unlike most compounds of this group the medicament is not usually prescribed to control psychotic states, but rather for its good anti-emetic action and to relieve moderately severe anxiety and tension. In combination with isopropamide, the drug may be of help in relieving the pain of peptic ulcer and other gastro-intestinal disorders. Side-effects are similar to those elicited by other phenothiazine derivatives, and may include nausea, oversedation, mental depression and parkinsonian reactions. These are, however, marked only at high doses. Prochlorperazine should not be prescribed for patients who are severely depressed as well as anxious. The drug has been found useful in controlling symptoms of Ménière's disease for a limited number of patients.

▲ To prevent or control nausea/vomiting: 10–50 mg two or three times daily. As an anxiolytic: 5–10 mg three times daily. For hospitalized patients up to a maximum of 200 mg/day.

★ Contra-indicated in severe depression, convulsive states, and for patients known to be hypersensitive to any phenothiazine compound. Concurrent use of antidepressants and of other centrally-depressant drugs, including strong analgesics and alcohol, must be under careful control.

➤ For further information, see Essay VI and Chart VI(B): Antipsychotic Tranquillizers.

◆ UK:
Prochlorperazine (Maleate) Tablets BPC
Prochlorperazine (Mesylate) Injection BPC &
Prochlorperazine (Maleate) Suppositories BPC: available as
Stemetil (May & Baker): Tabs 5 & 25 mg; Syr 5 mg/5 ml; Amps 12.5 mg/
1 ml; Suppos 5 & 25 mg
Vertigon (Smith Kline & French): SR Caps 10 & 25 mg
   USA:
Prochlorperazine Edisylate Oral Solution USP
Prochlorperazine Edisylate Injection USP
Prochlorperazine Maleate Tablets USP
Prochlorperazine Maleate Syrup USP 1974 &
Prochlorperazine Maleate Suppositories USP: available as
Compazine (Smith Kline & French): Tabs 5, 10 & 25 mg; SR Caps 10, 15,
30 & 75 mg; Soln 10 mg/1 ml; Syr 5 mg/5 ml; Amps 5 mg/1 ml; Suppos 2.5,
30 & 75 mg.
Combid (Smith Kline & French); SR Caps prochlorperazine 10 mg,
isopropamide 5 mg & 75 mg

PROLINTANE

● Prolintane is almost unique among central nervous system stimulants in that it enhances rather than decreases appetite. Thus, it may be of considerable benefit during convalescence following major surgery, when the medicament combats lassitude and fatigue and helps to improve concentration. Prolintane lacks the formidable potency of AMPHET-AMINE and some of its analogues. It is true that high doses may occasion restlessness, agitation, excitability, gastro-intestinal upsets or other unto-ward effects associated with amphetamines, but to a much lesser extent than, for example, PHENMETRAZINE or METHYLPHENIDATE. If euphoria is experienced this is apt to be mild. A study conducted among undergraduates about to sit an examination has demonstrated that prolintane was effective in increasing concentration. The drug has only slight potential for abuse and psychological dependency, but nevertheless long-term administration is seldom warranted.

▲ 20–80 mg daily: usually 10–20 mg at breakfast and a further dose of 10–20 mg at lunchtime. The last daily dose should be taken not later than 4 p.m. to obviate the risk of insomnia.

★ Not advised in epilepsy, thyrotoxicosis, agitated states, and severe hypertension. Concomitant prescription of antidepressants of any kind is contra-indicated.

➤ For further information, see Essay I and Chart I: Amphetamines.

◆ UK:
Villescon (Boehringer Ingelheim): Tabs prolintane hydrochloride 10 mg, thiamine 5 mg, riboflavine 3 mg, pyridoxine 1.5 mg, nicotinamide 15 mg, ascorbic acid 50 mg (i.e. B & C vitamins); Liq 20 ml equivalent to 1 Tab

PROMAZINE

● Promazine is a major tranquillizer prescribed chiefly to control symptoms of schizophrenia and other psychotic disorders. It is sometimes also given to control severe nausea and vomiting and to reduce agitation during alcoholic withdrawal. Like its close analogue CHLOR-PROMAZINE, it may cause oversedation, apathy, mental depression, parkinsonism and other unwanted effects typical of antipsychotic agents. Protracted administration, especially to psychiatric inpatients, brings with it the risk of tardive dyskinesia, a severe disturbance of motor and muscular co-ordination which may be irreversible. Promazine should not be prescribed in minor psychological and emotional problems, for which other medicaments are more appropriate and far less likely to provoke serious side-effects. In particular, the drug may considerably intensify pre-existing mental depression.

▲ Outpatients: 25–75 mg daily. Psychiatric inpatients may need up to 200 mg per day for relief of symptoms.

★ Contra-indicated in convulsive states, liver disorders, and known sensitivity to any other compound of the phenothiazine class. Effects of barbiturates, other tranquillizers, opiate analgesics and alcohol will be enhanced.

➤ For further information, see Essay VI and Chart VI(B): Antipsychotic Tranquillizers.

◆ UK:
Promazine (Hydrochloride) Tablets BPC
Promazine (Hydrochloride) Syrup BPC &
Promazine (Hydrochloride) Injection BPC: available as
Sparine (Wyeth): Tabs 25, 50 & 100 mg; Oral Susp 50 mg/5 ml: Amps 50 mg/1 ml
  USA:
Promazine Hydrochloride Tablets USP
Promazine Hydrochloride Syrup USP
Promazine Hydrochloride Oral Solution USP &
Promazine Hydrochloride Injection USP: available as
Sparine (Wyeth): Tabs 10, 50, 100 & 200 mg; Syr 10 mg/5 ml; Soln 30 mg/1 ml; Amps 100 mg/2 ml; Syrettes 25 mg/1 ml & 50 mg/2 ml; Vials 250 & 500 mg/10 ml
Hyzine (Hyrex): Vials 500 mg/10 ml

PROMETHAZINE

● Like PROMAZINE, the drug described in the preceding Entry, promethazine is a tranquillizer of the phenothiazine series, whose prototype is CHLORPROMAZINE. Promethazine, however, is virtually devoid of antipsychotic activity. Nonetheless it is an extremely versatile compound with a number of clinical applications: it is a strong antihistamine, and may be useful in allergic conditions. As a sedative, it has much to recommend it as an alternative to conventional remedies for insomnia. It has a low toxicity and no abuse potential, but is unlikely to be of benefit in refractory sleep disorders. Both orally and by injection promethazine is an excellent anti-emetic: given in conjunction with MORPHINE and other potent analgesics, it serves the dual function of enhancing their pain-relieving efficacy and preventing the nausea or vomiting commonly provoked by opiates. Side-effects are uncommon at therapeutic doses: drowsiness, dizziness, and a fall in blood-pressure may occur.

▲ As an anti-emetic (e.g. travel-sickness): 25–50 mg of the hydrochloride or theoclate salt. For children and the elderly in particular, to promote sleep: 10–75 mg. As an adjunct to MORPHINE, PETHIDINE (MEPERIDINE) and other narcotics: 25–50 mg by deep intramuscular injection. Promethazine ampoules are very sensitive to light and become green unless kept in a dark place. Because the solution is slightly viscous, injection can be painful, so use of the gluteal (buttock) muscles is indicated.

★ No absolute contra-indications, except known hypersensitivity to phenothiazines, and epilepsy. Caution in impaired liver function.

➤ For further information, see Essay VI and Chart VI(B): Antipsychotic Tranquillizers.

◆ UK:
Promethazine Hydrochloride Tablets BPC
Promethazine Hydrochloride Elixir BPC &
Promethazine Hydrochloride Injection BPC: available as
Phenergan (May & Baker): Tabs 10 & 25 mg; Elix 5 mg/5 ml; Amps 25 mg/1 ml & 50 mg/2 ml
Promethazine Theoclate Tablets BPC: available as
Avomine (May & Baker): Tabs 25 mg
   USA:
Promethazine Hydrochloride Tablets USP
Promethazine Hydrochloride Syrup USP &
Promethazine Hydrochloride Injection USP: available as
Phenergan (Wyeth): Tabs 12.5 & 25 mg; Syr 6.25 & 25 mg/5 ml; Amps 25 mg/1 ml & 50 mg/2 ml; Suppos 25 & 50 mg
see also under AMYLOBARBITONE (AMOBARBITAL), BUTO-BARBITONE and PETHIDINE (MEPERIDINE)

PROPIOMAZINE

● This phenothiazine derivative, like that described in the foregoing Entry, PROMETHAZINE, and some others of the same chemical class (e.g. METHOTRIMEPRAZINE), is administered as a sedative and anti-emetic prior to surgery and in conjunction with general anaesthetics during surgical procedures. Propiomazine has essentially the same anti-nauseant and calmative effect as the other drugs named, and is like these useful for increasing the clinical efficacy of potent analgesics of the MORPHINE and PETHIDINE type: concurrent administration both prevents the vomiting often provoked by narcotics and considerably enhances pain relief, to the extent that dosage of morphine may be reduced while the same effect is achieved. Nonetheless caution is required because the central and respiratory depressant action of opiates is also intensified. Side-effects include dry mouth, oversedation, fluctuations in blood-pressure and rapid heart-rate (tachycardia).

▲ 10–40 mg intravenously or intramuscularly, depending upon the clinical indication, the patient's likely response and other variables.

★ Contra-indicated in coma, convulsive states, delirium, impairment of liver function and known hypersensitivity to any drug of the phenothiazine class (including those with antipsychotic activity, e.g. CHLORPROMAZINE).

➤ For further information, see Essay VI and Chart VI(B): Antipsychotic Tranquillizers.

◆ USA:
Propiomazine Hydrochloride Injection USP: available as
Largon (Wyeth): Amps & Syrettes 20 mg/1 ml & 40 mg/2 ml

PROPRANOLOL

● Propranolol is a compound belonging to a series known as beta-blockers: these drugs are widely used to relieve hypertension, angina pectoris, and disturbances of heart rhythm. Over the past decade this medicament, the standard beta-blocker, has been tried as a tranquillizer. High blood-pressure indicates overactivity of the sympathetic nervous system. It was felt that if propranolol was effective in reversing this hyperactivity it would not only decrease blood-pressure but possess more generalized calming, tension-reducing properties. This is to simplify the rationale for prescription of beta-blockers as psychotropic agents. Attractive features of propranolol include the fact that tolerance does not seem to occur with regular administration and that neither psychological nor physical dependency arise with the drug. It is now clear that the compound is beneficial for some anxious patients; whether it is so in control of the symptoms of mania or schizophrenia has not been fully established. In psychotic illness very high doses must evidently be given: then adverse effects, which are mild and transient at anxiety-relieving dosage levels, may pose problems. Nausea/vomiting, lethargy, insomnia, diarrhoea, dry eyes, skin rashes and undesirable changes in heart rhythm can then be experienced. Propranolol may be a useful alternative to DIAZEPAM (Valium) and its numerous chemical relatives for certain patients.

▲ 40–160 mg daily in two or three doses. A sustained-release formulation is now marketed: in this case a single dose at breakfast. To control psychotic symptoms, far higher dosages have been given.

★ Contra-indicated in diabetes, bronchospasm, heart block, after fasting and during pregnancy. Beta-blockers interact with several other drugs prescribed in heart disease and hypertension, including clonidine and verapamil, and the anticonvulsant levodopa.

➤ For further information, see Essay VI and Chart VI(A): Tranquillizers.

◆ UK:
Propranolol (Hydrochloride) Tablets BPC: 40, 80 & 160 mg
Berkolol (Berk): Tabs 10, 40 & 80 mg
Inderal (ICI): Tabs 10, 40 & 80 mg; SR Caps & Tabs 160 mg
   USA:
Propranolol Hydrochloride Tablets USP: available as
Inderal (Ayerst): Tabs 10, 20, 40 & 80 mg

PROPYLHEXEDRINE

● This compound is a central stimulant derived from AMPHETAMINE, which is sometimes prescribed for symptomatic relief of sinusitis, allergic rhinitis, and generally as a nasal decongestant. It is presented in the form of an inhaler, as was its parent drug when this was first introduced. Side-effects of any kind are rare when propylhexedrine inhalers are used as directed; but abusers have been known to extract the wadding (which contains the active substance, a volatile liquid) from the plastic container tube and to consume much larger quantities than are appropriate. The effect of this is to produce an amphetamine-like 'high': even when considerable quantities of drug are taken relatively slight stimulant action is experienced, which cannot compare for intensity with amphetamine and its more potent analogues.

▲ Two inhalations (about 25–50 mg) through each nostril, not more than once hourly.

★ Caution in hypertension and heart disease.

> For further information, see Essay I and Chart I: Amphetamines.

◆ USA:
Propylhexedrine Inhalant USP: available as
Benzedrex (Menley & James): Inhalers 250 mg

PROTRIPTYLINE

● This drug has actions and uses typical of the tricyclic class of anti-depressants, and is similar in important respects to its chemical analogue AMITRIPTYLINE. It is prescribed to mitigate the symptoms of various types of depressive illness. For this purpose, like its alternatives, the compound must be taken regularly for 2–4 weeks before any effect on mood is noticed. Other actions, however, may be experienced only two or three days after commencement of therapy: sedation, dry mouth, blurred vision, gastro-intestinal disturbances and lessening of libido are among those frequently reported. These side-effects are common to all tricyclic antidepressants but appear to be slightly more marked with protriptyline than amitriptyline. Caution is essential if the drug is prescribed for a severely depressed patient because his symptoms may be enhanced. In this connection it is hardly possible to overemphasize the hazards of tricyclic antidepressants when taken in suicide attempts: such overdosages are difficult to treat and the incidence of fatalities is rising annually.

▲ 10–60 mg daily. Dosage must be adjusted to meet individual requirements, and depends on severity of symptoms and on response.

★ Contra-indicated in glaucoma, hyperthyroidism, urinary retention, prostatic enlargement; and for concurrent administration with MAO-inhibitor antidepressants, amphetamines and other central stimulants, and certain antihypertensive agents.

> For further information, see Essay II and Chart II: Antidepressants.

◆ UK:
Protriptyline (Hydrochloride) Tablets BPC: available as
Concordin (Merck Sharp & Dohme): Tabs 5 & 10 mg
　USA:
Protriptyline Hydrochloride Tablets USP: available as
Vivactil (Merck Sharp & Dohme): Tabs 5 & 10 mg

PSILOCIN and PSILOCYBIN R

● Psilocin and psilocybin, which possess similar attributes, are the principal active constituents (alkaloids) of the mushroom *Psilocybe mexicana* and other fungi of the same species, as well as of another, *Stropharia cubensis*. Like other 'hallucinogenic' substances, these are used by the indigenous inhabitants of Mexico, Cuba, and elsewhere in Central and

South America as part of a religious ritual. It was with psilocybin that Timothy Leary and his colleagues at Harvard first experimented during the late 1950s and early 1960s, when investigating 'psychedelic' effects in normal volunteers. The rest, one might say, is history. Leary and his co-workers were sacked from their posts and LYSERGIDE (LSD), psilocybin and other compounds which produced extraordinary altered states of consciousness were banned. The psychedelics are now the most rigorously controlled of all drugs under national and international legislation. In terms of psychological effects, the two mushroom alkaloids are similar, but not identical, to lysergide. The states induced are difficult, if not impossible, to describe accurately, and the terms commonly used to indicate them are inadequate. Visions may indeed be experienced: whether one should call them 'hallucinations' is questionable. Under psilocybin all the senses may seem to merge (synaesthesia), and the mental 'filter' which operates to control sensory input in ordinary conscious states no longer works, so that the subject is flooded with bizarre perceptions. Depersonalization, whereby one appears to lose one's identity while the drug is acting, may be frightening if not anticipated. The profundity of the psychological changes triggered by psychedelics is hard to overestimate. For this reason there must be strict criteria for medical or other use of psychedelic compounds: for instance, this is absolutely contra-indicated for persons who are other than very stable mentally, and, if an experiment is contemplated, this should take place under the supervision of a practitioner who is familiar with these drugs.

➤ For further information, see Essay V and Chart V: Psychedelics.

PYRIDOXINE

● Pyridoxine, or vitam B₆, is important in protein metabolism and is an essential component of human diet. The substance is included here because it has been found effective in combating depression in women who take the contraceptive Pill. Whether and how the vitamin achieves this effect is still uncertain. At least, with the recommended doses adverse reactions of any sort are unlikely and the margin of safety is extremely wide. Pyridoxine has been given as an anti-emetic for morning sickness during pregnancy and for irradiation sickness. The combination of the vitamin with L-TRYPTOPHAN appears to relieve depression in some cases for males as well as females.

▲ 50–100 mg daily as a single dose.

➤ See also under L-TRYPTOPHAN and Essay II and Chart II: Antidepressants.

◆ UK:
Pyridoxine (Hydrochloride) Tablets BPC: 10, 20 & 50 mg
Comploment (Napp): SR Tabs 100 mg

QUINALBARBITONE (SECOBARBITAL) and QUINALBARBITONE SODIUM

● Quinalbarbitone and its sodium salt are prescribed for daytime seda-tion and to promote sleep. They are typical of the intermediate-acting barbiturates, such as AMYLOBARBITONE (AMOBARBITAL) and PENTOBARBITONE. The prescription of these compounds has declined in recent years as equally effective and safer alternatives have become available (e.g. NITRAZEPAM and other analogues of DIAZEPAM [Valium]). Many practitioners now believe that the only justification for giving barbiturates is for the prevention and treatment of epileptic fits. Quinalbarbitone, called secobarbital in the USA, certainly provides sound sleep, but at a price. REM, or dreaming, sleep is suppressed by barbiturates: this can lead to nightmares and other reac-tions when the drug is discontinued. Tolerance to these compounds sets on readily in many cases, although some patients are apparently able to take barbiturate hypnotics regularly without increasing the dose. Such are, possibly, in a minority. Psychological and physical dependence are serious risks with all compounds of this type: therefore they should not be prescribed except on a shut-ended basis, for periods of a few days or weeks. For daytime sedation use of quinalbarbitone, as of its chemical relatives, is unwise, because oversedation, confusion, impairment of reflexes and other unwanted effects are frequently experienced. Again, the taking of barbiturates in conjunction with aspirin, paracetamol and other analgesics, in the hope of increasing their effectiveness, is unsound, as these sedatives antagonize the action of pain-relieving drugs.

▲ 50–300 mg at night: individual response is very variable. Much larger doses may be required by epileptic patients.

★ Barbiturates are contra-indicated in severe respiratory ailments, por-phyria, liver disorders and for patients hypersensitive to them. These agents enhance the CNS depressant effects of tranquillizers, potent analgesics, and alcohol. Among the more important interactions occur with oral anticoagulants and the contraceptive Pill.

➤ For further information, see Essay III and Chart III: Barbiturates.

◆ UK:
Quinalbarbitone Sodium Tablets BPC 1950: 100 mg
Quinalbarbitone Sodium Capsules BPC 1950: 100 mg
Seconal (Lilly): Caps 50 & 100 mg
see also under AMYLOBARBITONE (*Tuinal*)

USA:
Secobarbital Elixir USP
Sodium Secobarbital Capsules USP
Sodium Secobarbital Injection USP &
Sterile Secobarbital Sodium USP: available as
Seconal (Sodium) (Lilly): Tabs 100 mg; Caps 30, 50 & 100 mg; Dry Amps 250 mg; Syrettes 100 mg/2 ml; Vials 1 G/20 ml; Elix 22 mg/5 ml; Suppos 30, 60, 120 & 200 mg
Sec-Kap (Scrip): Caps 50 & 100 mg
Seco-8 (Fleming): Caps 100 mg
see also under AMYLOBARBITONE (*Tuinal*)

SECBUTOBARBITONE (BUTABARBITAL) and SECBUTOBARBITONE SODIUM

● For details of this compound's actions and uses, see preceding Entry (QUINALBARBITONE). NB: This drug should not be confused with BUTOBARBITONE (known in the USA as butethal).

▲ 50–250 mg at night.

◆ USA:
Butabarbital Tablets USNF 1975: 15, 30, 50 & 100 mg
Da-Sed (Sheryl): Tabs 30 mg
Medarsed (Medar): Tabs 15 & 60 mg; Elix 30 mg/5 ml
Cystospaz–SR (Webcon): SR Caps butabarbital 45 mg, hyoscyamine sulfate 0.375 mg
Butabarbital Sodium Tablets USP
Butabarbital Sodium Capsules USP &
Butabarbital Sodium Elixir USP: available as
Butal (Blaine): Tabs 15 & 30 mg
Butalan (Lannett): Elix 30 mg/5 ml
Butazem (Zemmer): Tabs 15, 30 & 100 mg
Buticaps (McNeil): Caps 15, 30, 50 & 100 mg
Butisol (McNeil): Tabs 15, 30 & 100 mg; SR Tabs 30 & 60 mg; Elix 30 mg/5 ml
Butte (Scrip): Tabs 15 & 30 mg; Elix 30 mg/5 ml
Expansatol (Merit): Caps 60 mg
Intasedol (Elder): Elix 30 mg/5 ml
Quiebar (Nevin): Tabs & Caps 15 & 30 mg; Tabs 100 mg; Elix 30 mg/5 ml
Renbu (Wren): Tabs 32.4 mg
Soduben (Arcum): Tabs 30 mg
Minotal (Carnrick): Tabs butabarbital sodium 15 mg, acetaminophen (paracetamol) 325 mg
Phrenilin (Carnrick): as above + caffeine 40 mg

TALBUTAL

● Talbutal is an intermediate-acting barbiturate sedative and hypnotic with essentially the same properties as QUINALBARBITONE (SECOBARBITAL).

▲ 120–360 mg at night.

➤ For further information, see Essay III and Chart III: Barbiturates.

◆ USA:
Talbutal Tablets USP: available as
Lotusate (Winthrop): Tabs 120 mg

TEMAZEPAM

● Temazepam was introduced for prescription in the UK in 1978 as a new sleep-inducing drug. The compound belongs to the same class as DIAZEPAM (Valium) and shares most of the characteristics of the benzodiazepines. A number of substances, similar to diazepam not only chemically but in terms of clinical effects, have been introduced as distinct entities to promote sleep. Temazepam has a particular advantage over other tranquillizer/hypnotics of this type: the duration of action of the drug itself and its by-products is considerably shorter than that of diazepam or NITRAZEPAM. This means that hangover, oversedation, and slowing of reflexes on the morning after a nocturnal dose are less likely to occur, although these after-effects have been reported. Transient gastro-intestinal upsets and skin rashes are less frequent adverse reactions. Despite the short half-life, i.e. the length of time required for 50% of the drug to be eliminated, there is little doubt that if temazepam, like other benzodiazepines, is taken repeatedly, tolerance will develop and the patient may become psychologically dependent on the drug. At the dosage levels recommended by the manufacturers, chronic sufferers from insomnia may find it relatively ineffective. In any case, individual response to Valium-like medicaments is extremely variable. Long-term prescription of temazepam as of other hypnotics is not recommended.

▲ In the range 10–60 mg at night. Because the available preparation is a liquid enclosed in gelatin capsules size is a limiting factor, and several capsules may need to be taken.

★ Like diazepam and other analogues, contra-indicated in severe respiratory disorders, during pregnancy, and in cases of hypersensitivity to any benzodiazepine, whether prescribed as a daytime tranquillizer or as a hypnotic.

➤ For further information, see Essay III and Chart III: Barbiturates, and Essay VI and Chart VI(A): Tranquillizers.

◆ UK:
Euhypnos (Farmitalia CE): Caps 10 & 20 mg
Normison (Wyeth): Caps 10 & 20 mg

$\triangle^9$-TETRAHYDROCANNABINOL (THC) **R**

● Attempts to discover the active principle or principles of CANNABIS (marijuana) began at the turn of the present century with the isolation of the oil cannabinol from cannabis resin. Not until the late 1930s, however, were additional compounds isolated: at this time cannabidiol and THC were identified and soon afterwards made synthetically. A. R. (now Lord) Todd, one of those responsible, noted the variations in concentration of alkaloids from cannabis grown in different countries. According to him, THC showed 'the typical physiological effects of hashish in rabbits, dogs, and in man', and he hoped that the synthesis of THC and other cannabinoids would 'lead to their clinical examination and possibly to the discovery of medical applications [for them]' (Todd, A. R., 'The hemp drugs', *Endeavour* 2: 69–72, 1943). R. Mechoulam and his colleagues in Israel have now identified some 35 different compounds which are present in cannabis, and he has made it clear that yet more remain to be isolated as laboratory techniques become further refined. For many years it has been assumed that THC is the substance responsible for most or all of the psychological and physical effects associated with cannabis. That this hypothesis has hardly been challenged is surprising, since there exist important differences between the activity of the single alkaloid and that of cannabis extract or resin: specifically, for example, at high doses THC reliably provokes 'psychotomimetic' effects, such as depersonalization and hallucinations, which are comparitively rare following ingestion of marijuana or hashish. A whole spectrum of interesting but not easily quantifiable reactions occurs in the latter case (see also under CANNABIS). Nonetheless, THC has been far more extensively studied than any other individual alkaloid of the herb. In man, doses of 5–25 mg orally, and 2–10 mg by smoking, produce psychological and other effects for roughly six hours. These are often found by seasoned cannabis users to be disagreeable. THC has been shown to have several potentially important medicinal indications, as Todd predicted. Some interesting experimental compounds have been derived from it, in attempts to separate evidently undesirable psychic effects from those of therapeutic benefit. Some success has been achieved in these ventures with a substance to which no name has yet been assigned (BRL-4664), which is under current investigation. Considerably more promising appear to be NABILONE and LEVONANTRADOL, the latter in particular demonstrating some remarkable properties.

➤ see also under CANNABIS; LEVONANTRADOL; NABILONE.

THIOPENTONE

● The above-named drug is included here as an example of very short-acting injectable barbiturates: these are not prescribed for night sedation (and rarely to relieve epileptic seizures) but as the sole general anaesthetic in short surgical procedures; to induce unconsciousness prior to administration of other anaesthetics in surgery of longer duration; and for 'narcoanalysis' in psychiatry. The latter is a technique in which mental patients, held in a twilight zone between sleep and wakefulness, may be enabled to answer questions or to 'regress' in a fashion which is not possible in ordinary waking states because of inhibitions and other constraints. The effect of narcoanalysis may be compared with that of hypnosis, in the sense of the practice of hypnotism. Thiopentone, more familiar perhaps as Pentothal, has also been given as a 'truth drug' to criminal suspects and others, with results that are questionable. Duration of effect of this and other ultra short-acting barbiturates (e.g. methohexitone sodium, thiamylal sodium) is only a few minutes following intravenous injection: therefore, if a longer span is required the drug is administered by infusion. Adverse effects may be unpleasant and are such that thiopentone should be administered only by physicians experienced in its use who have antidotes available: respiratory depression, irregularities in heart-rate, sneezing, coughing and bronchospasm, shivering and prolonged sleepiness are reactions which depend in part on dosage and also on individual idiosyncrasy.

▲ For narcoanalysis: 100 mg/minute of a 2.5% solution, intravenously.

★ Contra-indicated in hypersensitivity to any barbiturate, severe asthma, porphyria. Thiopentone may be given as a rectal suspension: this is contra-indicated in ulcerative or inflammatory bowel conditions. Interactions with other drugs are as for barbiturates generally.

➤ For further information, see Essay III and Chart III: Barbiturates.

◆ UK:
Thiopentone (Sodium) Injection BPC: available as
Intraval (May & Baker): Vials 500 mg, 1.5 G etc (powder)
　USA:
Thiopental Sodium for Injection USP: available as
Pentothal (Abbott): Amps 500 mg & 1 G; Vials 5 G etc (powder)

THIOPROPAZATE

● Thiopropazate is a major tranquillizer, or antipsychotic agent, derived from and similar to CHLORPROMAZINE (Largactil, Thorazine). While occasionally prescribed to relieve obsessional neuroses and other moderately severe non-psychotic conditions, the drug should normally be reserved for administration to sufferers from seriously disabling illnesses such as schizophrenias and other forms of psychotic illness. In extremely small doses the compound may be given to control severe nausea and vomiting, but alternatives are available which do not provoke such disagreeable side-effects (e.g. PROMETHAZINE, Phenergan). Frequent adverse effects are parkinsonism, mental depression, lethargy, and anticholinergic reactions (dry mouth, blurred vision). The medicament is unsuitable for treatment of minor psychological or emotional disturbances. Pre-existing depression may be intensified, and reflexes impaired.

▲ Outpatients: 10–30 mg daily, in 2 or 3 divided doses; for psychiatric inpatients, up to 100 mg/day.

★ Among the principal contra-indications are convulsive disorders (e.g. epilepsy), delirium, and severe liver and heart ailments. Thiopropazate should not be prescribed concurrently with amphetamines or other stimulants or appetite-suppressants, and only with utmost caution with MAO-inhibitor antidepressants.

➤ For further information, see Essay VI and Chart VI(B): Antipsychotic Tranquillizers.

◆ UK:
Thiopropazate (Hydrochloride) Tablets BPC 1973: available as
Dartalan (Searle): Tabs 5 & 10 mg
USA:
Thiopropazate Hydrochloride Tablets USNF 1970: available as
Dartal (Searle): Tabs 5 & 10 mg

THIORIDAZINE

● Thioridazine is a close analogue of CHLORPROMAZINE and its proper applications are in control of hyperagitation, delusions, and other symptoms of schizophrenia and other psychotic illnesses. The drug is also prescribed to alleviate anxiety and tension states. This, however, is seldom justified unless symptoms are very severe, because the depression which so often accompanies anxiety may be enhanced to a considerable extent, even at relatively low doses. Also, adverse effects typical of the phenothiazine class of drugs to which it belongs may be unacceptably unpleasant: apathy, indifference to surroundings, fall in blood-pressure, oversedation and particularly loss of libido are among those most frequently complained of. In general, with the availability of relatively safe and effective 'minor' tranquillizers, such as DIAZEPAM (Valium) and its analogues, thioridazine is inappropriate except in severe mental disturbances. Repeated use of the compound, as of other antipsychotics, may lead to the insidious and possibly irreversible form of Parkinson's disease known as tardive dyskinesia.

▲ Outpatients: 50–400 mg daily. For mental hospital inpatients, doses in excess of this may be required.

★ Contra-indications etc.: as for THIOPROPAZATE, see preceding Entry.

➤ For further information, see Essay VI and Chart VI(B): Antipsychotic Tranquillizers.

◆ UK:
Thioridazine (Hydrochloride) Tablets BPC: available as
Melleril (Sandoz): Tabs 10, 25, 50 & 100 mg; Syr 25 mg/5 ml; Susp 25 & 50 mg/5 ml
   USA:
Thioridazine Hydrochloride Tablets USP &
Thioridazine Hydrochloride Oral Solution USP: available as
Mellaril (Sandoz): Tabs 10, 15, 25, 50, 100, 150 & 200 mg; Oral Soln 30 & 100 mg/ml

THIOTHIXENE

● This medicament belongs to the thioxanthene group of antipsychotic agents, also referred to as major tranquillizers. It is administered to control delusions, hyperagitation, aggressiveness and other features of psychotic illnesses, including schizophrenia. Unlike CHLORPROM-AZINE and many of its analogues, the thioxanthenes do not tend to provoke mental depression or to exacerbate this if it is already present. Further, the unwanted effects common to most major tranquillizers are likely to be less severe with this particular class of drugs: while lethargy, sedation, and parkinsonian reactions may still arise, and overactivity has been reported in some patients, such effects are likely to be mild unless very high doses are administered. The use of oral neuroleptics of this class is declining now that long-acting (depôt) injectable formulations – a single dose of which may last 2–4 weeks – have become available: these are CLOPENTHIXOL and FLUPENTHIXOL.

▲ For psychiatric outpatients: up to 30 mg daily. Inpatients: 30–60 mg a day, usually in two or three doses.

★ Cross-sensitivity to other antipsychotic agents (e.g. phenothiazines) is a possibility. Caution in convulsive disorders, alcoholic withdrawal and severe liver disorders. The central depressant actions of other drugs, including strong analgesics and alcohol, are increased by thiothixene.

➤ For further information, see Essay VI and Chart VI(B): Antipsychotic Tranquillizers, also under CLOPENTHIXOL.

◆ USA:
Thiothixene Capsules USP

Thiothixene Hydrochloride Oral Solution USP &
Thiothixene Hydrochloride Injection USP: available as
Navane (Roerig): Caps 1, 2, 5, 10 & 20 mg; Oral Soln 5 mg/1 ml; Amps
4 mg/2 ml

TOFENACIN

● Tofenacin, one of the metabolic by-products of the analgesic and
antiparkinsonian drug ORPHENADRINE, is a compound with antidepressant activity. While chemically dissimilar to AMITRIPTYLINE
and IMIPRAMINE, it possesses the important characteristics of these
tricyclic antidepressive agents. Tofenacin has been specifically recommended for treatment of mild to moderate depression 'in the over fifties'.
Regular administration for 2–4 weeks is required before symptoms are
likely to be alleviated. Side-effects appear to be mild, with difficulty in
visual accommodation, dry mouth, vertigo, drowsiness and gastro-intestinal upsets tending to be experienced at the beginning of treatment. The
possibility that the drug may intensify severe depressive states should be
borne in mind, as also should its potential use in suicide attempts.

▲ Up to 240 mg a day in two or three doses.

★ Tofenacin has contra-indications like those for tricyclic antidepressants. It should not be prescribed for patients suffering from very severe
depression, nor in cases of glaucoma, enlargement of the prostate, or
urinary retention; and concomitant ECT (electro-convulsive therapy) is
not recommended.

➤ For further information, see Essay II and Chart II: Antidepressants.

◆ UK:
Elamol (Brocades): Caps 80 mg (hydrochloride)

TRANYLCYPROMINE

● The majority of antidepressant drugs prescribed today belong to the
tricyclic group of compounds, such as AMITRIPTYLINE and IMI-
PRAMINE. Only when amitriptyline or one of its analogues is ineffective
in relieving a depressive state do clinicians resort to prescription of
monoamine-oxidase (MAO) inhibitors, of which tranylcypromine is an
example. The greatest problem associated with the latter type of drugs is
that they interact, with serious and sometimes fatal consequences, with a
number of commonly taken foods and beverages: among those contra-
indicated for patients under MAO-inhibitor therapy are hard cheeses,
pickled herrings, bananas, caviare, and concentrated meat, yeast and soya
protein extracts. Such patients should be issued with a card which lists the
foods to be avoided. Alcohol, in particular some beers and Chianti wine,
may also be dangerous. In addition, MAO-inhibiting antidepressants may

produce severe interactions with a wide variety of other medications: concurrent administration of amphetamines and other stimulants (including those found in cough remedies), barbiturates, tricyclic antidepressants, narcotic pain-killers, antihistamines and antidiabetic agents can be hazardous. This is not a comprehensive list, but indicates the kind of limitations required in treatment of depression with tranylcypromine. When it is appropriate to prescribe the compound, relief of symptoms takes between 2 and 4 weeks to commence. Dry mouth, nausea, headache, fatigue, sweating, and restlessness are adverse reactions which occur principally during the early part of treatment, but one or more of these may persist. Some psychiatrists are surprised at the continued availability of a branded tablet which contains tranylcypromine together with the antipsychotic TRIFLUOPERAZINE: the aim of this combination, which is called Parstelin, is to alleviate anxiety and tension as well as depression. It is possible that this may occur; more probably, however, the adverse effects associated with each class of drugs (MAOIs and phenothiazines) will be intensified. After-effects from Parstelin may be especially distressing, and the product should be withdrawn slowly.

▲ Initially 10 mg twice daily, increasing if necessary to 10 mg thrice daily after 1–3 weeks, according to the patient's response.

★ Principal contra-indications (apart from those mentioned above) are liver disease, cardiac and cardiovascular ailments, and epilepsy.

➤ For further information, see Essay II and Chart II: Antidepressants.

◆ UK:
Tranylcypromine (Sulphate) Tablets BPC: available as
Parnate (Smith Kline & French): Tabs 10 mg
Parstelin (Smith Kline & French): Tabs tranylcypromine sulphate 10 mg, trifluoperazine hydrochloride 1 mg
    USA:
Tranylcypromine Sulfate Tablets USP: available as
Parnate (Smith Kline & French): Tabs 10 mg

TRAZODONE

● It is agreeable to be able to include here information about this most interesting antidepressant, which has been marketed in Italy for several years but which only now (December 1980) has become available for prescription in the UK. Trazodone is chemically unrelated to either of the two principal classes of antidepressive agents, the tricyclics (e.g. AMITRIPTYLINE) and the MAO-inhibitors (cf preceding Entry). It nevertheless shows a broad spectrum of activity, with significant anxiety-relieving, sedative and depression-lifting properties. According to some published studies the drug may be beneficial in controlling psychotic symptoms also.

It is characteristic of manufacturers to make considerable claims for new products, but it does genuinely appear that trazodone represents a significant advance over conventional antidepressants. The compound will not alleviate all depressive states – no drug can do that – but comparison with standard drugs, in particular AMITRIPTYLINE and IMIPRAMINE, favours trazodone in several published studies which seem unbiassed. Onset of action is likely to be more rapid with the new antidepressant: within 7–10 days vs up to four weeks for tricyclics. Reported side-effects include a 'spaced out' feeling, drowsiness, nausea, and headache: these are evidently not severe and tend to be transient. In particular, the anticholinergic actions of amitriptyline-like agents (blurred vision, dry mouth, gastro-intestinal disturbances) are either absent altogether or negligible with trazodone. One especially promising application for the drug appears to be to relieve tardive dyskinesia, a severe form of Parkinson's disease which often results from long-term treatment with antipsychotic tranquillizers: this condition has hitherto been regarded as irreversible or at least extremely difficult to mitigate. Although trazodone is very expensive compared with standard antidepressants, the cost may well be justified if therapeutic response is as good as some clinical studies so far conducted indicate.

▲ At first, 100–150 mg daily in two or three doses, after meals, to a maximum of 600 mg/day, depending on the patient's response.

★ Trazodone lacks the cardio-toxicity of other antidepressants and has a wide margin of safety. Caution in severe liver or kidney disease. Patients should be warned that reflexes may be slowed. Concurrent treatment with other antidepressants is not recommended. The drug may interact with some antihypertensive agents and enhance the effects of central depressants.

➤ For further information, see Essay II and Chart II: Antidepressants.

◆ UK:
Molipaxin (Roussel): Caps 50 & 100 mg (hydrochloride)

TRIAZOLAM

● A number of derivatives of the tranquillizer DIAZEPAM (Valium) have in recent years been marketed not simply to quell anxiety but to promote sleep. One example is NITRAZEPAM (Mogadon), which has become the most extensively prescribed hypnotic in the UK. Whether one of these benzodiazepine compounds is indicated for this purpose rather than for relief of anxiety and tension depends on dose, and diazepam could equally well be given to combat insomnia: as a single nightly dose not much in excess of that recommended for daytime use. Almost all drugs belonging to this class are interchangeable because they have such similar mechanisms of action and clinical effects. Most benzodiazepines, including nitrazepam, produce perceptible effects for periods of 12 hours or longer. Triazolam possesses the advantage over other diazepines used as hypnotics that it is much more quickly metabolized than its alternatives. In practical terms this means that, following a nightly dose, hangover, oversedation and consequent slowing of reflexes are much less likely to occur with triazolam than nitrazepam, flurazepam and other hypnotics. Recent reports from the continent indicate that high doses of triazolam may provoke hallucinations and other bizarre psychological effects: however, more potent dosage formulations are involved there than are marketed in the UK. Prolonged administration of any benzodiazepine, either to alleviate anxiety or aid sleep, is not recommended because tolerance develops readily and psychological habituation is a risk.

▲ 0.125–0.75 mg at night.

★ Contra-indicated in severe respiratory disorders and known hypersensitivity to diazepam or any of its analogues. The sedative effects of other CNS depressants, such as tranquillizers, potent analgesics and alcohol, are increased by triazolam.

➔ For further information, see Essay III and Chart III: Barbiturates, and Essay VI and Chart VI(A): Tranquillizers.

◆ UK:
Halcion (Upjohn): Tabs 0.125 & 0.25 mg

TRICLOFOS

● This compound is a derivative of the old-established sedative and sleep-inducing drug CHLORAL HYDRATE. Some practitioners believe that triclofos is slightly superior to chloral and it is often claimed that it is less likely to cause irritation of the stomach. Because the compound has a fairly wide margin of safety between therapeutic and toxic doses, it has been considered suitable for administration to children and the elderly. Like chloral it may possibly enhance the effectiveness of potent analgesics. Triclofos is not appropriate for daytime sedation. Occasionally, headache, gastro-intestinal upsets and allergic skin rashes occur. Hangover and oversedation may follow the morning after a dose of the drug if a large quantity has been taken. Repeated use can lead to psychological and, more rarely, physical dependency.

▲ 750 mg – 2.5 G at night (adults). For elderly and debilitated patients lower dosage levels are recommended.

★ Contra-indicated in porphyria; utmost caution in severe cardiac, liver and kidney ailments. Patients hypersensitive to chloral will be so to triclofos. The drug may alter the metabolism of anticoagulants and will enhance the effects of other CNS depressants, such as tranquillizers, barbiturates, opiate analgesics and alcohol.

➤ For further information, see Essay III and Chart III: Barbiturates.

◆ UK:
Triclofos Tablets BPC (not available)
Triclofos Elixir BPC: 500 mg/5 ml
  USA:
Triclos (Merrell-National): Caps 750 mg; Elix 500 mg/5 ml (sodium)

TRIFLUOPERAZINE

● This derivative of CHLORPROMAZINE is extensively prescribed: at low doses, in anxiety states, senile agitation and confusion, and to relieve some psychosomatic complaints; and at high doses in the management of schizophrenia and other psychoses. Although the manufacturers include depressive conditions among this drug's clinical applications, these may in fact be intensified. Trifluoperazine may be useful in severe cases of anxiety and tension but, because of its likely side-effects even at small doses, should not be regarded as the drug of first choice. It is prescribed as an alternative to DIAZEPAM (Valium) and related anxiety-relieving tranquillizers, probably less because it is superior (which is debatable) than because there is no risk of habituation. The adverse reactions provoked by trifluoperazine are similar to those of chlorpromazine (Largactil, Thorazine): lassitude, oversedation, dizziness, dry mouth, blurred vision, and psychological depression may occur. Parkinsonian effects are occasioned in some patients even at very low dosage. Generally unwanted effects are somewhat less severe than those of chlorpromazine at comparable doses.

▲ To alleviate anxiety: 2–4 mg daily in one or two doses. In control of hyperagitation and other symptoms of psychotic illness: outpatients 4–10 mg, psychiatric inpatients up to 60 mg daily.

★ Contra-indicated in liver dysfunction, blood disorders, and known hypersensitivity to any member of the phenothiazine class of tranquillizers. Potentially serious interactions may occur with amphetamines and other stimulants and sometimes with antidepressants.

➤ For further information, see Essay VI and Chart VI(B): Antipsychotic Tranquillizers.

◆ UK:
Trifluoperazine (Hydrochloride) Tablets BPC: available as
Stelazine (Smith Kline & French): Tabs 1 & 5 mg; SR Caps 2, 10 & 15 mg; Syr 1 mg/5 ml; Oral Conc 10 mg/1 ml; Amps 1 & 2 mg/1 ml & 3 mg/3 ml
see also under TRANYLCYPROMINE

USA:
Trifluoperazine Hydrochloride Tablets USP
Trifluoperazine Hydrochloride Syrup USP &
Trifluoperazine Hydrochloride Injection USP: available as
Stelazine (Smith Kline & French): Tabs 1, 2, 5 & 10 mg; Syr 1 mg/1 ml;
Oral Conc 10 mg/1 ml; Vials 20 mg/10 ml

TRIFLUPERIDOL

● Trifluperidol is one of the most potent neuroleptic, or antipsychotic, agents available. An analogue of HALOPERIDOL (Haldol, Serenace), the drug is prescribed in acute and chronic schizophrenia and to mitigate the manic phase of manic-depressive psychosis. It has been suggested in the treatment of children suffering from severe psychotic illnesses. Common adverse reactions are lethargy, mental depression, loss of motivation and apathy, profound sedation, and parkinsonian effects (which, say the manufacturers, can usually be controlled by anti-Parkinson drugs). Severe muscular spasms occur in some patients. This compound should never be prescribed to relieve minor psychological or emotional disturbances.

▲ 4–8 mg daily, according to response.

★ Side-effects may persist for three months or longer after treatment is discontinued. Because Parkinsonism so often arises it has been suggested that compounds such as ORPHENADRINE should be given from the start to prevent these occurring. Contra-indicated particularly in convulsive disorders and during pregnancy. Concurrent administration of barbiturates or opiate analgesics is inadvisable.

➔ For further information, see HALOPERIDOL and Essay VI and Chart VI (B): Antipsychotic Tranquillizers.

◆ UK:
Triperidol (Janssen): Tabs 0.5 & 1 mg (deleted 1981)

TRIFLUPROMAZINE

● This compound is a member of the large family of antipsychotic drugs of the phenothiazine group, whose exemplar is CHLORPROMAZINE (Largactil, Thorazine). Triflupromazine, however, has a narrower range of uses, and indeed should be confined to treatment of only the most severe psychotic illnesses, whether acute or chronic: the drug considerably lessens hyperagitation, hallucinations, aggression, and other symptoms of schizophrenias and other seriously disabling conditions. Side-effects are similar to those of chlorpromazine. This is yet another drug whose prescription is contra-indicated in non-psychotic anxiety and tension and in other mild or moderate psychological disturbances.

▲ Psychiatric inpatients may require up to a maximum of 150 mg daily, though the usual range is 20–60 mg.

➤ As for CHLORPROMAZINE and other potent antipsychotic agents. See Essay VI and Chart VI(B): Antipsychotic Tranquillizers.

◆ USA:
Triflupromazine Hydrochloride Tablets USP
Triflupromazine Oral Suspension USP &
Triflupromazine Hydrochloride Injection USP: available as
Vesprin (Squibb): Tabs 10, 25 & 50 mg; Oral Susp 50 mg/5 ml; Amps 20 mg/1 ml; Vials 100 mg/10 ml

TRIMEPRAZINE

● This compound has the same actions, uses and side-effects as METHOTRIMEPRAZINE: it is primarily given to control nausea and vomiting, severe itching (pruritus), and to enhance the effectiveness of strong pain-relieving drugs of the MORPHINE type. In very small doses it is combined with other agents to control severe cough.

▲ Usually 10 mg 3 or 4 times daily; maximum single dose 100 mg, orally or by injection. As a cough suppressant, 2.5–5 mg.

★ Drowsiness may occur and reflexes can be slowed. Caution in convulsive disorders, liver and heart disease. Trimeprazine increases the central depressant effects of other tranquillizers, barbiturates, and alcohol.

➤ For further information, see METHOTRIMEPRAZINE, and Essay VI and Chart VI(B): Antipsychotic Tranquillizers. The drug is classed with these because it belongs to the phenothiazine class of compounds, most of which are prescribed for their antipsychotic activity.

◆ UK:
Trimeprazine (Tartrate) Tablets BPC &
Trimeprazine (Tartrate) Injection BPC: available as
Vallergan (May & Baker): Tabs 10 mg; Syr 7.5 & 30 mg/5 ml; Amps 30 mg/2 ml
Valledrine (May & Baker): Linct trimeprazine tartrate 2.5 mg, ephedrine hydrochloride 7.5 mg, pholcodine citrate 5 mg/5 ml
Vallex (May & Baker): Linct trimeprazine tartrate 2.5 mg, menthol 1.2 mg, phenylpropanolamine hydrochloride 10 mg, guaiphenesin 25 mg, liquid extract of ipecacuanha 0.015 ml/5 ml
    USA:
Trimeprazine Tartrate Tablets USP &
Trimeprazine Tartrate Syrup USP: available as

Temaril (Smith Kline & French): Tabs 2.5 mg; SR Caps 5 mg; Syr 2.5 mg/5 ml

TRIMIPRAMINE

● Trimipramine is an antidepressant of the tricyclic type, similar to AMITRIPTYLINE. It is prescribed for relief of moderate to severe depression, and may be effective in some cases when this is accompanied by anxiety. Of the antidepressants of its class trimipramine is probably the most sedative: for this reason, once the proper dose has been established, a single tablet or capsule at night may be the most appropriate regimen. While in some patients depression may begin to lift within two weeks, therapeutic benefit may not be apparent for a longer period. Side-effects include dry mouth, disturbances of visual accommodation, oversedation, and changes in appetite and libido: these are especially common during the early part of treatment. Severe depressive conditions may be intensified, so due caution must be exercised; and the potential suicidal use of trimipramine, as of other tricyclic antidepressants, should be considered. Overdosages with these compounds are increasing annually and may be difficult to treat.

▲ 50–150 mg daily, adjusted according to the patient's response.

★ Contra-indicated in glaucoma, urinary retention, enlargement of the prostate, cases of known hypersensitivity to tricyclic antidepressants, and utmost caution in heart disease. Concomitant treatment with amphetamines and other stimulants and appetite-suppressants, and with MAO-inhibitor antidepressants, may be hazardous.

➤ For further information, see Essay II and Chart II: Antidepressants.

◆ UK:
Trimipramine (Acid Tartrate) Tablets BPC: available as
Surmontil (May & Baker): Tabs 10 & 25 mg; Caps 50 mg
   USA:
Surmontil (Ives): Caps 25 & 50 mg

TYBAMATE

● Tybamate is an obsolete sedative and muscle-relaxant, a chemical analogue of MEPROBAMATE (Equanil, Miltown). Its hypnotic effect is more potent than that of meprobamate. Regular use is not advised because of the availability of more selective and less dependence-producing tranquillizers and sleep-inducing drugs. Side-effects include drowsiness, dizziness, gastro-intestinal upsets and, at high doses, paradoxical excitement.

▲ 125–350 mg at night.

★ Contra-indicated in porphyria, convulsive disorders, and severe liver and kidney complaints.

➤ See also under MEPROBAMATE and cf Essay III and Chart III: Barbiturates.

◆ USA:
Tybamate Capsules USNF 1970: available as
Tybatran (Robins): Caps 125, 250 & 350 mg

VILOXAZINE

● Viloxazine is one of the more recently introduced antidepressant agents. It has been claimed to provide therapeutic benefit earlier than standard drugs such as AMITRIPTYLINE, i.e. within 7–10 days as against two weeks or longer for standard compounds. A number of clinical trials indicate that viloxazine is as effective in mild to moderate depressive states as older-established tricyclic antidepressants, while provoking side-effects that are mild and transient. Lethargy, insomnia, tension and nausea are among unwanted reactions which may tend to occur at the beginning of therapy but which in most cases wear off rapidly. On the available evidence this compound has less potential for intensifying pre-existing depression than some other antidepressants, and has a wider margin of safety between therapeutic and toxic doses.

▲ On average, 150–300 mg daily, in two or three divided doses, according to individual response.

★ Contra-indicated in glaucoma. Safety for use during pregnancy has not yet been established. Concurrent administration of phenytoin to epileptics may be hazardous, and use of antihypertensive drugs should be very carefully monitored.

➤ For further information, see Essay II and Chart II: Antidepressants.

◆ UK:
Vivalan (ICI): Tabs 50 mg (hydrochloride)

YOHIMBINE

● Yohimbine is the principal alkaloid found in the bark of the South American tree *Corynanthe yohimbi*. The substance is known to have mild anti-diuretic properties but it is for its supposed aphrodisiacal effects that preparations containing the drug are marketed. Large doses produce anxiety, tension, restlessness and central nervous system stimulation, but of a disagreeable kind. Administration to schizophrenics of 20–40 mg by intramuscular injection produced visual and auditory hallucinations in one study. At the dosages incorporated in certain products which are marketed in the UK and USA, which also contain the mild stimulant PEMOLINE and a small quantity of the male sex hormone methyltestosterone, yohimbine is most unlikely to have any effect on sexual function, and larger doses are certainly toxic.

▲ See the formulations listed below.

★ Contra-indicated in inflammatory conditions of the genitals and of the prostate.

◆ UK:
Potensan-Forte (Medo-Chemicals): Pills yohimbine hydrochloride 5 mg, pemoline 10 mg, strychnine hydrochloride 0.5 mg, methyltestosterone 5 mg (deleted 1981)
   USA:
Andro-Medicone (Medicone): Tabs yohimbine hydrochloride 5 mg, thyroid extract 5 mg, strychnine sulfate 1 mg

ZIMELIDINE

● This is one of a few newly developed compounds which do not fit conveniently into the usual categories. Chemically, zimelidine is a derivative of brompheniramine, an anti-allergic (antihistamine) drug commonly found as an ingredient in cough-mixtures, which itself has practically no psychotropic action. The new drug, however, has significant antidepressant effects, which are comparable with those produced by conventional mood-lifting agents such as AMITRIPTYLINE. Zimelidine apparently provokes fewer adverse reactions than most antidepressants, and appears to show anxiety-relieving and antipsychotic activity. Like another new drug, TRAZODONE, it seems to enhance the potency of strong analgesics of the PETHIDINE (MEPERIDINE) type: clearly much more research in this area would be valuable. Whereas amitriptyline and its analogues sometimes increase appetite, zimelidine apparently does the opposite. The substance exerts its psychotropic activity at least in part by inhibiting the reuptake of the neurotransmitter 5-hydroxytryptamine (serotonin), disturbances of which are associated with various forms of psychological illness, including depressive states. At this writing zimelidine has not yet been made available for prescription, and it should be regarded as being still experimental. However, a number of clinical studies have established its efficacy and indicated a low toxicity and remarkable paucity of side-effects. It seems likely, on the basis of published reports, that zimelidine will soon be added to the armamentarium of psychotropic agents.

◆ Under investigation: Astra Läkemedel AB, Södertälje, Sweden.

The compound is now available under the trade-name *Zelmid* (Astra): Tabs 100 & 200 mg (Republic of Ireland: monitored release). An average dose of 200 mg in the morning, as a single dose, is recommended.

Part Two

Drug Classes: Essays and Charts

I: The Amphetamines and Other Stimulants and Appetite-Suppressants

History

Amphetamine was first synthesized in the laboratory almost by accident. In 1927 the pharmacologist Gordon Alles, working in San Francisco, was seeking to make a drug or drugs which would provide an effective substitute for ephedrine, a standard remedy for bronchial asthma. A few years earlier a good deal of interest had been aroused when researchers isolated the active principle (to be known as ephedrine) from the leaves and stalks of the Chinese herb *Ephedra vulgaris*. Decoctions of ephedra, which was called *ma-huang*, had been used in Chinese traditional medicine for many centuries, and clearly their efficacy in the treatment of bronchial complaints had been long recognized. The important specific actions of ephedrine are the expansion of the bronchial muscles, constriction of the blood-vessels, contraction of the mucous membranes (particularly in the nose), and raising of the blood-pressure. These are referred to as 'sympathomimetic' effects because they mimic the natural activity of the sympathetic (autonomic) nervous system, which is responsible for reflexes not normally under control of the will, and arousal of which produces acceleration of heartbeat, rise in blood-pressure, erection of hair on the head, and a marked decrease in the involuntary muscular movements (peristalsis) of the gastro-intestinal system.

Such reflexes are provoked when the hormone adrenaline (epinephrine) flows into the bloodstream in situations of stress, excitement or fear: the so-called fight-or-flight reflex. Adrenaline itself was isolated a century ago and has for many decades been regarded as an essential part of the pharmacopoeia: it remains extremely valuable in medicine as a heart stimulant, to relieve respiratory distress due to impaired functioning of the lungs, and to reverse the effects of clinical, life-threatening shock. More routinely, adrenaline in the earlier 20th century was used to control the symptoms of bronchial asthma and had been very efficacious for this purpose. Its chief disadvantage was that it had to be given by injection, because if it were administered by mouth the drug would be de-activated by the stomach acids. Adrenaline nebulizers are now available for those suffering from certain types of asthma, but the aerosol principle was not known in the 1920s.

Ephedrine was useful in that it could be taken in tablet or capsule form, and because it has a significantly longer duration of action than adrenaline, which is advantageous in the prevention as well as the alleviation of asthmatic attacks. In spite of the fact that ephedrine produces some unpleasant adverse reactions at normal doses in quite a high proportion of patients, it has continued to be prescribed over the years, and there remain on the market numerous ephedrine-based medicinal products – tablets, capsules, elixirs, injections, sprays – which are now more often given to suppress cough than for use by asthma sufferers. At the time when Gordon Alles was conducting his research during the 1920s, supplies of *Ephedra* herb were difficult to obtain and extremely expensive. So he tried, and succeeded, in formulating a synthetic preparation which could be used instead with equal efficacy.

Alles noted that the basic form of amphetamine was a volatile liquid, and in collaboration with F. P. Nabenhauer, he produced a simple device for inhalation: the drug was soaked in a tight, cylindrical pad of cotton-wool or similar absorbent material. This was enclosed in a plastic tube with an opening at one end, so that the product could be inserted up the nostrils and the vapour inhaled. Patented by Smith Kline & French Laboratories of Philadelphia as the Benzedrine Inhaler, it was put on the market in 1932, and soon proved highly successful. The drug would act directly, by this means, to constrict the mucosa of the nose, giving relief of nasal congestion in influenza and colds, as well as rapidly providing relief from a bout of asthma. It was believed at that time that amphetamine lacked the unfortunate side-effects associated with ephedrine, such as stimulation of the central as well as the sympathetic nervous system, with resultant feelings of energy and excitability.

Terminology

Before proceeding to describe in detail the differences between each of the relevant drugs, one should explain that in the standard medical texts there are terms whose meaning may not be obvious. 'Amphetamines' strictly refers to three very closely related substances: laevo- or l-amphetamine (Benzedrine), dexamphetamine (dextroamphetamine; Dexedrine) and methylamphetamine (methamphetamine; Methedrine, Desoxyn). More generally, derivatives such as methylphenidate (Ritalin) and phenmetrazine (Preludin), as well as most of the drugs shown in Chart I, are so described. These compounds are highly potent stimulants with virtually identical effects and liability for abuse. The three original drugs whose names end with -amphetamine differ slightly in terms of

absolute potency, methylamphetamine being the strongest and
l-amphetamine the weakest. Weight for weight, 10 mg of l-amphetamine
are equivalent to 5 mg of dexamphetamine and 2.5 mg of methylamphetamine. Of the three agents, the last-named is the most widely
sought after for illicit use: until a few years ago this was marketed in
injectable form as well as in tablets and capsules. Now, because the drug is
easy to synthesize, black-market methylamphetamine and other
amphetamine powders have appeared on the scene in Britain, the USA
and several European countries. The legally-prescribed preparations
available may contain the phosphate, sulphate or hydrochloride salts, e.g.
of dexamphetamine: these are practically identical in effect.

The term 'stimulant', as employed here, indicates stimulation or
excitation of the central nervous system (CNS): this is manifested by the
sort of physical changes elicited by adrenaline (epinephrine) and by
psychological signs and symptoms (intense, vigorous sense of well-being,
desire for action) provoked by sympathomimetic drugs. Certain other
CNS stimulants cannot be appropriately classified with the amphetamines
(e.g. cocaine, amyl nitrite) and are dealt with individually in the
Alphabetical Entries section of this book: in the case of most of these,
psychic excitation occurs as an unwanted side-effect. Thus, cocaine is used
medically as a surface anaesthetic, chiefly in ear, nose and throat surgery,
and amyl nitrite to counteract the effects of cyanide poisoning. Central
stimulants, including amphetamines, are referred to by some practitioners
as 'analeptics' and those which are prescribed in appetite reduction as
'anorexiants'. The latter term indicates only anorexia, or loss of appetite
for food, and has nothing to do with the pathological condition anorexia
nervosa.

Principal Effects

By the mid 1930s it was realized that the amphetamines not only relieved
bronchospasm and congestion of the nose, but that what were originally
considered unfortunate side-effects – increased alertness, in particular,
and a diminished desire for food – could be put to good therapeutic use.
Subsequent modifications of the amphetamine molecule have yielded
more than a dozen drugs now available for prescription, of which the
earliest important examples are phenmetrazine (introduced in 1958) and
methylphenidate (1960). These all retain some amphetamine-like effects,
although the object was principally to devise compounds which had a
good anorexiant activity without excessive CNS stimulation. Such
amphetamine derivatives are described in detail below (p. 222) and in
Chart I.

Amphetamines are absorbed from the gut and from the mucous
membranes very readily, most being available in tablet or capsule form.

Injectable preparations of methylamphetamine and methylphenidate are manufactured. But there is seldom if ever any justification for their use, except possibly in the management of barbiturate overdosage or to reverse excessive dosage of an anaesthetic. For the past 12 years ampoule formulations of these two drugs, as well as powders which could be made up into injections, have been available only to hospitals. This is primarily because of what has been referred to as an 'epidemic' of intravenous methylamphetamine (Methedrine) abuse during the early and mid 1960s: a time when a few practitioners in the UK grossly overprescribed drugs for addicts. Then it was believed that amphetamine was less dangerous than cocaine, specifically in the context of concomitant use of heroin or morphine. At approximately the same time a similar boom in illicit and over-prescribed Methedrine occurred in the USA, as graphically described by William Burroughs Jr in his book *Speed*.

Onset of action from a single dose of dexamphetamine (e.g. a standard 5 mg tablet) occurs within 15–30 minutes, which is fast for any orally-active drug, and perceptible effects will be felt for 4–6 hours. There are, however, a number of preparations which are specially formulated so that a single dose will exert effect for a span of 12–14 hours. As the amphetamine tablet or capsule's effects begin to wear off, it is common for individuals to experience a 'come-down', which may manifest itself as depression, irritability and irrational, sometimes severe, anxiety. Reactions of this kind are undoubtedly a factor in the development of tolerance and dependency, because, among persons lacking in will-power or predisposed to abuse drugs, the temptation to consume further doses may be irresistible. This will be reinforced by amphetamine's primary mood-altering actions, such as increased alertness and wakefulness and a powerful energetic euphoria. The degree of these effects is to a considerable extent dose-related, but may be marked even after administration of the amounts recommended. Reactions to these compounds do vary greatly because of individual idiosyncrasy, but for some patients even 2.5 mg of dexamphetamine (half the standard-strength tablet) will provoke such effects, which may persist for several hours until the 'come-down' phase. One of the best-documented actions of amphetamines is their power to stimulate fatigued, idle or listless people to perform some kind of physical activity. For many years they were given (particularly during the Second World War) to enhance performance of tasks requiring mental or physical concentration and to improve endurance, objectives which may be important in the context of warfare.

Careful studies have been carried out in recent years to assess the influence of amphetamines on these faculties, but have given contradictory results: in some work, the drugs' effect on performance (qualitative and quantitative) has been found to be absent or negligible, while other researchers have recorded a definite improvement in the performance of psychologically or physically taxing tasks (e.g. completing mathematical problems; and in various sports such as running and swimming). Lassitude resulting from fatigue or boredom can certainly be overcome in the short term by amphetamines, and one of the hazards associated with their use is that such drugs can mask the effects even of chronic fatigue: they should never be taken if the person is already overtired unless the reasons are really compelling. Such situations arose during the Second World War: then Benzedrine was routinely given to military personnel who required to be in a state of combat-readiness for long periods of time, such as fighter pilots. In fact amphetamine was used by German and Japanese as well as British soldiers and airmen.

At that time Benzedrine tablets were issued to servicemen and others in a way that would now be regarded as careless and irresponsible; but then amphetamine was seen as a safe and effective remedy against sleepiness. A practitioner known to one of the present authors recalls that he dispensed Benzedrine on demand to aircrews during the war, as did many of his colleagues, *ad libitum*. Immediately the war ended, the alerting effects of these drugs were made known to various groups of people who were obliged to work long hours, and among whom truck drivers were signalized.

By the 1950s in Britain and the USA amphetamine tablets, called 'purple hearts' because of a popular preparation's shape and colour, began to be used non-medically by young people of the post-war generation. The association between such phenomena and the arrival of rock-and-roll music is well documented. If one wanted to dance all night, then this was facilitated by a fistful of 'hearts'. But at a price: the ruinous dangers of chronic amphetamine misuse were only gradually recognized, and not until the mid 1960s was the prescription of these compounds curtailed by legislation. Illegal use then began to increase vastly.

The characteristic anorexia, or loss of appetite, produced by amphetamine and its analogues has already been touched upon. Some of the available research has indicated that amphetamines act directly on those portions of the brain which are concerned with appetite control, but the mechanism whereby this is supposed to happen is not properly understood. It is possible that the anorexia is a by-product of the drugs' psychic effects (i.e. one is too much occupied with the task in hand to want to eat), and of their adrenaline-like action, which is bound to preclude or at any rate greatly lessen feelings of hunger. Over the past two decades it has become quite clear that this appetite-suppressant effect lasts only a few weeks, as many chronic amphetamine-takers have discovered for themselves: it is one aspect of tolerance to amphetamines' principal actions. Within a period of, probably, two months the drugs will still provide central stimulation, yet their influence on food consumption will almost always be negligible. But with the development of tolerance the degree of alerting euphoria promoted by a constant dose lessens, thus giving encouragement for individuals wishing to maintain their enjoyment of this effect to increase the dose, and continue increasing it. Eventually a substantial number of people, some prescribed amphetamines 'legitimately' to promote weight loss and some using them for fun, were consuming far in excess of the therapeutic dose. Immediately before the 1967 ban (see below), doses of 0.5 G or more (orally or intravenously) were not uncommon among abusers.

In 1973, the distinguished pharmacologist Louis Lasagna found that 50% of a large sample of physicians prescribed anorexiants, 25% of these being willing to prescribe them for 3 months or longer. The most popular drugs given were: diethylpropion (Tenuate: 55% of the total sample), phenmetrazine (Preludin) 30%, and products containing dexamphetamine 13–17%. ('Attitudes toward Appetite Suppressants: a survey of US physicians', *Journal of the American Medical Association* 225:46, 1973).

Many thousands of unwitting patients, in America, Britain, Western Europe and elsewhere, discovered that they had become dependent on amphetamine preparations, which had been repeat-prescribed (typically for middle-aged, overweight women), often over periods of years. This is a classic example of iatrogenic, or doctor-created, disease. One of the most unsavoury aspects of this situation, as it occurred in the mid to late 1960s, was the fact that when amphetamines came under legal restriction many GPs simply refused to prescribe them any more, even for patients who had been receiving them regularly, often making no attempt to mitigate the distress which abrupt discontinuation of the tablets was bound to cause.

We have noted the main sympathomimetic properties of this category of drugs. These also include a marked influence on muscle tone: for instance, the sphincter muscle of the bladder tends to become contracted, so that difficulty with or pain on urination may occur. This observation led to the use of amphetamine to control enuresis (bed-wetting) in children, however with very variable and unpredictable results. This is one of the many historical indications for amphetamine administration which have become discredited.

Because the amphetamines and analogues were known to stimulate the respiratory centre, which is situated in the medulla of the brain, they were for many years popular in the treatment of overdosage with drugs which depress the central nervous system, such as barbiturates, anaesthetics, and narcotic pain-killers. Reversal of breathing difficulties in patients thus overdosed could be accomplished, and injectable amphetamines are still sometimes given for this purpose: they are likely to be within the anaesthetist's reach if he requires them. Still, there now exist more reliable and safe alternatives, such as doxapram (Dopram) and ethamivan

(Clairvan, Emivan) which are specific respiratory stimulants. And in poisoning with a narcotic of the morphine type, the recently (1976) introduced compound naloxone, a pure opiate antagonist, has been spectacularly successful. So the use of amphetamines in connection with the emergency room and in anaesthesia has naturally declined. It may be worth observing that, rather surprisingly, CNS stimulants do possess a definite, if not very strong, analgesic activity. This may account for the fact that until a few years ago several products were marketed which contained the typical APC (aspirin, phenacetin and caffeine) mixture, together with a small amount of amphetamine (see below, p. 221).

Adverse Reactions

Most of the unwanted effects of these drugs are closely related to their basic sympathomimetic activity. Obviously, if amphetamines are prescribed to increase alertness, such symptoms as hyperexcitability, loquaciousness and insomnia can be anticipated in a number of cases. It must be stressed that individual response to these stimulants is extremely variable. So, one patient, following ingestion of dexamphetamine 10 mg, may feel a mild, rather agreeable alerting effect with little or no change in pulse, heart-rate, or blood-pressure, and without any peripheral reactions which he would describe as troublesome. But a second person (of the same age, sex, weight, etc.) may find that as little as 2.5 mg of the same substance provokes intense nervousness, irritability, and tension, with palpitations, gastric upsets and other highly unpleasant sensations. The important adverse effects of amphetamines are listed in probable order of frequency in the Chart which accompanies this Essay.

A topic about which little can be found in the clinical literature is the influence of psychic stimulants on sexual desire and capacity. *A priori*, it might be supposed that amphetamines would enhance both libido and performance. In fact, this is the case for only a minority of persons, although a few individuals report that even at a low dose of dexamphetamine sexuality is always aroused, that in men penile erection is facilitated and that orgasm, while delayed, is heightened. On the other hand, most patients, if they are affected at all in this area, find not only a diminution in desire but partial or complete loss of potency as well. Except in chronic amphetamine abusers, who tend to be sexually inactive, normal functioning will resume on discontinuation of the drug.

Toxicity

For a group of medicaments with such potent physical and psychological effects, the level of acute toxicity is remarkably low. That is to say, the lethal dose in humans is usually many times greater than the therapeutic dose, and it will be much higher still in long-term amphetamine habitués. There is one case on record of a 36-year-old man who ingested 20 × 5 mg dexamphetamine tablets and, after routine supportive measures in hospital, recovered completely within 3 days. However, another instance may be cited of a man aged 22 who died after taking 28 × 5 mg methylamphetamine tablets, with acute kidney failure, fever, jaundice, and circulatory collapse. Fatal overdosage with amphetamines is actually rare: during the last year for which statistics are available in the UK (1977), no cases are recorded in which amphetamines were responsible for either accidental or deliberately suicidal death. But such data should not lead the reader to suppose that amphetamines are not dangerous drugs. Even if they are unlikely to kill directly, at high dosages they may affect you seriously, by precipitating an episode of confusion, irrationality, and a kind of persecution complex. Among inexperienced users, such reactions subside spontaneously after a short time.

In considering dosages of these drugs, it should be borne in mind that persons who abuse stimulants and take them without medical supervision for prolonged periods may require regular, and sometimes enormous, increments. Within a few weeks, with the supervention of tolerance and psychological dependency, up to ten times the maximum accepted therapeutic dose may be needed to maintain the abuser, or 'speed freak', in a state of relative equilibrium. The manufacturers of amphetamine products now (rather belatedly) warn, in their literature addressed to prescribers, that all such drugs are contra-indicated for (i.e. should never be given to) persons considered susceptible to, or with a history of, drug abuse. Nevertheless, a great many patients initially prescribed amphetamines for reasons considered legitimate at the time, and falling into neither of the above categories, have in the event become dependent on these compounds.

Chronic Effects

The long-term effects of amphetamines may be so severe that, except in very special circumstances, prolonged administration of them is considered medically unacceptable. Even in those unusual conditions which do require such medication, dosage must be carefully monitored and adjusted according to individual response. It must be admitted that there are a relatively few individuals who have used amphetamines on a non-medical basis for periods of years without apparent adverse consequences. Such persons require immense amounts of will-power in order to keep the dose at a reasonable level and to retain their place in society.

Much more likely to develop among illicit users, apart from their dependency on the drug and the direct problems which this will cause, is what has been called 'amphetamine psychosis'. This may manifest itself so similarly to spontaneous psychotic behaviour that the expression has real justification, and it may mimic classic paranoid schizophrenia. Such states have been elicited in experimental subjects (e.g. medical students) following only a few days' administration of heavy doses of dex- or methylamphetamine, but lasted only as long as the drug was taken. Amphetamine psychosis is typified by two important elements, only one of which may be apparent and both of which may coexist: first, irrational fear ('paranoia' in the jargon), associated with a belief that one is being watched, or persecuted, or punished, unremittingly. Again, delusions may be experienced which may take all manner of bizarre forms, including auditory (seldom visual) hallucinations. The expressions of amphetamine psychosis can often be distinguished from 'genuine' paranoid schizophrenia in that sufferers from the former maintain some self-consciousness or sense of identity: indeed, were this not so, the habitué would evidently be unable to undertake regular purchasing ('scoring') of drug.

This type of reaction, which may sooner or later require hospitalization, is especially likely to occur among very long-term amphetamine abusers who inject the drug intravenously, though it is not exclusive to this group. Other features of chronic amphetaminism are similar to the secondary consequences of opiate abuse. The victim of such dependency has his life centred upon obtaining and then taking supplies of the drug; food and hygiene are neglected, and self-respect is lost. In the case of other than very careful injectors, the results of non-aseptic techniques will be found: apart from track-marks on the arms, following the lines of the superficial veins, abscesses will develop at injection sites, and hepatitis and septicaemia (blood-poisoning) are common hazards if unsterile syringes, needles, drugs or diluents are used. Additionally, compulsive stereotyped behaviour, such as arranging and re-arranging the contents of a room or a shelf, bruxism (involuntary gnashing of the teeth) and formication (a feeling that insects are crawling under the skin) are frequently experienced: these closely resemble some of the manifestations of chronic cocainism.

Thus far we have not written of amphetamine 'addiction'. Most authorities now reserve that term for types of drug dependency in which, when the particular drug is abruptly discontinued, a clearly-defined set of withdrawal symptoms occurs (e.g. in habituation to narcotics of the morphine type, and to barbiturates). Although some authorities are doubtful, the consensus is that even among people who have abused amphetamines for prolonged periods, when sudden abstinence is enforced or chosen, none of the painful, even life-threatening reactions such as obtain on heroin withdrawal, develop. Instead, the habitué of stimulants may become very lethargic, fatigued, and depressed and go to sleep, often for many hours. Significant physiological and biochemical disruption such as typifies the opiate withdrawal syndrome occurs but signs of it are few. There is relatively little 'physical' suffering associated with amphetamine withdrawal, and substitute drugs (such as tranquillizers or methadone to ease the agonies of heroin abstinence) are not required. Long-term abuse of sympathomimetics is referred to not as 'addiction' but as 'dependency' or 'habituation', despite the fact that craving for repeated doses of drug may be just as strong among amphetaminists as among narcotic addicts.

Uses: Historical

It has already been recounted how extensively Benzedrine was used during the Second World War: indeed, according to one source (1946), this drug 'played a vitally important part' in its conduct. According to official figures from the Admiralty, more than 72 million Benzedrine tablets were supplied to the British forces. No doubt comparable quantities were dispensed to American and certainly to Japanese troops and airmen. Immediately the war ended, vast stockpiles of amphetamine tablets (along with much other army surplus material) flooded the market in Japan, where at that time the drug was considered harmless and possession of it was not illegal. A social problem of considerable scale developed in that country because young people in particular suddenly discovered a new way to get 'high': similar phenomena occurred later in Europe and America, but not then to the same extent as in Japan. The now classical signs and symptoms of amphetamine psychosis were evident among large numbers of Japanese youth, who were avidly consuming the new 'pep pills', and many had to be detained in psychiatric hospitals. Non-medical amphetamine abuse by intravenous injection proved to be a problem there for the first time. The authorities, amazed and shocked, responded to the situation by enacting draconian laws with stiff penalties for possession and use of amphetamines. The Japanese experience was either disregarded in the West or dismissed as a freak phenomenon. Medical champions of amphetamines would aver that the Japanese youngsters concerned already had pre-psychotic personalities, with the drug merely triggering in their florid form mental disturbances which would have manifested themselves in due course anyway. This opinion has been demonstrated to be incorrect by a number of careful experiments on 'normal' volunteers, in whom amphetamine psychosis has been provoked, but in the late 1940s and 1950s the view generally held by clinicians was that amphetamines were exceedingly valuable medicinal agents, the benefits conferred by them far surpassing any detrimental effects. Reading reviews and articles from the medical journals of this period, one is struck by the uncritical enthusiasm for sympathomimetic drugs which was obviously widespread in the profession.

Until about the mid 1960s, physicians in the USA, Canada, the UK, continental Europe and elsewhere were prescribing amphetamines, and some amphetamine derivatives which had been lately synthesized, for a remarkable range of complaints: unquestionably their most popular use was as appetite-suppressants, but they were also given to relieve such diverse conditions as Parkinson's disease, epilepsy, nocturnal enuresis, mental depression, and even in withdrawal from opiate or alcohol dependency. In 1946 W. R. Bett published an exhaustive survey of the clinical indications for amphetamine prescription and was able to list no fewer than 39 different disorders in which Benzedrine was the recommended treatment, among them migraine, seasickness, night blindness, and impotence. A decade later, the distinguished pharmacologist, Chauncey D. Leake, in his book on amphetamines, waxed lyrical about their individual and social benefits. By the 1960s most responsible researchers, if not practising GPs, had realized that for all, or almost all, the maladies which the manufacturers of amphetamine products claimed to relieve or cure, other, more effective and less hazardous forms of treatment were available.

Uses: Current

Because the risks of amphetamine preparations are now recognized not only by physicians but by legislators, there are considered to be only three conditions for which it is legitimate to prescribe the three original compounds, l-amphetamine (Benzedrine), dexamphetamine (Dexedrine), and methylamphetamine (Desoxyn, Methedrine). They are given in obesity, to diminish food intake. Now, at last, pharmaceutical manufacturers warn that stimulants should in this case be prescribed only for a maximum period of a few weeks, and only as an adjunct to strict dieting, exercise and other forms of appetite control, the drugs providing no substitute for will-power. It is in fact questionable whether amphetamines themselves, rather than one or two of their much less centrally-stimulant derivatives, should ever be prescribed in obesity, as their anorexiant effect is so transient and the hazard of misuse so great.

The single medical complaint for which most authorities would agree that amphetamine prescription, and that on a long-term basis, is justifiable is narcolepsy. This is an extremely rare disorder, in which the affected person has recurrent attacks of drowsiness and sleep during the day, despite normal sleeping at night: narcolepsy is chronic and, so far, incurable. The patient is unable to control these episodes of somnolence, which may be accompanied by cataplexy, a state in some respects analogous to a *grand mal* fit. The cause of this unfortunate illness remains completely obscure, and all that the medical profession can offer is some relief of symptoms: it appears that only amphetamine or a stimulant of comparable potency will achieve this object. It is probable that narcolepsy is over-diagnosed, which is easy because the symptomatology is not precise, but it is sufficiently uncommon that many general practitioners will not see a case in their working lives. That remarkable and iconoclastic entertainer, the late Lenny Bruce, is the only famous figure whom the present writers can call to mind as suffering from narcolepsy: for many years he was obliged to take intravenous doses of methylamphetamine to keep the condition under control. It has been suggested that the mental overstimulation which this produced was so great that Bruce resorted to opiates.

Vincent Zarcone, in an exhaustive review of narcolepsy and its treatment, notes that 'amphetamines disturb nocturnal sleep and cause a vicious circle of taking more drugs in the daytime to ward off sleep attacks, which occur more frequently because of the disturbed nocturnal sleep'. ('Narcolepsy', *New England Journal of Medicine* 288:1164, 1973). Partly because of this problem, this specialist has found that a combination of methylphenidate, a less potent stimulant (5–10 mg) with the antidepressant imipramine (25 mg), each taken three times daily, is the most successful type of regimen. Normally concurrent administration of these two drugs is contra-indicated, but in these special circumstances and with careful observation of the patient seems to be justified.

The third ailment in which some authorities advocate the use of amphetamines is the so-called 'hyperkinetic syndrome' (HKS) of some children and adolescents, also referred to as 'minimal brain dysfunction' (MBD), and, more recently, as the 'attention deficit disorder' (ADD). HKS is not at all well defined, but its typical manifestations are said to be restlessness, hyperactivity, easy distractability, poor attention span, the affected children in some cases being very easily frustrated and unduly prone to aggressiveness. Hyperkinesis (hyper + kinēsis) literally means excessive movement: however, the term has come to be applied to youngsters (principally boys) who display some or all of the traits listed above, who are obstreperous in class and who, despite normal intelligence as judged by IQ, find learning difficult. Tests have been devised to differentiate HKS from dyslexia and other disorders (and indeed from the characteristics of normal children) but these are inevitably unreliable. The cause of HKS is also difficult to ascertain: sometimes it seems to be associated with injury (trauma) immediately before, during, or after birth (e.g. slight damage to the brain produced by pressure in forceps delivery); more often HKS appears to arise spontaneously between the ages of five and twelve. Some paediatricians and psychiatrists distinguish between 'organic' and 'non-organic' HKS: however, the treatment they recommend may well be the same.

The treatment in question is prolonged administration of, usually, dexamphetamine, often at a dose which would be regarded as high for an adult (10–20 mg per day). Alternative medicaments are methylphenidate

(Ritalin) and magnesium pemoline (Kethamed, Cylert), the former having a slightly less and the latter having a much less potent stimulant action when given to adults. These compounds act, or appear to act, on children in a surprising fashion: whereas if they were administered to a hyperactive or aggressive adult, these traits would be aggravated, if given to children or young adolescents they tend to (but do not invariably) calm them down. This type of drug action is known as a paradoxical effect, and it might be similar to a phenomenon which adults experience: sometimes an individual, after taking an unusually heavy dose of sleeping-pills, finds that instead of dropping off he feels quite wakeful, even alert. Conversely, very high dosages of amphetamines in adults occasionally produce drowsiness rather than stimulation. Nobody has yet explained why these paradoxical effects occur, but perhaps they are comparable to a situation in which a person, having already consumed a great deal of alcohol, then imbibes yet more to 'drink himself sober'. As far as amphetamines are concerned, however, they cannot be relied on to calm or tranquillize every hyperkinetic child: for some youngsters they produce the stimulant effect expected in adults, thereby exacerbating the condition.

There is not sufficient space here to argue in detail the pros and cons of this type of treatment, nor to deal at length with the vexed question of the diagnosis of HKS. Still, it must be said that the practice, increasingly favoured in the USA and apparently gaining ground elsewhere, of prescribing amphetamine-like agents for children has severe critics. A number of researchers claim that HKS is heavily over-diagnosed, and that the condition does not exist at all as a clinical entity. Certainly the criteria used to define it are extremely imprecise. The pertinent question is asked: Where do you draw the line between a child who is naturally, even appropriately, very active, rebellious and recalcitrant, and one who is suffering from a genuine illness, be it physical, psychic or psychosomatic? The answer is that the point of demarcation is bound to be somewhat arbitrary. Some critics suspect that in the USA amphetamines are being used on children unethically, particularly if the subjects are black and/or poor, in order to manipulate them into conforming to the norms of white society: in effect, that the drugs are 'brainwashing' young people; or at least that their administration is a substitute for adequate standards of individual care by parents, teachers and others in authority, especially in the context of overcrowded, understaffed schools in the inner-city ghettos of America.

It is surely right that, before what is essentially still experimental prescription of such potent substances can be justified, strict criteria should be adhered to. In no sense ought use of these drugs to replace help for the individual, whose greater need may be to know that he is loved and worthwhile. The risks of all centrally-acting drugs, important to consider in adults, should be taken into consideration even more where children are concerned. The weight of evidence suggests that a small proportion of children originally regarded as having HKS, notably in cases where persistent hyperactivity is present, will benefit from treatment with stimulants. However, psychiatrists and paediatricians are not agreed on the length of time, in terms of months or years, during which amphetamines or methylphenidate should be given: some favour continuous, others intermittent, administration. Neither is there a consensus on daily dosage levels.

It is estimated that in the USA, at the present time, some 600,000 children with 'HKS' are under treatment with amphetamines or methylphenidate. Reviewing the field, Gabriella Weiss and Lily Hechtman consider that there is 'unwarranted enthusiasm about the efficacy of stimulants in affecting outcome of hyperactive children, and that stimulants should be used more conservatively and their use should be accompanied by careful monitoring. In our opinion, stimulants should not generally be used when there is evidence that the source of the problem *lies primarily in a poor school or home situation* [our emphasis]. A careful ˙assessment does much to avoid indiscriminate use of medication' ('The Hyperactive Child Syndrome', *Science* 205: 1351, 1979). It is only at the time of this writing (1980) that the first comparative study of the effects of dexamphetamine in normal and hyperactive children and in normal adults has been published. Judith L. Rapoport and her colleagues considered the following questions: Is response to the drug different in normal and hyperactive children? Is the decreased motor activity in hyperactive children a 'paradoxical effect' in respect of their illness and age? Does the mood alteration that is provoked by the drug differ between children and adults?

These authors report: 'Both groups of boys and men showed decreased motor activity, increased vigilance and improvement on a learning task after taking the stimulant. The men reported euphoria while the boys reported feeling . . . "tired" . . . or . . . "different" . . . after taking (dexamphetamine). It is not clear whether this difference is due to differing experience with drugs, ability to report effects or a true pharmacologic age-related effect.' They conclude that stimulants act similarly on children and on adults, but perhaps they give undue weight to quantifiable differences.* We believe that the fact that children reported 'tiredness' rather than 'euphoria' supports the notion of a paradoxical effect.

---

* J. L. Rapoport et al., 'Dextroamphetamine: its cognitive and behavioral effects in normal and hyperactive boys and normal men', *Archives of General Psychiatry*, 37: 933–43 (1980).

Preparations of Amphetamines

The only actual amphetamine products currently available for prescription in the UK are dexamphetamine (tablets: 'Dexamed' and 'Dexedrine'), and a delayed release capsule containing laevo- and dexamphetamine in a 1:3 ratio ('Durophet', 'Durophet-M'). Methylamphetamine ('Methedrine') tablets and ampoules were withdrawn from official listings 12 years ago but are still manufactured, although restricted for hospital use only.

Until a few years ago numerous products could be supplied whose principal ingredient was one of the three amphetamine compounds but which contained other drugs in the same tablet or capsule. Widely used preparations included dexamphetamine in conjunction with one or more simple pain-killers (e.g. aspirin, phenacetin) or with a strong sedative agent, usually the barbiturate amylobarbitone. The analgesic combinations were prescribed for people with mild to moderate, acute or recurrent, pain states: the purported aim of these was to enhance analgesia with small amounts of amphetamine, which would at the same time give the patient a 'lift'. Many individuals unknowingly became dependent on CNS stimulants by regularly taking these preparations (see above p. 212). Last year (1979) saw the deletion in Britain of the notorious 'Drinamyl' tablets and capsules (dexamphetamine + amylobarbitone): once extensively prescribed here, and still used in the USA as Dexamyl, Drinamyl was given to promote weight loss in obesity. It was believed that the barbiturate component of the capsule would prevent, or reduce the degree of, excitation produced by the amphetamine. In fact the two drugs combine to give a peculiar type of euphoria which is much enjoyed by certain drug abusers: hence there is still a black-market in amphetamine/barbiturate products, which are now illegally imported. Chronic use, even that sanctioned by physicians, of these formulations could result in engendering dependency on both types of drug. Long-term use of barbiturates in whatever form can result in physical addiction, as many GPs found when the alarm began to be raised about these strong soporific agents. It is now generally agreed that there is no therapeutic justification for prescribing amphetamines and barbiturates concurrently.

Some amphetamine preparations are manufactured in such a way that the drug is released over a longer period than is possible with simple tablets, one dose of which will last for approximately 4–5 hours. The sustained- or delayed-release capsules (or more rarely tablets) are so formulated that a single dose will act for the whole day (i.e. 12–14 hours): this is accomplished in a variety of ways, including the production of tablets in several layers or capsules containing small granules. The best-known of these long-acting formulations are the 'Spansules' manufactured by Smith, Kline & French Ltd. On the face of it such products should be very useful, in that the need for multiple daily doses of a drug is obviated. However, their principal disadvantage is that their duration of action may exceed the desired period, continuing to exert perceptible effects for up to 20 hours in some cases. Also, with Spansule-type capsules there tends to be 'peaking and troughing', i.e. the drug is not released at a constant rate: when this occurs, a person may believe at a given time that the dosage unit has ceased to work, only to find some hours later that the drug is beginning to affect him with renewed force. Pharmacologists tend to dislike sustained-release formulations of drugs, except when they are essential, because of the variability of effect.

Amphetamine Derivatives and Analogues

Knowledge of the amphetamines' various unwanted effects as well as their potential for abuse led pharmacologists to make a number of modifications to the basic amphetamine structure, in the hope of separating the therapeutic actions from the undesirable ones: for example, to prepare a substance which would diminish appetite without CNS stimulation. To this end many new compounds were synthesized, some of which were marketed commercially. Most of the latter were introduced in the 1950s and early 1960s. All those at present available for prescription in the USA and UK are described in the accompanying Chart. Of the drugs listed, only one is not a central stimulant (fenfluramine), despite its being derived from amphetamine, while another (mazindol), though chemically quite unrelated to the rest, certainly has stimulatory effects.

The most potent of these amphetamine analogues are undoubtedly phenmetrazine ('Preludin') and methylphenidate ('Ritalin'). Both are now under the same legal restrictions in America, the UK and some European countries as the parent compounds. Phenmetrazine is used solely for its appetite-suppressing action. While early studies appeared to indicate fewer untoward effects, it is now realized that this drug is only marginally less stimulant than amphetamine and hardly less liable to abuse: nevertheless Preludin is still often prescribed in the USA, and in Britain, Germany, France and elsewhere a product called Filon, or Cafilon, whose main ingredient is phenmetrazine, remains on the list of prescribable drugs. In Europe the illicit use and sale of Filon and Cafilon are limited, but in the USA Preludin, particularly in the stronger formulations (50 mg and 75 mg tablets), is much sought after on the black market.

Methylphenidate, available almost world-wide under the trade-name Ritalin, was introduced just two years after Preludin, in 1960. Its characteristics are essentially those of amphetamines and probably most closely resemble those of phenmetrazine. Despite its definite anorexiant effect, this drug is not marketed to control obesity, but is recommended by its manufacturers to reverse physical and mental lethargy and fatigue, both when associated with chronic illness or during convalescence, and also, less justifiably, to mitigate symptoms of 'mild depression'. The American prescribing literature indicates Ritalin for use in narcolepsy and in the childhood hyperkinetic syndrome (see above, pp. 217–8): in addition, it is heavily promoted by means of advertisements in the medical journals to 'bring your elderly patient out of his apathetic/withdrawn senile behaviour'. The US Food and Drug Administration has stated that methylphenidate is 'possibly' effective for this latter purpose, but convincing evidence is lacking. In any event, Ritalin's potential benefits must be balanced against its hazards, which are well documented and substantially the same as those of amphetamine. Tolerance to and dependence on both Preludin and Ritalin will occur with repeated use, and the protracted administration of high doses of either drug may lead to 'amphetamine psychosis'. The relative potential for misuse and habituation of all compounds of this type is indicated in Column Three of Chart I.

The other available appetite-depressant drugs shown in the Chart are benzphetamine, chlorphentermine, clortermine, diethylpropion, fenfluramine, mazindol, phendimetrazine and phentermine. All except fenfluramine are stimulant to some degree, some markedly so (benzphetamine, clortermine) and some only to a marginal, dose-related, extent (diethylpropion, phentermine). Fenfluramine in fact tends to sedate, a surprising attribute of an amphetamine-derived compound, and it appears to be neither more nor less effective as an anorexiant than the amphetamines themselves. However, various cases of its abuse have been recorded, presumably because some patients (by no means all) find it euphoriant. Mazindol, which has a chemical structure totally different from amphetamine, nevertheless exerts an excitatory effect, albeit an unpredictable one, at the higher dosage ranges. Both these drugs are of recent introduction and much about them remains unclear, including their specific mode of action, their long-term effects, and their abuse potential. It is important to underscore the point that none of these compounds, except possibly diethylpropion and phentermine, should be prescribed for more than a few weeks, and then only as part of a total programme aimed at weight loss: no drug by itself obviates the need for will-power and determination in the fight against physical inflation.

We have already described how methylphenidate (Ritalin) has been indicated to help overcome fatigue and lassitude, such as may occur during convalescence. There exist other drugs which will perform this function quite adequately, but with less likelihood of adverse reactions. Pemoline (marketed as Cylert in the USA, and as Volital, Kethamed and Ronyl in the UK) is especially valuable in such situations and has until lately been under-utilized: it does induce a sense of well-being and increased energy, but not so powerfully as to make abuse likely. Very similar to pemoline in most respects is fencamfamin (Reactivan); this useful agent, unavailable in North America, has been prescribed in Germany for several years and has recently been reintroduced to the UK. Reactivan tablets contain, in addition to fencamfamin, ascorbic acid (vitamin C) and vitamins of the B complex. Pemoline and fencamfamin are about equally effective in counteracting somnolence, e.g. that likely to be experienced by those who must take regular doses of morphine or other strong analgesics. We have found that 1–2 tablets of either drug, given ½-hour after IM injection of morphine, once or twice daily, will often restore clarity of thought to the patient. However, recent (1981) reports from the UK indicate that some persons are abusing pemoline, if amphetamines become unavailable.

Of the remaining substances listed in Chart I, prolintane is probably unique among central stimulants in that it tends to enhance rather than diminish appetite. Pipradol has been prescribed primarily to alleviate depression: it is no longer given because of its unreliable action and the advent of more modern, specific antidepressant drugs. It will be remembered that amphetamine was first advertised as a nasal decongestant: propylhexedrine, a derivative, is now the only compound of this type used for this purpose. Propylhexedrine (Benzedrex) is presented just as was the original Benzedrine, as an inhaler. Its stimulant effect, though, is negligible.

Interactions with Other Drugs

In these days of multiple prescribing, when a single patient may be receiving several types of medication concurrently, the importance of drug interactions has been realized, although much still needs to be learned about the subject. Amphetamines and their analogues can affect or be affected by various other medicaments. One of the most significant interactions occurs with certain drugs prescribed to control high blood-pressure, in particular guanethidine (Ismelin), methyldopa (Aldomet), and acetazolamide (Diamox), whose activity is decreased by amphetamine. Stimulants should not be given concurrently with anti-depressants, especially those of the MAO-inhibitor group (see Chart II), such as tranylcypromine (Parnate), nialamide (Nardil), isocarboxazid (Marplan) and iproniazid (Marsilid). Fatalities have resulted from this combination: it may provoke a hypertensive crisis, in which the blood-pressure soars uncontrollably and severe fever ensues. Amphetamine-like drugs should be avoided if anti-epileptic medication must be given: this applies to phenytoin (diphenylhydantoin: Epanutin) and generally to barbiturates. Insulin requirements of diabetics may be affected by con-sumption of amphetamines and blood-sugar should be regularly moni-tored. Other possibly dangerous interactions may arise with antipsychotic drugs: haloperidol (Haldol, Serenace) and lithium carbonate (Eskalith, Priadel, Phasal) have been signalized in this respect. A very recent, and most interesting, finding is that the stimulatory activity of amphetamines and similar drugs is completely blocked by two of the newest antipsychotic agents, pimozide (Orap) and fluspirilene (Redeptin). Important interactions are summarized in the Chart.

Warnings and Contra-indications

Most of the contra-indications usually cited for drugs of the amphetamine type involve the degree to which the compound in question stimulates not only the CNS, but respiration, blood-pressure and other functions. Thus, methylamphetamine is absolutely contra-indicated in hypertension, but for an agent with mild excitatory effect such as diethylpropion this is not necessarily so. In general, this class of drugs ought to be avoided in cases of hyperthyroidism (overactivity of the thyroid gland); glaucoma; urinary retention; hypertension, particularly if severe; and advanced arteriosclerosis and heart disease. Individuals prone to agitation or hyperexcitability should obviously not receive amphetamines, nor should persons with a known hypersensitivity to their effects. The administration of highly euphoriant drugs such as the amphetamines themselves, phenmetrazine, and methylphenidate is not advisable to patients who have a history of alcoholism or drug abuse or who are considered to be susceptible to this – a diagnosis which is by no means always easy. Stimulants are absolutely contra-indicated during pregnancy.

The above warnings apply chiefly to the more potent amphetamine-like drugs, but if the physician or the patient is in any doubt, then one should err on the side of safety. Sympathomimetics should be given with the utmost caution, if at all, in cases of liver or kidney disorder, and their use is seldom if ever justified in individuals who are neurotic or psychotic, or who suffer from severe depression, anxiety or insomnia, as amphetamines are likely to aggravate all these states. If there are compelling reasons for prescribing an appetite-suppressant in such a case, one with the least stimulant effect (phentermine, diethylpropion) should be selected. Whichever drug is used and whatever the circumstances, the smallest effective dose should be prescribed: this will naturally vary according to age, weight, idiosyncrasy and other factors and will have to be determined empirically. Dosage regimens which are judged to be acceptable are listed.

Illicit Use

Many physicians in Britain, and an increasing number elsewhere, have in recent years agreed to a voluntary ban on the prescription of all powerful stimulants. It is argued that the cases in which amphetamines are clinically necessary, if indeed such exist, are extremely rare, and that their hazards far outweigh their doubtful benefits. Partly as a consequence, a black market in these drugs thrives as never before, with a single tablet of dexamphetamine now (1981) costing £1 ($2) or more. Amphetamine is easy for any competent chemist to synthesize, the raw materials and equipment not difficult to obtain, and illicit manufacturers produce large amounts of the drug in powdered or finely crystalline form. Relatively pure amphetamine is seen more often than might be expected, considering the extent to which black-market heroin, for example, is 'cut' with lactose and other bulking agents.

During the early and mid 1960s a handful of unscrupulous practitioners, operating mainly in London, overprescribed amphetamines (notably ampoules of methylamphetamine) along with opiates and cocaine. At that time injectable preparations of amphetamine were not subject to special legal control, so some prescribers felt free to give out scores of ampoules at a time, a few in the belief that methylamphetamine was less dangerous than cocaine when injected together with an opiate. By 1967 so many cases of amphetamine psychosis and heavy dependency had occurred that the manufacturers of injectable amphetamines undertook to withdraw these products and only to provide hospitals directly with supplies. It was immediately following this ban that illicitly manufactured amphetamine powder entered the market.

Numerically, amphetamine habitués (or 'speed-freaks' as they are known) probably far outnumber narcotic addicts in the UK. In spite of this, only one treatment centre exists in the entire country which has special facilities for dealing with these individuals, whereas over 30 centres have been established since 1968 for the treatment of opiate users.

The dangers of amphetamine abuse having been so firmly stated, it is appropriate to add that the taking of these drugs other than on a prescription does not necessarily constitute abuse or misuse. Apart from medical practitioners, including some surgeons, who work very long hours in conditions of considerable stress, there are persons belonging to other professions who use Dexedrine or Ritalin on an occasional basis: for instance, authors, especially when working to meet deadlines, and truckers, who have already been mentioned. For the most part, such individuals take stimulants in reasonable dosage and ought not to be classed as 'drug abusers'. We consider this very occasional use of amphetamines to be not illegitimate, but any reader who falls into the category described should be aware that the desired effects – increased concentration, lessened fatigue – can be accomplished quite adequately by therapeutic doses of fencamfamin or pemoline, for instance. Neither of these two drugs possesses so powerful a stimulatory action as dexamphetamine, nor do they provoke any but the mildest euphoria. Yet they both produce the required effects without serious risk of habituation and without the psychologically very unpleasant depression of an amphetamine 'come-down' as their action wears off. It is obviously desirable that, other things being equal, potent psychotropic drugs should be taken under medical supervision.

A number of celebrated (or notorious) people have lately been shown to have been dependent on amphetamines. It appears that Adolf Hitler received regular intravenous doses of amphetamine or some similar substance, which some scholars hold to be partly responsible for the dictator's irrational behaviour. Sir Anthony Eden, Prime Minister of Britain at the time of the Suez crisis of 1952, was apparently 'living on Benzedrine'. And there is more than a suspicion that John F. Kennedy made regular use of injectable methylamphetamine.

In Britain, each year, more individuals are arrested for offences involving amphetamines than for any other drug or drug type except cannabis. The scale of stimulant use, abuse and misuse on both sides of the Atlantic has resulted in very little effective action on the part of the authorities. The scheduling of amphetamines, with Ritalin and Preludin, on the British Misuse of Drugs Act and corresponding American legislation, and the imposition of harsh penalties for illegal possession and supply, has not reduced the volume of traffic: indeed, this has been increasing year by year. Facilities exist at some centres in the USA for treating amphetamine habitués, but these are virtually non-existent in Britain. The basic approach to the problem has remained fundamentally punitive rather than rehabilitative. This is an odd state of affairs in view of the fact that abuse of stimulants is considerably more widespread than that of opiates, for the treatment of which there are various techniques available in specialized psychiatric clinics. That there are still practitioners, admittedly few in the UK but many in America, who prescribe strong stimulants irresponsibly is unfortunate, and those concerned with regulating prescribing practices must campaign more vigorously. The dangers associated with amphetamine use, legal or illegal, are now so far beyond question that it may be appropriate to prohibit by law administration of amphetamine, dexamphetamine and methylamphetamine, except for the treatment of narcolepsy and perhaps the childhood hyperkinetic syndrome. Nevertheless, as long as the demand for such substances exists, and for whatever reason is not met by the medical profession, means of supply will always be found. The only effective approach to the problem today lies in educating the public about the hazards of all potent psychotropic drugs in specific, accurate and detailed terms.

Suggestions For Further Reading

Unfortunately, no full account of the amphetamine class of drugs has been published which (a) is not rather difficult for the layperson and (b) is accurate and up to date. The determined reader, however, will find material of interest in the following works:

Leake, Chauncey D.: *The Amphetamines: their actions and uses*. Springfield, Ill., 1958 (American Lecture Series, no.338)
  The first book-length study of the subject, Dr Leake's work is not very technical, but it suffers from the disadvantages that it is dated (e.g. amphetamine psychosis is not considered adequately) and that the author, who himself helped to develop the amphetamines, is too enthusiastic about their properties and uses. Nevertheless, an interesting study, chiefly from the historical point of view.

Costa, A. and Garattini, S. (editors): *The Amphetamines and related compounds*. Amsterdam & New York, 1973 (Monograph of the Mario Negri Institute for Pharmacological Research, Milan)
  This is a symposium containing numerous research reports from different centres. The bulk of this heavy volume deals with the results of experiments on laboratory animals, but there are several papers which concern the effects of amphetamines in man, including their use in children with the 'hyperkinetic syndrome'.

Connell, P. H.: *Amphetamine Psychosis*. London, 1973.
  The only book-length study of this subject. Though somewhat technical, it may be useful for people having to deal with amphetamine habitués.

Bray, G. A. (editor): *Obesity in Perspective*. Washington, 1975. (Proceedings of the Conference, J. E. Fogarty International Center, National Institutes of Health, USA)
  This work contains a very lucid account of the various treatments for obesity, including stimulants. Considerable detail will be found on the less hazardous of the amphetamine derivatives.

Goodman, Louis S., Gilman, Alfred, Gilman, Alfred G. and Koelle, George B. (editors): *The Pharmacological Basis of Therapeutics*, ed.6. New York, 1980.
  Chapter 18: 'Central Nervous System Stimulants' by D. N. Franz and T. W. Rawl pp. 585–607.
  The blue bible of pharmacology, this book is both authoritative and very detailed. Its contents may not always be readily comprehensible to those without a medical or scientific background, though some of the vast mass of material is summarized in a less formidable style.

Chart I: The Amphetamines and Other Stimulants
and Appetite-Suppressants: *overleaf*

CHART I: THE AMPHETAMINES AND OTHER STIMULANTS AND APPETITE-SUPPRESSANTS

IMPORTANT NOTE: If any of the drugs here listed are to be prescribed in cases of obesity to reduce appetite, they should be given (a) for a

Where Available	Name of Drug & Brand Name(s)	Dependence Liability	Indications	Usual Daily Dose (Oral)
UK,USA	*AMPHETAMINE (L-AMPHETAMINE) (Benzedrine)	++(+)	Narcolepsy (bronchial asthma; nocturnal enuresis; hyperkinesis in children; psychomotor epilepsy; reduction of appetite in obesity; adjunct in psychotherapy; treatment of mild transient depression. By injection: treatment of barbiturate etc overdose)	5 – 20 mg
UK,USA	*DEX-AMPHETAMINE (DEXTRO-AMPHETAMINE; Dexedrine)	+++		2.5 – 15 mg
UK,USA	*METHYL-AMPHETAMINE (METH-AMPHETAMINE; Methedrine)	+++(+)		2.5 – 15 mg
USA	†BENZPHETAMINE (Didrex)	++	Reduction of appetite in obesity	25 – 100 mg
USA	†CHLORPHEN-TERMINE (Pre-State)	++	Reduction of appetite in obesity	65 – 130 mg
USA	CLORTERMINE (Voranil)	++	Reduction of appetite in obesity	50 – 100 mg
UK,USA	DIETHYLPROPION (Tenuate)	+(+)	Reduction of appetite in obesity	50 – 150 mg
UK	FENCAMFAMIN (Reactivan)	+(+)	Relief of fatigue and lassitude, especially in convalescence	20 – 60 mg

lımited period only, say 4–6 weeks, and (b) only as an adjunct to diet and exercise: they should never be given continuously for long periods. None of these drugs should be taken during pregnancy. Indications which are historical (see Essay I) are given in parentheses.

Adverse Effects	Warnings and Contra-Indications	Interactions With Other Drugs
Common: Restlessness, nervousness, overstimulation, insomnia, loss of appetite, gastro-intestinal upset (e.g. diarrhoea), psychological depression 'let-down' as drug begins to wear off *Occasional:* Palpitations, tremors, elevation of blood-pressure, altered libido/sexual potency (either way), angina and disturbances of heart rhythm, depression *Uncommon:* Psychosis, especially of paranoid type (chronic abusers), delusions, auditory hallucinations, stereotyped behaviour, formication (abusers chiefly)	*Contra-indicated in:* hypertension, glaucoma, urinary retention, agitated states, arteriosclerosis, cardio-vascular disease, hyperthyroidism, during pregnancy, hypersensitivity to stimulants, persons prone to or with a history of drug abuse. *Greatest caution:* liver or kidney disorders, insomnia, depression, most neurotic and *all* psychotic states. DEPENDENCE IS LIKELY TO OCCUR EVEN AT THERAPEUTIC DOSAGE IF DRUGS PRESCRIBED FOR MORE THAN VERY SHORT PERIODS.	Amphetamines and similar drugs must NOT be given in conjunction with, or within at least 14 days of cessation of, treatment with, antidepressants of the MAO-inhibitor type, e.g. Parnate (tranylcypromine), Nardil (phenelzine), Marplan (isocarboxazid), and Marsilid (iproniazid). They should also not be taken concurrently with: the diuretic acatazolamide (Diamox); certain blood-pressure-lowering drugs such as guanethidine (Ismelin) and methyldopa (Aldomet); haloperidol (Haldol, Serenace) and other antipsychotic agents, including lithium (Eskalith, Priadel); barbiturates; ALCOHOL; sodium bicarbonate. Insulin use in diabetics *must* be carefully monitored. Effect of amphetamines on blood-pressure is enhanced by atropine. NOTE: Major tranquillizer/antipsychotics of the dibutylphenylpiperidine class, pimozide (Orap) and fluspirilene (Redeptin) completely block the stimulant action of amphetamines.
As for amphetamine but less pronounced	As for amphetamine	As for amphetamine
As for amphetamine but less pronounced	As for amphetamine	As for amphetamine
As for amphetamine but less pronounced	As for amphetamine	As for amphetamine
As for amphetamine but considerably less pronounced	*Contra-indicated* in hypertension, agitation, concurrent use with most antidepressants (see Drug Interactions). *Not recommended* in severe cardiac disease, arteriosclerosis, insomnia, for persons liable to drug abuse	As for amphetamine
Dry mouth, headache, dizziness, euphoria, dysphoria (mild), overstimulation, irritability, insomnia, gastro-intestinal upsets (e.g. nausea, diarrhoea)	*Not recommended* in severe cardiac disease, hypertension, hyperexcitability, glaucoma, hyperthyroidism	Probably as for amphetamine

Where Available	Name of Drug & Brand Name(s)	Dependence Liability	Indications	Usual Daily Dose (Oral)
UK,USA	FENFLURAMINE (Ponderax, Pondimin)	+?	Reduction of appetite in obesity	20 – 60 mg
UK,USA	MAZINDOL (Teronac, Sanorex)	+?	Reduction of appetite in obesity	1 – 4 mg
UK,USA	†METHYLPHENI-DATE (Ritalin)	++(+)	Narcolepsy (relief of fatigue and lethargy in chronic illness, hyper-kinesis in children; to counter senile apathy)	5 – 30 mg
UK,USA	PEMOLINE (Kethamed, Cylert)	+(+)	Drug-induced lethargy and somnolence e.g. patients in severe pain treated with narcotics; fatigue in con-valescence; hyperkinesis in children	40 – 70 mg
USA	†PHENDIMET-RAZINE (Plegine)	++	Reduction of appetite in obesity	25 – 70 mg
UK,USA	*PHENMETRAZINE (Filon, Preludin)	++(+)	Reduction of appetite in obesity	25 – 75 mg
UK,USA	PHENTERMINE (Duromine, Ionamin)	+	Reduction of appetite in obesity	15 – 45 mg
USA	†PIPRADOL (Meratran)	+(+)	Relief of fatigue and las-situde in convalescence; hyperkinesis in children; transient depression	2.5 – 7.5 mg
UK	PROLINTANE (Villescon)	+	Relief of fatigue and lethargy after radiotherapy, in convalescence etc; to counter senile apathy; to *stimulate* appetite	20 – 80 mg
USA	PROPYL-HEXEDRINE (Benzedrex)	+(+)	Nasal decongestant (sinusitis, hay fever); relief of Eustachian tube blockage in air travellers	2 inhalations 2–3 hourly

*indicates a Schedule 2 Controlled Drug (UK) = Class II restricted drug (USA)
†indicates a Schedule 3 Controlled Drug (UK)

+ = slight;   ++ = moderate;   +++ = high

Adverse Effects	Warnings and Contra-Indications	Interactions With Other Drugs
Sedation (common), dizziness, diarrhoea (frequent), euphoria or dysphoria, palpitations, facial flush; dependency of type not well documented	*Contra-indicated* in patients taking antidepressants (see next column), concurrently with other appetite-suppressants, glaucoma, hypersensitivity to amphetamines, hyperexcitability. *Caution:* Persons with a history of alcoholism or drug abuse	In addition to the interactions given for amphetamine, fenfluramine's effects may be enhanced by other depressants of the central nervous system (e.g. tranquillizers of any type, barbiturates, narcotic pain-killers) and it should not be taken concurrently with any of these
Dry mouth, insomnia, constipation, nervousness, headache, dizziness, skin rashes, disturbances of sexual function (usually negative), palpitations (dose-related); dependency (?)	As for fenfluramine	As for amphetamine, but somewhat less significant
Common: Nervousness, overstimulation, insomnia *Occasional:* Loss of appetite, dizziness, elevation of blood-pressure, headache, rashes, euphoria *Uncommon:* psychotic behaviour, delusions, formication etc (chiefly chronic abusers)	As for amphetamine	As for amphetamine
As for fencamfamin	As for fencamfamin	As for amphetamine
As for amphetamine but much less pronounced	As for amphetamine	As for amphetamine
As for amphetamine but slightly less pronounced	As for amphetamine	As for amphetamine
Dry mouth, insomnia, elevation of blood-pressure (dose-related)	As for diethylpropion	As for amphetamine, but less significant
As for fencamfamin	As for fencamfamin	As for amphetamine, but less significant
Palpitations, nausea, abdominal pain, overstimulation (dose-related)	As for fencamfamin	As for amphetamine, but only in cases of real abuse at substantial dosage levels
Irritation of mucous membranes (not common), amphetamine-like effects, though less severe, if very large doses abused	As for diethylpropion	

NOTE: Amphetamine/barbiturate combinations have been deliberately omitted from the above Table: see accompanying Essay I. Several of the formulations listed are available as sustained-release tablets or capsules: in the case of these, a single daily dose is taken in the morning (to last 8–12 hours). There is no clinical justification for the prescription of amphetamine/barbiturate or amphetamine/analgesic combination products (see Essay).

II: Antidepressants

How Antidepressant Drugs were Developed

Serendipity – happy accident – has often been responsible for advances in medical treatment: a chance observation, followed up by intelligent, original investigation. The classic example of this was the discovery of penicillin by Alexander Fleming, on to whose laboratory dish a few spores had happened to land. Subsequent research by Florey, Chain, S. A. Waksman and others yielded the magic bullets – antibiotics – which inaugurated a revolution in the treatment of bacterial infections.

It was Waksman who developed streptomycin, the first proper treatment for tuberculosis, formerly one of the major killing diseases, effectively and with relative safety. By the 1950s two other drugs were also being used with excellent results: isoniazid and its close chemical relative, iproniazid. Physicians noticed that patients for whom iproniazid was prescribed not only tended to be cured of their tuberculosis but became unexpectedly cheerful, even euphoric, whereas isoniazid produced no mood changes. A few years elapsed before the questions why and how the two drugs differed in this respect were pursued. Careful research was eventually conducted into the effect of these compounds on catecholamines, which are substances affecting the central nervous system and other systems in a variety of ways. Not only do they influence muscle-tone and temperature but they are also responsible for mood changes. These are found principally in the brain. The discovery was made that iproniazid blocked the production of one of these, monoamine oxidase (MAO), high concentrations of which were associated with the symptoms of depression.

By 1959 iproniazid (Marsilid) was being tested, occasionally with spectacular results, to see whether it would improve the mood of severely depressed individuals. The discovery that the drug did so in a proportion of cases led pharmacologists to devise other compounds, mostly based on iproniazid, which would be still more effective. Those which were developed and are still in clinical use are isocarboxazid (Marplan), phenelzine (Nardil) and tranylcypromine (Parnate). It is arguable whether any of these can be regarded as superior to the parent drug, although tranylcypromine is considered by many psychiatrists to be the most useful of the monoamine-oxidase inhibitors, or MAOIs as they are commonly known. Concurrently with the development of the MAOIs research was proceeding along another path. Pharmacologists working with piperazine, a drug widely used to kill tapeworms, hookworms and similar infestive organisms, found that a particular adaptation of its chemistry resulted in a series of compounds (phenothiazines) with profoundly tranquillizing, antipsychotic activity (for a description of which see Essay VIB). Further modifications of the structures of certain of these phenothiazines were discovered to be ineffective as tranquillizers but useful as antidepressants. The first of these tricyclic antidepressants, amitriptyline and imipramine, became available in 1960. Tricyclics are so named because their basic chemical configuration consists of three conjoined rings. These drugs offered a number of advantages over the MAO inhibitors, which will be considered presently.

Before the advent of the MAOIs and the tricyclics, physical treatments for depressive illness were to say the least inadequate. True, the snakeroot *Rauwolfia serpentina* (sarpagandha) had been employed for many centuries in the traditional Ayurvedic herbal medicine of India, to control manifestations of psychosis such as hyperagitation and delirium. But when the active principle of *rauwolfia*, reserpine, was isolated and used in Western psychiatry as a tranquillizer, it was found markedly to increase depression as well as to produce other undesirable side-effects. Although reserpine (Serpasil) and other *rauwolfia* alkaloids continue to be extensively prescribed to control high blood-pressure, their use in psychiatry has been all but abandoned.

Before the arrival of specific antidepressives, among the most popular remedies were amphetamines, especially dexamphetamine (Dexedrine), often together with a barbiturate. In the very short term, these potent stimulants do indeed improve mood, but as the effects of the drug begin to wear off the initial depression returns, commonly at heightened intensity. Because the amphetamines' antidepressant activity tended to be unpredictable, and when present ephemeral, and the danger of abuse and dependency was so considerable, they were seen to be quite unsatisfactory. A few psychiatrists still maintain that dexamphetamine has a limited role in the treatment of depression; however, the overwhelming majority believe drugs of this type to be obsolete in treatment of depression.

Electro-convulsive therapy (ECT) has now been available for some 40 years and continues to be regarded as an orthodox technique for alleviating many types of psychological disorder. Some practitioners argue, the arrival of antidepressant drugs notwithstanding, that ECT is still the quickest, safest, and most effective means of treating depression. The fact that nobody knows how this medically-induced epileptic-type fit works is considered to be hardly relevant, so long as it does the job. However, for some years there has been vocal opposition from some members of the psychiatric profession to its use at all, let alone its (as they see it) indiscriminate administration. This is not the place to argue the pros and cons of such methods, but there is no doubt (a) that ECT is not invariably successful in making people less depressed and (b) that after-effects, of which the most common is probably partial amnesia, can be severe. It might be supposed that with the advent of the tricyclics and the MAOIs the use of ECT would decline. This is not so, and indeed it is now often administered concurrently with antidepressant drugs.

The Meaning and Prevalence of Clinical Depression

A standard medical dictionary defines depression as: 'a mental state characterized by dejection, lack of hope, and absence of cheerfulness. Observed in manic-depressive psychoses. Depression is to be differentiated from grief which is realistic and is proportionate to that which has been lost.' We are not concerned in this Essay with manic-depression and other conditions which are regarded as psychotic, such as the different forms of schizophrenia, which are considered elsewhere in this book (pp. 349–53): depression is but one of several symptoms and signs in these profound and often very disabling psychological illnesses, which may require long-term hospitalization.

Between the poles of 'psychotic' depression and that which is regarded as 'normal' or 'appropriate' there exists a large grey area which has not been, and perhaps cannot be, completely defined. Numerous attempts have been made to classify clinical depression, or melancholia as some prefer to term it, by means of lengthy questionnaires (known as projective tests). Among those in current use are the Minnesota Multiphasic Personality Inventory (MMPI), the Eysenck or Maudsley Personality Inventory (EPI), the *Befindlichkeits-Skala* (B-S), and the Hamilton Rating Scale. The last-named of them is among those most frequently applied by psychiatrists in assessing the symptoms of depression: it will be seen from Table 1 that this is extremely detailed, and should be administered by therapists with skill as well as experience. The patient's scores for each symptom are totalled and the final figures subjected to complicated statistical analysis.

The cause (aetiology) or causes of melancholia are often difficult to establish, with both genetic and environmental factors playing a part. Also, the biochemical changes which occur in the patient's brain may be numerous and as yet are not by any means fully understood. It was at first believed that depressive states arose simply from excessive levels of monoamine oxidase (MAO), which seemed reasonable because drugs which suppressed the production of this enzyme often also could abolish depression. On the other hand, the much more widely prescribed tricyclic antidepressants do not appear to affect MAO, whereas they do block the re-uptake of catecholamines and other neurotransmitters, chemicals which conduct nerve impulses in the brain. Among the most important of these substances are noradrenaline (norepinephrine), serotonin (5-hydroxytryptamine), dopamine, and γ-amino-butyric acid (GABA). The means whereby antidepressants act on these chemicals, and what is their precise function in terms of mood alteration, is not yet fully known.

There exist a number of techniques for classifying depressive symptoms, but these are bound to be somewhat arbitrary and to overlap. Each individual's problems are unique, in the sense that they will not be exactly the same as for someone else. However, broad definitions can be of help, provided that their limitations are recognized. Apart from psychotic conditions, such as manic-depression, the various types of clinical depression can be roughly distinguished as follows:

Table 1: THE HAMILTON RATING SYSTEM FOR DEPRESSION

Item No.	Range of Scores	Symptom
1	0–4	*Depressed Mood* Gloomy attitude, pessimism about the future Feeling of sadness Tendency to weep Sadness, etc .... 1 Occasional weeping .... 2 Frequent weeping .... 3 Extreme symptoms 4
2	0–4	*Guilt* Self-reproach, feels he has let people down Ideas of guilt Present illness is a punishment Delusions of guilt Hallucinations of guilt
3	0–4	*Suicide* Feels life is not worth living Wishes he were dead Suicidal ideas Attempts at suicide
4	0–2	*Insomnia, initial* Difficulty in falling asleep
5	0–2	*Insomnia, middle* Patient restless and disturbed during the night

Item No.	Range of Scores	Symptom
		Waking during the night
6	0–2	*Insomnia, delayed*
		Waking in early hours of the morning and unable to fall asleep again
7	0–4	*Work and Interests*
		Feelings of incapacity
		Listlessness, indecision and vacillation
		Loss of interest in hobbies
		Decreased social activities
		Productivity decreased
		Unable to work

Stopped working because of present illness only 4

(Absence from work after treatment or recovery may rate a lower score.)

8	0–4	*Retardation*
		Slowness of thought, speech and activity
		Apathy
		Stupor

Slight retardation at interview 1
Obvious retardation at interview 2
Interview difficult 3
Complete stupor 4

9	0–2	*Agitation*
		Restlessness associated with anxiety
10	0–4	*Anxiety, psychic*
		Tension and irritability
		Worrying about minor matters
		Apprehensive attitude
		Fears
11	0	*Anxiety, somatic*
		Gastrointestinal, wind, indigestion
		Cardiovascular, palpitations, headaches
		Respiratory, genito-urinary, etc.
12	0–2	*Somatic Symptoms, Gastrointestinal*
		Loss of appetite
		Heavy feelings in abdomen
		Constipation
13	0–2	*Somatic Symptoms, General*
		Heaviness in limbs, back, or head
		Diffuse backache

Item No.	Range of Scores	Symptom
		Loss of energy and fatiguability
14	0–2	*Genital Symptoms*
		Loss of libido
		Menstrual disturbances
15	0–4	*Hypochondriasis*
		Self-absorption (bodily)
		Preoccupation with health
		Querulous attitude
		Hypochondriacal delusions
16	0–2	*Loss of Weight*
17	2–0	*Insight*

Loss of insight 2
Partial or doubtful loss 1
No loss 0
(Insight must be interpreted in terms of
patient's understanding and background.)

18	0–2	*Diurnal Variation*
		Symptoms worse in morning or evening
		Note which it is
19	0–4	*Depersonalization and Derealization*

Feelings of unreality ⎱ Specify
Nihilistic ideas   ⎰

| 20 | 0–4 | *Paranoid Symptoms* |

Suspicious
Ideas of reference   ⎱ Not with a
Delusions of reference and persecution   ⎰ depressive
Hallucinations, persecutory   quality

| 21 | 0–2 | *Obsessional Symptoms* |

Obsessive thoughts and compulsions
against which the patient struggles

from: M. Hamilton, 'A rating scale for depression' in *Journal of Neurology and Neurosurgical Psychiatry* vol. 23 (1960) p. 62. (reproduced by kind permission)

---

(1) Endogenous depression: This is held to arise from inner psychological conflicts for which no external cause can be found. It may be accompanied by anxiety, tension, and an overwhelming feeling of pessimism. Such conditions may occur during adolescence, when severe problems of identity can arise, and in women at the age of menopause, but can be manifested at any time during a person's life.

(2) Reactive depression: The onset of this is triggered, or brought to the

surface, by some external event, such as bereavement, severe physical illness, breaking with one's emotional partner, loss of livelihood. It may be secondary to some other psychiatric disturbance.

(3) Involutional melancholia is regarded by some therapists as distinct from endogenous depression, though the edges are blurred. This term describes a feeling of deep despondency, and lack of personal worth, which causes the sufferer to become passive and withdrawn, perhaps even unable to continue working or to seek social outlets. Involutional melancholia is probably found more often among the elderly than in other age groups.

(4) 'Drug' depression: Several classes of drug specifically produce depression. Major tranquillizers of the chlorpromazine (Largactil, Thorazine) and haloperidol (Haldol, Serenace) types are especially likely to do so, very profoundly in some cases. Other drugs of which depression may be a side-effect are barbiturates, alcohol, anti-hypertensives (agents which lower blood-pressure, e.g. reserpine [Serpasil], methyldopa [Aldomet]); steroids, e.g. cortisone and oral contraceptives (the Pill); and potent pain-killers, such as morphine at high dosages, and pentazocine (Fortral, Talwin) even in low doses. This type of depression may immediately follow withdrawal from narcotics (e.g. heroin, morphine, methadone) or from alcohol.

Antidepressant drugs are not uniformly successful in alleviating all such types and sub-types of melancholic symptoms: reactive depression, in particular, is very often not helped by their use, whereas both tricyclics and MAOIs may benefit sufferers from endogenous depression.

Amongst the enormous mass of literature, in books and articles from the medical journals, there will be found very few studies on the prevalence of clinical depression. H. Helmchen, contributing to a German symposium on an interesting new antidepressant, nomifensine (see below, p. 252), has lately reviewed what little work has been done on the condition's epidemiology in various countries.* Whereas the incidence of depression has been cited as 3% to 4% of the adult populations of Westernized countries, a survey of the inhabitants of midtown Manhattan indicated that 23.6% of these had clearly defined depressive symptoms. A careful study of the population of Iceland showed 6.8% of adults thus afflicted (5.2% of men, 8.32% of women). It is reckoned that people in the 15–34 age-range are the most prone to melancholia: this seems probable as suicide is the third leading cause of death among this group. Approximately 50,000 Americans commit suicide each year, although only one in eight or ten attempts is successful. The proportion is likely to be similar in Britain, where, in a survey by P. Bebbington (1979) of a

* H. Helmchen, 'Häufigkeit depressiver Erkrankungen' in *Alival (Nomifensin): Symposium über Ergebnisse der experimentellen und klinischen Prüfung*, ed. E. Lindenlaub (Stuttgart, 1977) pp. 19–29.

London borough, 5.9% of men and 11.9% of women manifested some kind of psychological problem requiring medical help, most complaints involving depression.

The figures quoted above illustrate the ubiquity of the condition. Even allowing for different criteria being used by investigators, the prevalence of clinical depression is certainly high. In the UK, more than 8 million NHS prescriptions are now filled annually for antidepressant drugs alone (and more than 20 million for tranquillizers) at a cost to the taxpayer of about £8 million, with the sum rising year by year. Antidepressants account now for 15% of all prescriptions written in the UK.

Tricylic Antidepressants

Because MAO inhibitors interact dangerously with a remarkable number of other drugs and with several types of foods (see below, p. 246), their use has declined considerably, although some psychiatrists are beginning to turn back to them after a decade or more of desuetude. The reason for this decline, which continues in most countries, is certainly attributable to the introduction of the tricyclic antidepressants. The accepted practice is now to prescribe MAOIs only in carefully selected cases, and when the patients concerned have failed to respond to tricyclics or to ECT.

The first two tricyclic compounds to become available in the early 1960s, amitriptyline (Tryptizol, Elavil) and imipramine (Tofranil), remain the most often prescribed. Advantages claimed for drugs of their group over the MAOIs are that they are more effective, their side-effects are fewer, and they are more compatible with other medication given concurrently. The dozen or so tricyclics now marketed do not seem to differ much from the two parent drugs, amitriptyline and imipramine, and all represent minor chemical modifications of their basic structure. The only significant difference between them appears to be that some are rather sedative (e.g. dothiepin [Prothiaden] and trimipramine [Surmontil]), while others, such as clomipramine (Anafranil) and nortriptyline (Aventyl), are not. The statement made by certain psychiatrists that some of the tricyclics have a 'stimulant' action is misleading, as the term suggests some amphetamine-like effect which is wholly absent with these drugs.

Imipramine and amitriptyline account for a very high proportion of prescriptions for mood-modifying drugs. More recently introduced derivatives, the latest of which was butriptyline (1977), are in some cases several times the cost of amitriptyline. Each manufacturer of tricyclics seems to vie with the rest (as in the case of other drug types), claiming that its product is superior to the others by virtue of greater effectiveness, fewer adverse reactions, etc. Some makers assert that their product will relieve anxiety and tension as well as depression. In fact the tricyclics may be effective in controlling such symptoms in some cases, but among patients whose principal problem is anxiety, with depression only a minor component, tranquillizers of the benzodiazepine type (e.g. diazepam, ['Valium']) are more likely to help. Nor are amitriptyline and its analogues panaceas for depression itself: 'endogenous' melancholic states appear to respond more readily to treatment with these than the other classes of depression, but by no means all such sufferers find these drugs useful.

It is important to realize that antidepressants, whether tricyclics or MAOIs, are not immediately effective in relieving symptoms. Some of the tricyclics (e.g. butriptyline) are said to begin working more rapidly than others: however, whichever of the available drugs is chosen, it must be taken at least once daily for two to four weeks before the patient begins to feel relief. If there is no therapeutic response after four weeks, either the drug will not work at all or dosage is too low. Long before the tricyclics exert any perceptible activity on the mind, side-effects may be noticeable. Sedation, one of the commonest of these, can be negated by giving the drug in a single dose regimen at night: virtually all amitriptyline-like antidepressants have a duration of action of 24 hours or more, so the traditional 'one three times a day' routine is usually unnecessary with them. Taking the drug at night has the advantage that side-effects can be minimized, such as slowing of reflexes, which may otherwise make it risky to drive or operate machinery. Other adverse reactions which tend to be experienced after one or two days' treatment with tricyclics are of the anticholinergic type, typically including dry mouth, blurred vision, and gastro-intestinal upsets (see below, p. 248).

The range of appropriate dosages for these antidepressants is wide, as can be seen from the accompanying Chart II. Individual variation to a given dose is considerable: a few patients may be helped by amitriptyline 20 mg per day, while others will require 300 mg or even more. A sensible procedure for amitriptyline, and *mutatis mutandis* for other drugs of the group, has been suggested by Leo Hollister (see Table 2):

Psychiatrists and general practitioners have their own favourite antidepressant, their choices being influenced sometimes as much by advertising material, whose volume is enormous, as by their clinical experience. Many would, we believe, agree that the tricyclic agents are almost interchangeable so far as antidepressive effect is concerned, and that if a patient has not responded to treatment with, say, nortriptyline, he is very unlikely to benefit from trimipramine or any other drugs of this class. Others disagree with this view.

The tricyclics in general are used entirely for their mood-enhancing properties, but amitriptyline is also prescribed for children who suffer from nocturnal enuresis (bed-wetting), obviously at much smaller dosages than those required to treat adults. The tendency of these antidepressants

Table 2: GUIDE TO DOSAGE OF TRICYCLIC ANTIDEPRESS-
ANTS (AMITRIPTYLINE)

Day 1: 50 mg three hours before bedtime, if well tolerated

Day 2: 75 mg three hours before bedtime, if well tolerated

Days 3–6: 100 mg three hours before bedtime, if well tolerated

Days 7–14: 150 mg three hours before bedtime; evaluate at
the end of 14–21 days. If response is less than
desired, continue basic dose in evening and add
progressive 25 mg increments every 2–3 days in
afternoon or evening to maximum dose of 300 mg
daily

Day 28: 300 mg. Re-evaluate if no response. Consider
another diagnosis, or use of a MAO inhibitor

from : L. E. Hollister, *Clinical Pharmacology of Psychotherapeutic Drugs*, New
York, 1978, p.103 (reproduced by kind permission).

to cause urinary retention in some cases led to researchers putting what
would ordinarily be considered a troublesome adverse effect to positive
use. Amitriptyline is generally prescribed for this purpose because, as the
prototype, it has been far more extensively studied than other tricyclics.
This drug is not universally effective in controlling enuresis but is certainly
worth trying when other (e.g. mechanical) means have failed.

Amitriptyline and its chemical relatives are most often taken by mouth
in the form of tablets or capsules, a few being also available as elixirs or
syrups for those who find solid-dose preparations difficult to swallow.
Three of the tricyclics are additionally marketed as injectable solutions
(amitriptyline, imipramine, and clomipramine): these are normally
reserved for hospital inpatients who initially are unable to take oral
medication. In these circumstances the drug is given at a dose of 20–30 mg
three or four times daily by the intramuscular or, more rarely, the
intravenous route. Marked relaxation usually follows such an injection.
Tablets, capsules or a syrup are substituted as soon as practicable.

Monoamine-Oxidase Inhibitors (MAOIs)

As can be seen from the Chart, only four of the antidepressants belonging
to this category are now marketed: the original MAOI, iproniazid
(Marsilid), is now seldom prescribed, and has been deleted from the US

listings. Isocarboxazid (Marplan) and phenelzine (Nardil) are given a little more frequently, while tranylcypromine (Parnate) is relatively more popular, certainly in Europe. This last-named drug has been termed a 'psychic energizer', possibly because it was originally derived from amphetamine: the expression is imprecise and should not lead the reader to believe that tranylcypromine has central stimulant activity, which is not the case.

Like amitriptyline and the other tricyclics, MAO inhibitors do not exert their antidepressive effect immediately. The length of time required for the lifting of symptoms varies between individuals but is generally not less than two weeks, and some patients may not experience any relief for three or even four weeks. Whereas most of the tricyclic antidepressants can be taken in only one daily dose, thus helping to obviate side-effects, of the MAOIs only iproniazid (Marsilid) is specifically recommended to be taken in this way. Isocarboxazid (Marplan) may be adequate for some patients with a single daily dose, but a twice-daily regimen is more likely to be required. Phenelzine and tranylcypromine must ordinarily be taken twice or three times each day.

The procedure for prescribing MAOIs is essentially similar to that indicated for tricyclic antidepressants, i.e. beginning with a moderate dose, increasing until the best response is obtained or side-effects become troublesome, then lowering the dose for maintenance therapy (see Table 2). As in the case of other drugs for depression, the range of dose levels required by different patients is considerable (see Chart II).

When a practitioner first prescribes a drug of the MAO inhibitor type, either he or the pharmacist should issue the patient with a special card: failure to do this, which both the present writers have encountered, constitutes gross negligence, because MAOIs interact in a toxic and potentially lethal fashion with numerous other drugs, including perhaps tricyclic antidepressants, as well as with several quite commonly used foodstuffs. The Treatment Card used in the UK is reproduced overleaf (Table 3).

It can be seen from Chart II that the standard MAOI Card does not include all of the foods and drinks which can be dangerous if taken by a patient under MAOI therapy: in particular, yoghurt, caviare and bananas should be avoided. As far as drinks are concerned, it is advisable to avoid all alcohol, as it is not only Chianti wine which is contra-indicated: sherry and various types of beer may also be hazardous. The many drugs that are incompatible with MAO inhibitors are listed in the Chart and described below (p. 250). Failure to observe the necessary restrictions can result in a hypertensive crisis. This syndrome, which can be precipitated when some of the listed foods have been consumed, commonly involves a rise in body temperature, very steep elevation of blood-pressure, and severe headache. In the early days of MAOI prescription deaths from hyperten-

Table 3: MAOI ANTIDEPRESSANT TREATMENT CARD

TREATMENT CARD

Carry this card with you at all times. Show it to any doctor who may treat you other than the doctor who prescribed this medicine, and to your dentist if you require dental treatment.

INSTRUCTIONS TO PATIENTS

Please read carefully

While taking this medicine and for 10 days after your treatment finishes you must observe the following simple instructions:-

1 Do not eat CHEESE, PICKLED HERRING OR BROAD BEAN PODS.

2 Do not eat or drink BOVRIL, OXO, MARMITE or ANY SIMILAR MEAT OR YEAST EXTRACT.

3 Do not take any other MEDICINES (including tablets, capsules, nose drops, inhalations or suppositories) whether purchased by you or previously prescribed by your doctor, without first consulting him.

   NB *Cough and cold cures, pain relievers and tonics are medicines.*

4 Drink ALCOHOL only in moderation and avoid CHIANTI WINE completely.

Report any severe symptoms to your doctor and follow any other advice given by him.

Prepared by The Pharmaceutical Society and the British Medical Association on behalf of the Health Departments of the United Kingdom.

7332/4567L D8038784 125M 7/79 TP Gp 3628/2

sive crises were not particularly rare, but each year still a few individuals die from this condition. Unless the rapidly rising blood-pressure can be brought under control quickly, usually by intravenous injection of phentolamine (Rogitine), risk of fatality is high.

Antidepressant/Tranquillizer Combination Products

Depression occurs much more frequently with symptoms of anxiety and tension than on its own. Antidepressant drugs, whether tricyclic or MAOI, may be highly efficacious in controlling the melancholic element in an individual's condition, but they do not always exert much effect on agitated, anxious and tense states. Some of the tricyclics and a few antidepressants of more recent introduction (Chart II, C) are claimed to relieve the whole triad of symptoms: these might have mild anti-anxiety properties but if taken alone are often inadequate to meet the patient's needs. Therefore some practitioners prescribe a strong anxiety-relieving agent ('minor' tranquillizer) such as diazepam (Valium) to be taken concurrently with the chosen antidepressant.

In an attempt to circumvent this problem, a few pharmaceutical manufacturers have produced tablets and capsules which contain both an antidepressant and a tranquillizer. Four such combinations are currently marketed:

amitriptyline + chlordiazepoxide (Limbitrol)
amitriptyline + perphenazine (Triptafen, Etrafon, Triavil)
nortriptyline + fluphenazine (Motival, Motipress)
tranylcypromine + trifluoperazine (Parstelin).

Parstelin combines a MAO inhibitor with a potent tranquillizer of the phenothiazine type, whose prototype is chlorpromazine (Largactil, Thorazine). In most reference texts it is stated that MAOIs should not be given in association with strong tranquillizers, and the justification for prescribing Parstelin is hard to see, particularly since the commonly-experienced adverse effects of MAOIs are thereby added to those of chlorpromazine-like drugs. The authors have seen a number of cases in which the use of Parstelin, even for limited periods, has severely aggravated patients' mental conditions.

The prescribing of a tricyclic antidepressant (amitriptyline, nortriptyline) with a tranquillizer may be easier to justify. Limbitrol (amitriptyline + chlordiazepoxide) may be regarded as reasonably safe, because chlordiazepoxide (Librium) is an anti-anxiety agent with a wide margin of safety and few adverse effects. On the other hand, perphenazine and especially fluphenazine are basically antipsychotic drugs, like chlorpromazine (Largactil). They should not be given too freely to dispel mild to moderate anxiety, although their effectiveness in controlling psychotic agitation and hyperexcitability cannot be challenged. When taken alone, antipsychotic tranquillizers tend to enhance depression and to provoke in many cases a wide range of other adverse reactions (see Essay VI and Chart VIB). It is doubtful whether the association of perphenazine or fluphenazine with a tricyclic antidepressant will lessen the likelihood of unpleasant side-effects, though such a combination may indeed relieve tension, anxiety, and depression too. The Triptafen preparations (known as Etrafon and Triavil in the USA) have been extensively used in psychiatry for several years, and they do benefit some patients. As with all medications, individual or combined, the likely benefits must be assessed against the possible hazards.

It is noticeable that pharmacopoeias, in which medicaments are given the official imprimatur of the relevant national commissions, contain only a small handful of drug combinations. None of those listed in either the UK or the US formularies are antidepressants, tranquillizers, or indeed any other combined preparations of psychotropic drugs. Medical students are being taught, rather belatedly, that products of the Parstelin type, referred to as fixed-dose combinations, should usually be avoided. The rationale of this is chiefly that such tablets are unlikely to contain the optimum dose of both, rather than of one or other, of their ingredients: given the considerable variability of individual response to a drug, dosage regimens need to be flexible, and it is difficult to achieve this with combined products. Naturally they are more convenient for the doctor to prescribe, and this is their only real advantage. Many modern psychiatrists believe that such preparations should be eschewed altogether.

Antidepressant Drugs: side effects and interactions with other drugs

The incidence and severity of side-effects attributable to antidepressants are such that it is not easy to generalize. To what extent such reactions may be troublesome is not completely known, and any assessment of these must be based at least in part on the practitioner's experience. However, in a major survey involving many thousands of American patients (the Boston Collaborative Drug Surveillance Program) it was shown that side-effects of sufficient severity to deserve documentation occurred in 15.4% of persons treated with antidepressants, while 4.6% suffered major adverse reactions, such as hallucinations, disorientation, hyperagitation and the manifestation of other symptoms of a 'psychotic' type. Any unwanted action of a drug will depend on a patient's age, sex, body-weight, idiosyncrasy, dosage, and other factors, some of which are hard to quantify.

To take the tricyclic antidepressants first: side-effects may be categorized in two ways. One relates to those which may occur throughout a course of treatment, and Chart II lists them in terms of probable incidence (i.e. common; occasional; less common). The other technique differentiates between those reactions which are likely to be experienced at the beginning of therapy with amitriptyline and similar drugs (the first couple of weeks) and those which may either persist or only become apparent after a period of several weeks or months. Within 24–48 hours of the commencement of tricyclics the patient may notice any of the following signs and symptoms: oversedation, dry mouth, blurred vision, abdominal upsets, difficulty in urination, and rapid fall in blood-pressure upon movement (postural hypotension). The patient may be asked to put up with such disturbances while dosage of the drug is adjusted. A high dose may be prescribed initially, until a person's response is gauged, and in many cases dosage can be much reduced: this itself will tend to abolish the above adverse effects in most patients. When the tricyclic drug has started to achieve its mood-modifying activity, certain other disagreeable phenomena may arise: trembling, weight gain, hallucinations, epileptiform fits, paralytic ileus (paralysis of the abdominal muscles), hyperexcitability, and, importantly, cardiac effects. It should be stressed that only a relatively small minority of patients are thus affected.

One probable effect of long-term tricyclic use will, although virtually unknown as such, we hope be recognized before long. Amitriptyline and the other tricyclics do, as has been stated, tend to cause dryness of the mouth. In fact a Danish researcher is at present studying this phenomenon in detail, and has found that these drugs decrease production of saliva by 50% or more. Dentists in that country are worried about the increased risk of tooth decay which absence or paucity of saliva appears to promote.

More seriously, there have appeared recently several reports indicating that these antidepressants can have significant effects on the heart even at ordinary dosage levels. Tachycardia (increased heart-rate) and palpitations are not uncommon reactions, while some unfortunately susceptible patients (not all of whom can be identified in advance) have been found to go into heart failure or suffer a myocardial infarction (coronary thrombosis) during tricyclic therapy. Clearly individuals who already have cardiovascular disorders are particularly at risk from such effects, as also are the elderly. Studies indicate that in terms of cardio-toxicity there is little to choose between any of the tricyclic range of compounds. One or two of the newer antidepressants (Chart II C), e.g. mianserin and nomifensine, seem less likely to affect the heart adversely. The Boston survey, to which reference has already been made, found that the mortality rate from cardiac disease was no higher among patients who had received tricyclic antidepressants than among a control group who had not. Given this information, it has been suggested that the cardio-toxicity of these drugs has been overestimated. Nevertheless, other well-researched clinical trials have demonstrated a higher incidence of morbidity and death due to cardiac disorders among patients for whom tricyclics were prescribed.

It is a fact that tricyclic antidepressants are numerically second only to barbiturates as the cause of death from accidental and deliberate suicidal overdosage, and each year the former take a greater toll of lives. In many cases doses which might be thought only slightly hazardous have proved to be lethal: death occurs with disturbance of cardiac rhythm in such cases. Iproniazid (Marsilid) and the other MAO inhibitors provoke many of the same untoward effects as tricyclic antidepressants: these are summarized in the Chart. Like amitriptyline and its relatives, MAOIs may during the first few weeks of treatment deepen, rather than relieve, depression, most often in cases where the pre-existing depression is very severe. The possibility of a patient's becoming suicidal should therefore be watched for as closely as is practicable. Apart from their being almost certainly less cardio-toxic, the adverse reactions attributable to MAOIs are various: some patients experience faintness, tingling in the extremities (acroparaesthesiae), swelling (oedema) of the ankles and, commonly, disturbances of visual accommodation. Psychological effects are troublesome in a minority of cases: a few patients become pathologically overactive (hypomanic) and find that their mind becomes clouded. Lack of desire and/or capacity for sex is not infrequent among patients on MAOI or tricyclic drugs. The 'hypertensive crisis', resulting from a toxic interaction between an MAOI and a tyramine- or serotonin-containing food, or other drugs, has already been described.

The kinds of medicaments which interact in a potentially serious way with MAO inhibitors are shown in the accompanying Chart. J. P. Griffin and P. F. D'Arcy, in their fundamental work on drug interactions (1979), tell us that these are probably more numerous than for any other class of drug and devote considerable space to detailing such instances of incompatibility. In the case of both MAOIs and tricyclics, the main types of drugs to avoid are: alcohol; antihistamines; some antihypertensives (drugs to lower blood-pressure); all stimulants and appetite-suppressants; anticonvulsants; pethidine and other narcotics (MAOIs); tranquillizers of the antipsychotic type; coumarin anticoagulants; barbiturates; and xanthines, i.e. material containing caffeine (MAOIs). Examples from these categories are shown in the Chart. Tricyclic antidepressants should not be prescribed concurrently, or within 14 days of cessation of, MAO inhibitors: a few psychiatrists do use these together in refractory cases, but most would contra-indicate such a practice.

The patient, especially if being treated with MAO inhibitors, may find it difficult to observe the necessary restrictions so far as some incompatible drugs are concerned. One has in mind over-the-counter products, for example cough syrups, which often contain several ingredients. Many of these contain diphenhydramine or another antihistamine, and/or a stimulant, such as ephedrine or phenylpropanolamine. If it proves necessary to take a cough suppressant, one composed of a single active ingredient, not belonging to either of the above categories, should be chosen, e.g. Pholcodine Linctus BPC or Dextromethorphan Syrup (Cosylan). The pharmacist's advice is often invaluable in such circumstances.

The principal contra-indications to the use of most antidepressants are: known hypersensitivity to a particular drug (patients hypersensitive to amitriptyline, for instance, will be so also to any other tricyclic); enlargement of the prostate; urinary retention; the eye disorder glaucoma; following myocardial infarction ('coronary'), stroke or other serious cardiovascular illness; and pregnancy. Antidepressants should not be given to children, except a well-studied drug like amitriptyline to relieve enuresis. It is worth repeating that in cases of very severe depression, symptoms may be exaggerated by antidepressants and the hazards associated with ECT increased. Conditions in which tricyclic and MAOI drugs are not absolutely contra-indicated, but in which they should be prescribed with utmost caution, with regular monitoring of the patient, are indicated in Chart II. Because antidepressants may affect reflexes, driving or operating machinery should be undertaken with extra care.

New Antidepressants

A group of antidepressant drugs which do not belong either to the tricyclic or the MAO inhibitor classes is listed in Section C of the Chart. Most of these have been introduced only during the past 5–10 years. Benzoctamine (Tacitin) has been available for a considerable time, and, although some therapists regard it as obsolete, others maintain that it is useful in handling mild to moderate depression. Benzoctamine also appears to be more effective than some more popular antidepressants in reducing anxiety. This compound may be quite valuable, insofar as side-effects from its use are generally mild and contra-indications few. Also structurally distinct from the tricyclics is tofenacin (Elamol), which has some anxiety-relieving as well as antidepressive activity. This compound should be regarded as being similar to amitriptyline and the other tricyclics in most important respects. Oxypertine (Integrin) has been variously classified as a tranquillizer and as an antidepressant, as it possesses both types of effect. Fuller information on these drugs is provided in the alphabetical formulary of this book.

Among the chemical treatments for depressive illness which are still experimental is L-tryptophan (Pacitron, Optimax), a natural precursor of the neurotransmitter 5-hydroxytryptamine (serotonin). Being a 'natural' substance, L-tryptophan has been thought to combine the advantages of safety and efficacy. It is marketed both on its own and in combination with the B vitamin pyridoxine, itself believed to have antidepressant activity. In some clinical trials the usefulness of L-tryptophan has apparently been demonstrated, while other studies indicate that the chemical has no more antidepressive effect than a placebo. The effectiveness of pyridoxine is likewise in dispute. Discussion of other drugs which in treatment of depression remain unproven or equivocal, such as thyroxine (thyroid hormone) and the anti-Parkinsonian agent levodopa (L-dopa, Larodopa), is outside the scope of this work.

Among the most important treatments for certain psychotic illnesses such as manic-depression is lithium (prescribed principally as the carbonate salt in the USA and UK): this and flupenthixol, another major addition to the range of antipsychotic drugs, are considered in the individual Alphabetical Entries and in the Essay on Tranquillizers (VIB). Lithium is a relatively toxic drug and for this reason is prescribed only to control severely psychotic symptoms: it does appear to be beneficial in relieving both manic and depressive phases of the manic-depressive cycle, being almost the only psychotropic agent to do so.

Between 1975 and 1977 four new antidepressants made their appearance in Britain. Since then additional dosage forms for three of these have been introduced. Maprotiline (Ludiomil) and mianserin (Bolvidon, Norval) are similar in chemical structure to the tricyclics, but with a fourth ring added: they are thus referred to as tetracyclics. The respective manufacturers of both these compounds assert that, while maprotiline and mianserin resemble amitriptyline and the other tricyclics in some ways, the newer drugs (1) begin to show antidepressant activity more rapidly i.e. within one to two weeks, and (2) provoke fewer unwanted reactions. These claims are not wholly convincing. Such evidence as exists at present, in the form of results from experiments (new drug compared with a standard, e.g. amitriptyline), strongly suggests that maprotiline and mianserin provide only marginal advantages over conventional tricyclic antidepressants, all or almost all of whose significant characteristics, benefits and risks they too possess.

The other two recent additions to the range of antidepressants are viloxazine (Vivalan) and nomifensine (Merital). Both are chemically quite unlike the tricyclics or tetracyclics, and indeed each other. The claims made for them include the supposed advantages of maprotiline and mianserin: viloxazine and nomifensine are held to have useful anxiety- as well as depression-relieving properties. The latter drugs do seem to be responsible for fewer side-effects and to be generally well tolerated by patients. Their antidepressant effectiveness has been established, and they may apparently be safely prescribed for patients with cardiac complaints, epilepsy and perhaps other conditions in which the use of MAOIs or tricyclics are contra-indicated or not recommended.

Further details about maprotiline, mianserin, nomifensine and viloxazine will be found in the Alphabetical Entries. Of the four, nomifensine shows the most promise: it has been available in continental Europe for some years and has perhaps been subjected to the most rigorous study. All these compounds have been produced in the hope of surmounting the problems associated with the MAO inhibitors and the tricyclics, such as intolerable side-effects, low patient compliance, misuse and, notably, their toxicity, which has led to so many suicidal deaths. It is clear that substantial progress has been made, nomifensine and viloxazine apparently having a much wider margin of safety than amitriptyline and its analogues, but that pharmacologists have not yet found the ideal antidepressant, if such can exist.

In the United Kingdom most patients are insulated against the real cost of medicaments, because the prescription charges which are levied are likely to represent only a fraction of their true cost. Antidepressants are among the most expensive items. Now that amitriptyline and imipramine can be obtained as unbranded formulations, as opposed to branded products, prices of these standard drugs are not high: unbranded amitriptyline tablets 25 mg (which are identical in quality) have a trade price of £1.00 per 100 tablets, against £1.92 for 100 of the same drug marketed as 'Tryptizol'. The more recent additions to the antidepressant armamentarium, available only as branded products under patent, are all very expensive: examples (cost per 100 units) are maprotiline 50 mg (Ludiomil) £9.66, mianserin 20 mg (Bolvidon) £12.10, nomifensine 50 mg (Merital) £15.85. Viloxazine (Vivalan) comes relatively cheap at £5.50. Note that these are wholesale prices: the price of a private prescription to a patient will be about half as much again. The pharmaceutical houses naturally assert that such prices must reflect the cost of research and development as well as actual production. However, in the case of minor chemical modifications of imipramine, for example clomipramine (Anafranil), is the trade price of £6.11 per 100 25 mg capsules justified? The present authors are not suggesting that certain drugs rather than others should be prescribed solely because they are cheaper: only that, if there is no real evidence of greater benefit than can be provided by a standard compound, cost should be a consideration not to be overlooked.

Given such a plethora of drugs from which the practitioner can choose, it may reasonably be wondered why not everybody afflicted with melancholia will respond to treatment with one or other of the compounds available. Some argue that when the neurophysiology of depressive illnesses is clearly understood, and the precise mechanisms of action of psychotropic drugs are known, it should be possible to banish such afflictions altogether. However, there exist some specific reasons why certain people fail to derive relief from antidepressants. In a concise guide to the subject Dr John Pollitt has listed six factors which may be relevant:
(1) The patient is using night sedatives, minor tranquillizers (e.g. diazepam [Valium]) or analgesics that deepen the depressive illness or prevent response;
(2) The patient, although not addicted, uses alcohol moderately, or heavily or regularly;
(3) A female patient may suffer from a marked premenstrual syndrome associated with a regular monthly recrudescence of depressive symptoms;
(4) The patient is taking a drug as part of specific treatment for another disorder, for example methyldopa (Aldomet), a compound used to treat hypertension, which has for him a depressant action;
(5) A physical illness such as glandular fever, myxoedema or intracranial disease (e.g. a brain tumour) has been missed;
(6) The patient is using an oral contraceptive and is sensitive to its depressant effects. (J. Pollitt, *The Practitioner*, vol.220, 1978, p.212)
Many question-marks surround the current, and ever-expanding, use of

antidepressants, particularly the prescribing of these in general practice. We have stated that some individuals do not respond to MAOIs, tricyclics, tetracyclics, or any other such medication; indeed that certain severely depressed patients find such agents aggravate their symptoms. In describing the side-effects, interactions, and other undesirable properties of these potent substances, we have tried to present a balanced picture. Opinions as to the usefulness of antidepressants, as of other mood-modifying drugs, among psychiatrists are many and various: at one pole, an appreciable number of practitioners hold that these agents are a *sine qua non* in the treatment of psychological disorders. Such doctors are likely to be behaviouristic in outlook. At the other extreme, the 'anti-psychiatrists' such as R. D. Laing, few in number but vocal and articulate, on principle never prescribe antidepressants, arguing that personal con-frontation between the therapist and patient provides the most effective, as well as the more ethically sound, technique of allaying the condition concerned. Between these extreme standpoints lie the judgments of most practitioners.

The routine prescription of psychotropic agents, as at present practised by many thousands of members of the medical profession, occurs as much in general practice as in the specialist psychiatric clinic. Frequently repeat prescriptions continue to be issued for months or years, often when these have long ceased to be necessary, if they were in the first place, with the doctor failing to see the patient often for very long periods of time. Of course antidepressants have legitimate indications: many people who previously would be condemned to states of severe intermittent or constant despair are now, with the accessibility of these drugs, able to take gainful employment. Whether such individuals comprise the majority of those treated with antidepressants is open to question. In a surprisingly high proportion of depressed patients treated by the authors of this book, medication proved unnecessary when the practitioner was prepared to expend time and energy in listening to the person's problems, to advise on difficulties arising from work or relationships, or even just to pledge moral support.

Virtually all the effective antidepressants, as we have seen, carry risks of one sort or another: in the case of MAO inhibitors, of toxic reactions from eating the wrong foods or taking the wrong drugs concurrently, and in the case of amitriptyline, imipramine and their relatives, of potentially life-threatening cardio-toxicity and the lethality of accidental or deliberate overdosage. The subject of after-effects when patients have completed a course of antidepressant therapy has hardly ever been discussed in the clinical literature: sometimes a whole range of 'psychotic'-type reactions manifests itself weeks or months after an antidepressant (particularly a MAOI) has been discontinued. The subject of duration of such treatment has also not been settled, some practitioners favouring intermittent, relatively short courses of antidepressants, others deeming it appropriate to maintain the drug regimen indefinitely.

It may not be wholly platitudinous to remind our readers that melancholia, like other emotions, is a quintessential element in the human condition. Even in the stressful conditions which obtain today, depression may not be completely negative. Periods of downheartedness, of despair – what St John of the Cross called the *noche obscura del alma* (dark night of the soul) – may prove, in retrospect, to be important in some respect, in terms of emotional development, in some cases even a source of creativity. The poet Arthur Rimbaud, in moods of deep psychic turmoil, composed the magnificent *Une Saison en Enfer*. Professor A. W. Woodruff has recently presented a fascinating paper on the medical condition of the painter J. M. W. Turner and other artists (D. G. Rossetti, Vincent Van Gogh), in which he concludes: 'Depressive states in particular appear to encourage this [creative] process *and to be helped by it* [our italics]. A remarkably large proportion of great artists have suffered from moderate or severe degrees of depression' (in *Journal of the Royal Society of Medicine* vol.73, 1980, pp.391f).

Of course we are not all artists or poets, and depression, like physical pain, may be degrading rather than ennobling, particularly if the symptoms are protracted and severe. Perhaps the main question which should be posed is this: when, how and why may it be ethical, or just good medical practice, to obtund or otherwise interfere with the processes of consciousness, more especially now that we have drugs which act so powerfully on the brain? Is it proper for patients to expect, and physicians to provide, chemical palliatives, often at the first twinge of anxiety or melancholia or whenever fluctuations of mood are found disagreeable? In this book we do not seek to answer such basically philosophical issues; but we feel that they ought to be at least raised.

Suggestions for Further Reading

Unfortunately, after an exhaustive search, the present writers have been unable to find any adequate, detailed account of depression and its treatment which is not technical to some extent. The following references may, however, be helpful.

Kornetsky, Conan: *Pharmacology: drugs affecting behavior*. New York, 1976. pp. 103–16.
A very reasonable, if too short, résumé of the subject, written intelligently but not too abstrusely.

Biel, J. H. and Bopp, B. 'Antidepressant drugs' in *Psychopharmacological Agents*, ed. Maxwell Gordon, vol.3 (New York, 1974) pp.283–341.
For the reader who has some knowledge of chemistry, this is an

excellent account, densely packed with information on the history,
actions, and uses of antidepressants.

Hollister, Leo E.: *Clinical Pharmacology of Psychotherapeutic Drugs.*
New York, 1978. pp.68–130.

This is the most up-to-date survey of antidepressants and one of the
most detailed to be found between hard covers. The author, eminent as
he is, occasionally allows his own opinions to affect what is essentially a
useful work of reference. The lay reader will find little difficulty with
most of the material as presented, even though a few headings may
need to be skipped.

Baldessarini, R. L. 'Drugs in the treatment of psychiatric disorders' in
Pharmacological Basis of Therapeutics, ed. L. G. Goodman & A.
Gilman, *op. cit.,* pp.391–447.

A comprehensive, if somewhat technical, account, from one of the most
respected of pharmacological textbooks.

Griffin, J. P. and D'Arcy, P. F.: *A Manual of Adverse Drug Interactions*,
ed.2. Bristol, 1979. pp.144–68.

Since interactions with other drugs are so important in the case of
antidepressants (especially MAO inhibitors, but tricyclics as well), this,
the most up-to-date and informative work on the subject, is recommended.

Chart II: Antidepressants: *overleaf*

CHART II: ANTIDEPRESSANTS

NOTE: The dosage ranges given here are those for *maintenance*, i.e. when the patient's response to a given drug is known. Initial doses may be higher. * indicates that the drug may be given in two or three divided doses daily, and † that a single daily dose (usually taken at bedtime) may be appropriate.

DRUG

Generic Name	Brand name(s)	Usual Dosage Range (daily, oral)	Tablet/Capsule Strength(s)
(a) **Tricyclic Antidepressants**			
AMITRIPTYLINE	UK: Domical, Lentizol, Saroten, Tryptizol US: Amitid, Amitril, Elavil	50 – 300 mg †	UK: 10,25,50 & 75 mg US: 10,25,50,75,100 & 150 mg
IMIPRAMINE	UK: Berkomine, Tofranil US: Tofranil, Imavate, Janimine, Presamine	50 – 300 mg †	UK: 10 & 25 mg US: 10,25 & 50 mg (hydroch-loride 75,100,125 & 150 mg (pamoate)
BUTRIPTYLINE	UK: Evadyne	75 – 150 mg *	UK: 25 & 50 mg
CLOMIPRAMINE	UK: Anafranil	25 – 100 mg *†	UK: 10,25 & 50 mg
DESIPRAMINE	UK: Pertofran US: Pertofrane, Norpramin	75 – 300 mg *	UK: 25 mg US: 25 & 50 mg
DIBENZEPIN	UK: Noveril	240 – 480 mg†	UK: 80 mg
DOTHIEPIN	UK: Prothiaden	75 – 150 mg †	UK: 25 & 75 mg
DOXEPIN	UK: Sinequan US: Sinequan, Adapin	10 – 100 mg †	UK: 10,25,50 & 75 mg US: 10,25,50 & 100 mg
IPRINDOLE	UK: Prondol	45 – 180 mg *	UK: 15 & 30 mg
NORTRIPTYLINE	UK: Allegron, Aventyl US: Aventyl, Pamelor	20 – 200 mg *	UK: 10 & 25 mg US: 10 & 25 mg
OPIPRAMOL	UK: Insidon	150 – 300 mg †	UK: 50 mg
PROTRIPTYLINE	UK: Concordin US: Vivactil	10 – 60 mg †	UK: 5 & 10 mg US: 5 & 10 mg
TRIMIPRAMINE	UK: Surmontil US: Surmontil	50 – 150 mg *†	UK: 10,25 & 50 mg US: 25 & 50 mg

Side-Effects
Common: Dry mouth, blurred vision, dizziness, lowering of blood-pressure, appetite changes
Occasional: Drowsiness, hyperexcitability, constipation, urinary retention, jaundice, trembling, skin rashes, cardiac effects, insomnia, perspiration, disturbances of sexual function
Less common: Epileptiform fits, fatigue, weight gain, severe cardiac effects (see also accompanying Text), enhancing of depression
Also reported: High blood-pressure, palpitations, stroke, coronary thrombosis; confusion, delusions, hallucinations, nightmares, tinnitus, paralytic ileus, nausea, black tongue; swelling of testes, development of breasts (men), milk secretion from breasts.

Interactions with other Drugs   Tricyclics & MAO-Inhibitors
Avoid altogether: Adrenaline (epinephrine), noradrenaline (norepinephrine, Neo-Synephrine); Antihistamines, Motion Sickness remedies e.g. promethazine (Phenergan), atropine, hyoscine (scopolamine, Buscopan); Certain Anti-Hypertensives (drugs to lower blood-pressure), including guanethidine (Ismelin), methyldopa (Aldomet), bethanidine (Esbatal), clonidine (Catapres), propranolol (Inderal); MAO-Inhibitor Antidepressants – see below; Barbiturates, e.g. amylobarbitone (Amytal), butobarbitone (Soneryl), phenobarbitone; Alcohol; Amphetamines and ALL other appetite-suppressants, including fenfluramine (Ponderax, Pondimin), mazindol (Teronac, Sanorex)
Great caution with: Analgesics, especially phenylbutazone (Butazolidin), and narcotics (e.g. pethidine), Anticoagulants of the coumarin type; Anticonvulsants e.g. phenytoin (Epanutin); Tranquillizers of the antipsychotic type, e.g. chlorpromazine (Largactil, Thorazine), haloperidol (Haldol, Serenace).

Additionally for MAO-Inhibitors:
Avoid altogether: As for Tricyclics, and also Anticoagulants, e.g. dicoumarol (Marcoumar), warfarin (Panwarfin); pethidine (meperidine, Demerol) and other narcotics; Anti-Parkinsonian Drugs, e.g. levodopa (l-dopa, Larodopa), orphenadrine (Disipal), procyclidine (Kemadrin); Tricyclic Antidepressants (see above)
Great caution with: As for Tricyclics, and also Diuretics (drugs to increase urine flow) e.g. hydrochlorothiazide (Esidrex, Oretic); Caffeine (coffee)

FOODS AND DRINKS WHICH MUST UNDER NO CIRCUMSTANCES BE TAKEN WHILE UNDER TREATMENT WITH MAO-INHIBITORS:
Tyramine-containing: broad bean pods, beers, Chianti wine, sherry, canned figs, caviar, most cheeses, game, meat, vegetable and yeast extracts (Marmite, Bovril, Oxo); Serotonin-containing: bananas. Pickled herrings, yoghurt, and chocolate may also be dangerous. Failure to observe these precautions CAN BE FATAL.

Contra-Indications to the use of Antidepressants:
Known hypersensitivity to any of these drugs; following coronary thrombosis; enlargement of prostate; urinary retention; during pregnancy; for administration to children (except amitriptyline for nocturnal enuresis).
Particularly for MAO-Inhibitors: Stroke, hypertension; phaeochromocytoma; epilepsy, diabetes

UTMOST CAUTION IF DRUGS ARE USED WHERE THERE IS:
Epilepsy, kidney disorders; impaired liver function; hyperthyroidism; glaucoma; any cardiac ailment. Depression may be exacerbated in persons already severely depressed, when the risk of suicide may be great. Signs and symptoms of psychotic illnesses, including schizophrenia, may be aggravated. Use of antidepressant drugs may increase the hazards of electro-convulsive therapy (ECT).

ANTIDEPRESSANTS MAY INTERFERE WITH REFLEXES, SO CAUTION IF DRIVING OR OPERATING MACHINERY.

CONCURRENT ADMINISTRATION OF TRICYCLIC AND MAO-INHIBITOR ANTIDEPRESSANTS SHOULD BE AVOIDED EXCEPT IN VERY REFRACTORY CONDITIONS AND WHEN FREQUENT MONITORING OF THE PATIENT CAN BE CARRIED OUT.

260

(b) **Monoamine-Oxidase Inhibitor (MAOI) Compounds**

IPRONIAZID	UK: Marsilid	25 – 150 mg *	UK: 25 & 50 mg
ISOCARBOXAZID	UK,US: Marplan	10 – 40 mg *†	UK,US: 10 mg
PHENELZINE	UK,US: Nardil	15 – 75 mg †	UK,US: 15 mg
TRANYL-CYPROMINE	UK,US: Parnate	10 – 40 mg †	UK,US: 10 mg

(c) **Others**

BENZOCTAMINE	UK: Tacitin	20 – 60 mg †	UK: 10 mg
L-TRYPTOPHAN	UK: Optimax, Pacitron	2 – 6 G †	UK: 500 mg
MAPROTILINE	UK: Ludiomil	25 – 150 mg *†	UK: 10,25,50,75 & 150 mg
MIANSERIN	UK: Bolvidon, Norval	30 – 180 mg *†	UK: 10,20 & 30 mg
NOMIFENSINE	UK: Merital	50 – 200 mg †	UK: 25 & 50 mg
OXYPERTINE	UK: Integrin	30 – 120 mg †	UK: 10 & 40 mg
TOFENACIN	UK: Elamol	80 – 240 mg †	UK: 80 mg
VILOXAZINE	UK: Vivalan	100 – 300 mg†	UK: 50 mg

261

Side-Effects

Common: Dry mouth, nausea, headache, dizziness, restlessness, fatigue
Occasional: Palpitations, constipation, blurred vision, abdominal pain, urinary retention
Less common: Double vision, hepatitis (jaundice), skin rashes, tinnitus, muscular spasms, trembling, numbness in extremities, enhanced depression
Also reported: See under Tricyclics, above, and also Text
Cf also above: interactions with other drugs and foods

Dry mouth, oversedation, nausea, gastro-intestinal upsets

Uncommonly, nausea, drowsiness. Very rarely, fatigue, restlessness, headache

As for Tricyclics but possibly less severe

Probably as for Tricyclics but less severe

Probably similar to Tricyclics but much less severe

Sedation, dizziness, nausea/vomiting, fall in blood-pressure, extra-pyramidal reactions (Parkinsonian effects, e.g. muscular disco-ordination), enhanced depression

As for Tricyclics

As for Tricyclics but less severe

Interactions, Contra-Indications: generally as for Tricyclics: see above

ADDITIONAL NOTES: Antidepressants used in the treatment of psychotic illnesses (e.g. manic-depression) are considered under TRANQUILLIZERS (ANTIPSYCHOTIC) in Chart V(b) and Essay V: such are lithium and flupenthixol.

Products in which an Antidepressant is combined with a Tranquillizer are described in the accompanying Text.
These are:
Amitriptyline + Perphenazine (UK: Triptafen, US: Etrafon, Triavil)
Amitriptyline + Chlordiazepoxide (UK & US: Limbitrol)
Nortriptyline + Fluphenazine (UK: Motival, Motipress)
Tranylcypromine + Trifluoperazine (UK: Parstelin)

III: The Barbiturates and Other Sedative and Hypnotic (Sleep-Inducing) Drugs

Introduction

According to reliable estimates, in England every tenth night's sleep is induced by a hypnotic drug. The term 'hypnotic', derived from the Greek *hypnos* (sleep), has in medical parlance nothing to do with the practice of hypnotism, and refers to that category of medicaments which has soporific effects. Even before the boom in the introduction of psychotropic drugs which began in the late 1950s there existed many remedies for insomnia, apart from the now notorious barbiturates, including various bromide salts, chloral, paraldehyde, and some which would not today be regarded primarily as hypnotics, such as cannabis and opium. Still, the past two decades have seen the development of yet more sleep-inducing agents. All of these were promoted as safer alternatives to the barbiturates and other older remedies. In some cases the new drug turned out instead to be if anything more dangerous (e.g. methaqualone, Quaalude, Mandrax) than traditional hypnotics, while others (e.g. triazolam, Halcion) do appear to be not only effective but relatively safe. It is, of course, ultimately for the prescriber and the patient to judge which of the available soporifics best meets the needs of the individual case. The adjoining Chart III shows the principal alternatives.

This Essay is concerned with drugs which are prescribed chiefly, or exclusively, to promote sleep. Of the many other compounds which have sedative properties but are administered for other indications, three principal classes are considered in this book under different headings. Such are the antipsychotic or major tranquillizers of the chlorpromazine (Largactil, Thorazine) and haloperidol (Haldol, Serenace) type (see Essay VI(B): Antipsychotic Tranquillizers); some of the tricyclic antidepressants, e.g. amitriptyline (Elavil, Tryptizol; see Essay II: Antidepressants); and various tranquillizing and anxiety-relieving drugs like diazepam (Valium) and meprobamate (Miltown, Equanil) (see Chart VIA and VIC). There is inevitably some overlapping between such categories, more especially now that certain drugs, antidepressants for instance, may be prescribed to aid sleep and to relieve the depression which may be responsible for insomnia.

The Barbiturates: actions – use – abuse

It was in 1865 that a German chemist condensed urea, the principal non-liquid component of urine, and malonic acid, derived from a substance found in apples, to produce barbituric acid. From this, in the first few years of this century, Fischer and von Mering obtained a potent sleep-inducer, barbitone (barbital, diethylbarbituric acid). Soon thereafter phenobarbitone, first marketed in 1912, was introduced, and many other barbiturates were synthesized between then and 1950. Phenobarbitone is still prescribed all over the world under its original trade name Luminal. The most extensively used of the numerous other derivatives of barbituric acid are amylobarbitone (Amytal), known in the USA as amobarbital, pentobarbitone (Nembutal), and quinalbarbitone (secobarbital, Seconal), all of these available both as the basic compounds and their more rapidly absorbed sodium salts (e.g. amylobarbitone sodium, Sodium Amytal).

The barbiturates are commonly classified according to their duration of action: this may be only a few minutes, in the case of injectable barbiturates such as methohexitone (Brietal) and thiopentone (Pentothal), which are used exclusively to provide anaesthesia during surgical operations. (Since these ultra-short-acting agents are not prescribed otherwise they are not considered further here.) At the other end of the scale barbitone itself, phenobarbitone, metharbitone and methyl-phenobarbitone (mephobarbital) exert perceptible effects for up to 24 hours, and a single dose of any of these long-acting barbiturates may not be completely eliminated from the body for several days. Phenobarbitone and the other compounds mentioned, being slowly absorbed and excreted, are still prescribed by some practitioners for night sedation, but are more often taken because of their anticonvulsant properties, to protect against the occurrence of epileptic fits. Many thousands of people with symptoms of epilepsy must consume tablets or capsules of seizure-preventing agents every day for life. Although more modern anticonvulsant drugs have been developed, such as clonazepam (Rivotril), and sodium valproate (Epilim), all of which are less toxic than barbiturates, some epileptics do not find them effective and hence remain on phenobarbitone or one of its analogues.

Those barbiturates, such as amylobarbitone and pentobarbitone, whose duration of action is considerably less than that of phenobarbitone, are distinguished in many pharmacological texts as being 'intermediate-' or 'short-acting'. Hence amylobarbitone is assigned to the former, pentobarbitone to the latter category. According to modern evidence, however, these compounds and the others listed in Chart III(B) are virtually identical in terms of length of activity and in all other important respects too. Thus these are quite interchangeable; for example, butobarbitone (Soneryl) will fully substitute for quinalbarbitone (Seconal). Any of these compounds, taken to promote sleep, will begin to act within 20 to 40 minutes, allowing sleep for between 4 and 8 hours. One difference between them has significance: they are not all equipotent, i.e. effective at the same milligramme dosage. Butobarbitone 100 mg is approximately equivalent to 200 mg of cyclobarbitone or heptabarbitone (Medomin). The relative strength of each drug is indicated by the usual range of dosage, as shown in Chart III. About the only indication for preferring one formulation to another is that those barbiturates which are available as the sodium (in the case of cyclobarbitone the calcium) salt are, as already stated, more quickly absorbed and eliminated from the system more rapidly. Preparations in which two (or even more) barbiturates are combined, such as Tuinal (amylobarbitone sodium + quinalbarbitone sodium) and Evidorm (cyclobarbitone + hexobarbitone) have no medical justification: these are no more effective than a dosage unit of one barbiturate brought up to the appropriate number of milligrammes.

Anybody who has tried a barbiturate tablet or capsule will say that it promoted sound sleep: for several decades phenobarbitone in particular received high praise for its efficacy. But this and the other long-acting compounds, though traditional, cannot be recommended as hypnotics because they and their metabolites (by-products) linger in the system for so long. A figure much used by pharmacologists is the plasma $t_{1/2}$(half-life) of a given drug, i.e. the length of time for 50% of a dose to be eliminated from the bloodstream. (Perceptible effects may last a longer or shorter time than this, for various reasons.) In the case of phenobarbitone, the $t_{1/2}$ is approximately 80 to 100 hours. The practical implication of this knowledge may be that if the drug is taken daily, even for a relatively short period, amounts of it which will accumulate in the body can reach toxic levels: delirium, confusion, and even convulsions may then ensue.

All barbiturates have a general damping-down effect on the central nervous system, which far exceeds that required to produce sleep. The typical hangover reaction experienced the morning after taking one of these hypnotics – a feeling of being dopey and sluggish – testifies to the profundity of such action. Barbiturates also suppress REM (rapid eye-movement) sleep (paradoxical sleep), during which we dream: episodes of 'normal' and REM-sleep alternate throughout the night, and the latter phases are known to be psychologically and physically important. If REM sleep is attenuated or abolished for other than a short period of time, a phenomenon known as 'REM rebound' occurs: this state is characterized by intense, often horrifying, nightmares.

Regular use of any barbituric acid derivative is likely to produce immediate side- and after-effects; tolerance; and psychological and/or physical dependency. The present writers are aware, as are some readers, that certain individuals who have regularly consumed, say, 2 tablets of Soneryl at night for many years feel no adverse reactions, do not suffer

Table 4: 'MASKED BARBITURATES': PREPARATIONS
AVAILABLE FOR PRESCRIPTION IN THE UK

1 Sedative/Analgesics, migraine remedies etc.

BELLERGAL tabs	phenobarbitone 20 mg + belladonna + ergotamine
BELLERGAL RETARD tabs	phenobarbitone 40 mg + belladonna + ergotamine
BEPLETE elixir	phenobarbitone 20 mg/5 ml + B vitamins
CAFERGOT suppos	butalbital 100 mg + ergotamine + belladonna + caffeine
BUDALE tabs*	butobarbitone 60 mg + codeine + paracetamol
SONALGIN tabs*	butobarbitone 60 mg + codeine + paracetamol
SONERGAN tabs*	butobarbitone 75 mg + promethazine

2 Preparations for asthma, chronic bronchitis and cough

AMESEC caps	amylobarbitone 25 mg + ephedrine + theophylline
ASMAL tabs	phenobarbitone 7.5 mg + ephedrine + theophylline
FRANOL tabs	phenobarbitone 8 mg + ephedrine + theophylline
FRANOL PLUS tabs	phenobarbitone 8 mg + ephedrine + theophylline + thenyldiamine
FRANOL expectorant	phenobarbitone 4 mg/5 ml + ephedrine + theophylline + guaiphenesin
TEDRAL tabs	phenobarbitone 8 mg + ephedrine + theophylline
TEDRAL-SA tabs	phenobarbitone 25 mg + ephedrine + theophylline
TEDRAL suspension	phenobarbitone 4 mg/5 ml + ephedrine + diprophylline + guaiphenesin

3 Preparations for angina and hypertension

CARDIACAP-A caps	amylobarbitone 50 mg + pentaerythritol tetranitrate
HYPERTANE CO tabs	amylobarbitone 15 mg + rauwolfia
SEOMINAL tabs	phenobarbitone 10 mg + reserpine + theobromine

THEOGARDENAL tabs	phenobarbitone 30 mg + theobromine
THEOMINAL tabs	phenobarbitone 30 mg + theobromine
VERILOID-VP tabs*	phenobarbitone 15 mg + veratrum alkaloids

4 Antacids and gastro-intestinal sedatives

ACTONORM tabs	phenobarbitone 5 mg + antacids etc.
ACTONORM-SED gel	phenobarbitone 8 mg/5 ml + antacids etc.
APP-STOMACH tabs	phenobarbitone 15 mg + antacids
ALUHYDE tabs	quinalbarbitone 32.5 mg + belladonna + antacids
BELLOBARB tabs	phenobarbitone 15 mg + belladonna + antacids
ALUDROX-SA susp	secbutobarbitone 8 mg/5 ml + ambutonium + antacid
NEUTRADONNA-SED	amylobarbitone 5 mg/5 ml + hyoscyamine + antacid
BELLADENAL tabs	phenobarbitone 50 mg + belladonna
BELLADENAL-RETARD tabs	phenobarbitone 50 mg + belladonna
DONNATAL tabs & elix	phenobarbitone 16.2 mg + belladonna
DONNATAL-LA tabs	phenobarbitone 48.6 mg + belladonna
FENOBELLADINE tabs	phenobarbitone 15 mg + belladonna

5 Hormone preparations

| HORMOFEMIN-Co tabs | phenobarbitone 10 mg + dienoestrol etc. |
| POTENSAN tabs* | amylobarbitone 15 mg + yohimbine + strychnine |

*indicates that the product will be discontinued shortly

adapted from: *Drug & Therapeutics Bulletin* vol. 18 (1980) pp. 10–11

---

from hangovers, do not require periodic increments in dose, and are (apparently) not dependent on the drug. If a high proportion of such persons were physically addicted, one would have expected an enormous number of cases in which, with the sharp decline in barbiturate prescription in recent years, withdrawal symptoms would be experienced. And barbiturate withdrawal reactions, when they do occur, may be more severe, indeed more life-threatening, than opiate abstinence. It must be said, though, that serious symptoms are much more likely to arise when the individual is a chronic drug abuser, accustomed to taking very large doses.

Immediate side-effects from amylobarbitone and its congeners will be absent in many cases, for the obvious reason that sleep has supervened. But before this happens, dizziness may be felt, an allergic skin rash may develop, or, when a high dose has been taken, paradoxical excitement may occur: a state of talkativeness and excitability similar to that seen after consumption of excessive amounts of alcohol. Indeed, barbiturate intoxication in this sense quite closely resembles drunkenness.

Both long- and intermediate-acting barbiturates are incorporated, generally at low dosage, in tablets and capsules which are marketed (1) with aspirin or other simple analgesics, to control pain; (2) with theophylline, ephedrine and other bronchodilators to relieve asthma, bronchitis or cough; (3) with reserpine in the treatment of hypertension; and (4) with antacids, belladonna etc. as gastro-intestinal sedatives. Table 4 lists the so-called 'masked barbiturate' preparations which are available for prescription in the UK. In the USA well over 100 such products are marketed. Most of these have brand names which give no hint that a barbiturate constitutes one of the ingredients. There are several cogent reasons for avoiding masked barbiturate products. The most important is that these drugs are without value in the treatment of respiratory disorders (and indeed can exacerbate them), hypertension and cardiac complaints, and in gastro-intestinal upsets. Worse, barbiturates antagonize the effects of analgesics, perhaps simple pain-killers like paracetamol and certainly potent drugs of the morphine type. Therefore products containing even small amounts of phenobarbitone and similar compounds are altogether contra-indicated in pain states, particularly the chronic ones (such as arthritis and related conditions) for which a barbiturate combination product is most often prescribed. With all these preparations, if they are taken repeatedly, the patient runs the risk of insidious dependency. Combinations of amylobarbitone with amphetamines are extremely dangerous, and these have no legitimate clinical indications (see Essay I: Amphetamines).

In 1980 the British Committee on the Review of Medicines (CRM) issued a set of recommendations concerning barbiturates, which it had been studying at length. The CRM's findings are easily summarized, and these agree generally with current medical opinion and with the judgment of the authors of this book. Predictably, the Committee takes the view that combination products of the type shown in Table 4 should be withdrawn by their respective manufacturers for the reasons indicated above. So far as barbiturates as hypnotics are concerned, these should be prescribed only for 'intractable insomnia'. A rather cautious statement, it probably represents a sop to those practitioners who are still convinced of the drugs' effectiveness and supposed relative safety and who will go on prescribing them come what may. The CRM also contra-indicates the use of barbiturates to relieve pain states or anxiety or for daytime sedation (see *Drug and Therapeutics Bulletin* vol. 18 no. 3, February 1, 1980). The evidence on which these judgments have been formulated has been familiar to clinical pharmacologists for a number of years: even though the CRM's recommendations should be welcomed, since they have almost the status of a *nihil obstat*, they come belatedly. As the body asserts, barbiturates are readily habit-forming and easily produce physical addiction. The latter is manifested by a severe withdrawal syndrome, marked by delirium, convulsions and hyperagitation, which if left untreated can be fatal. In the UK and other countries there are almost certainly far more people physically or psychologically habituated to barbiturates than to morphine, heroin and other narcotics. The problem remains largely hidden, in part because these hypnotics are not yet subject to the Misuse of Drugs Regulations. We understand that amylobarbitone and its congeners will soon be thus legally restricted along with opiates, amphetamines and other dangerous drugs.

A further significant point made by the CRM relates to the fact that barbiturates are far more frequently responsible for inducing death, accidental or deliberate, than any other drug class: in 1978, of the 2,900 British cases of death caused by drugs, they were cited in 27% of cases.

Among the other hazardous properties of these compounds, they stimulate their own metabolism (enzyme induction) if administered chronically, which in practical terms means that duration of action of a given dose is decreased and that tolerance to their effects develops swiftly. Barbiturates also decrease the efficacy of several other drugs: the most important interactions are shown in column 5 of Chart III. Those which give the greatest cause for concern are with the anti-epileptic drug phenytoin (Epanutin); griseofulvin (Grisovin, Fulvicin), which is used to treat fungal infections; anticoagulant agents of the coumarin type, such as warfarin (Marevan, Coumadin); and corticosteroids, notably all types of contraceptive Pill as well as cortisone, hydrocortisone, prednisone and similar agents prescribed chiefly to relieve inflammatory (e.g. arthritic) and allergic conditions. It may, rarely, be necessary to give a barbiturate concomitantly with one of these, but in that event the physician should be aware of the likely interaction and adjust the dosage regimen accordingly. Alcohol should be avoided altogether by patients receiving barbiturates: this combination can be lethal.

Brief mention should be made of a series of amylo-, buto-, cyclo- and phenobarbitone tablet preparations which incorporate a small quantity of ipecacuanha. This is, with the possible exception of apomorphine, the most powerful inducer of vomiting known in medicine. A typical example of these barbemets, as they are called, is Butomet, a tablet comprising butobarbitone 100 mg and emetine (the main alkaloid of ipecac) 0.6 mg. If taken at appropriate dosage for night sedation, only the hypnotic will be effective; however, if an overdose is attempted, the ipecacuanha will cause vomiting before serious harm can be done. For some obscure reason the barbemets are prescribed only rarely. We believe that, in cases where night sedation with a barbiturate is really required, the use of such preparations could provide a valuable safeguard.

As indicated in the Chart, barbituric acid derivatives are contra-indicated in porphyria variegata, an uncommon but severe metabolic disorder which can itself be brought on by long-term use of these hypnotics. Because barbiturates so profoundly depress respiration, they obviously ought not to be given in cases of other than mild bronchial disorders. They should also be avoided in serious liver ailments and in cases of known hypersensitivity: a person sensitive, say, to phenobarbitone will be so additionally to all chemically related drugs. The general practitioner should watch for the patient (who may not necessarily be young) who tries to insist on a prescription for such products as Tuinal, Nembutal, Amytal and Seconal. This may be a person who has a history of drug abuse, and the aforementioned tablets and capsules are those most frequently requested for illegitimate purposes.

A new and still experimental application for pentobarbitone has been described by Harvey M. Shapiro of the University of California, San Diego. This anaesthesiologist and his colleagues have found that patients who suffer serious head injury respond well to this drug: it is administered intravenously for several days in addition to the usual resuscitative measures. Apparently morbidity and mortality are reduced with this technique, although it is uncertain why. Part of the explanation is probably that barbiturates reduce intra-cranial pressure, which after trauma to the head may be considerably raised, and constrict the brain's blood cells. Shapiro and his team are currently testing intravenous pentobarbitone on patients who have suffered stroke, cardiac arrest and other conditions involving swelling of the brain: so far, the results appear promising.

Habituation to barbiturates has been mentioned: despite campaigns in Britain to reduce their availability on prescription, the numbers of individuals affected have for the past decade been rising alarmingly. In the USA treatment facilities are relatively well developed: there most addicts to heroin and other narcotics also take barbiturates, which are effective in staving off withdrawal symptoms when opiates become unavailable on the black market. At the Addiction Research Institute at Lexington, Ky, and similar institutions, it is assumed that barbiturate and narcotic dependency coexist and appropriate steps are taken to ensure safe withdrawal from both types of drug.

Since the considerable restriction in the legal availability of opiates in Britain, which began a decade ago with a statute forbidding almost all doctors to prescribe heroin to addicts, the situation here has more closely resembled that obtaining in the USA. At present British opiate addicts, if they are to obtain any supplies legally, must present at hospital Drug

Dependency Clinics where they may be offered methadone (a heroin substitute) in the form of syrup: heroin and other injectable drugs are prescribed increasingly rarely. For this reason many addicts take their chances with illicit sources of supply, but as heroin is ruinously expensive and at times virtually unobtainable, barbiturates are used as a stand-by. Often the contents of a Nembutal or Tuinal capsule are dissolved and injected intravenously: a highly dangerous practice which can cause abscesses, gangrene and septicaemia (blood-poisoning). A. F. Teggin and Thomas Bewley have recently reported on a series of 120 patients admitted to a London psychiatric hospital over a 6-month period. These were suspected barbiturate addicts, of whom 75 needed treatment for abstinence reactions. Common signs and symptoms of withdrawal included restlessness, trembling, insomnia, increased muscle tone, convulsions, delusions, confusion and delirium. The patients were given pentobarbitone elixir, at an average dose of 250 mg four times daily, for 3 days, after which dosage was reduced by 100 mg per day until withdrawal was complete. The authors of this paper observe that the numbers of persons presenting with barbiturate addiction are increasing annually: some of these are poly-drug abusers, and some concurrent opiate habitués, relatively few using barbiturates alone. (*The Practitioner* vol. 223, 1979, pp. 106f.) In the UK at present facilities for treating such cases are woefully inadequate: the paper by Teggin and Bewley indicates how extensive is the problem.

Given all their hazards, adverse effects, and so on, it may be wondered why barbiturates are ever prescribed as a remedy for insomnia. It will be seen from the Chart, and from the following pages, that equally effective, and safer, hypnotics have been available for some years. Many practitioners would go further than the CRM and ban the prescription of these compounds altogether except in the relatively few cases of epilepsy when other anticonvulsant medication is unsuitable. Reviewing American prescriptions of soporifics, Jan Koch-Weser and David Greenblatt conclude: 'The barbiturate hypnotics have been rendered obsolete by pharmacologic progress and deserve speedy oblivion' ('The Archaic Barbiturate Hypnotics', *New England Journal of Medicine* vol. 291 [1974] 791).

Other Old-Generation Hypnotics

Still in most cases manufactured, but seldom prescribed, are a few soporifics which have been known for a century or more. These include the bromides (e.g. potassium bromide) whose hypnotic and anticonvulsant properties were recognized in the 1860s. Despite the bromides' high toxicity, their tendency to irritate the stomach and other undesirable attributes, they are still present in many composite preparations used in

France and other European countries. Because of their very slow (12 + days) elimination from the body, accumulation occurs with repeated bromide usage and dangerous levels in the system are soon reached: the intoxication thus produced is referred to as bromism. Derived from these obsolete compounds were carbromal, acetylcarbromal and bromisovalum: prescription of medicines containing any of these is extinct in the UK and has dwindled in the USA. There, and in some other countries, the Carbrital capsule (carbromal + pentobarbitone) in particular remains unaccountably popular. Carbromal and its two analogues have a wider margin of safety than the original bromides: still, they have a potential for dependency that matches that of the barbiturates.

Paraldehyde, chemically similar to alcohol, is a volatile liquid. First prepared in 1882, it is still listed in the major pharmacopoeias. While rarely given as a hypnotic, paraldehyde is considered a safe and efficacious remedy in delirium tremens, tetanus and the repeated seizures of status epilepticus. Paraldehyde draught has an indescribably vile taste, and injection (which must be deeply into muscular tissue) is painful. Glass syringes must be used because the drug causes standard, disposable polypropylene ones to disintegrate. Another unpleasant feature is that paraldehyde is excreted partly through the respiratory tract, and the breath odour of someone who has taken the drug is nauseating and unmistakable at a considerable distance. Habituation to the substance has been recorded, but not recently.

Of the old-generation hypnotics, apart from the barbiturates, only chloral hydrate and its derivatives are regularly administered nowadays. First produced in 1869, chloral has been used ever since and appears in all pharmacopoeias. Advantages of chloral hydrate over barbiturates appear to be a slightly shorter duration of action (than, say, amylobarbitone), and a lower toxicity. In other respects it does resemble the barbitones, in that it suppresses REM sleep and its repeated use may lead to habituation. Since chloral hydrate, like other old-fashioned hypnotics, tends to upset the stomach, other related compounds have been devised with the object of overcoming this problem: hence we now have dichloralphenazone (Welldorm), chloral betaine (Beta-Chlor) and triclofos sodium (Triclos). These do not usually provoke gastric irritation and, because the margin of safety between effective and toxic doses is fairly high, they are considered suitable for insomniac children. Chloral hydrate itself is a foul-tasting volatile liquid, which the standard pharmaceutical Chloral Mixture does little to conceal. Unfortunately it is not practicable to prepare the drug in tablet form, but a few years ago E. R. Squibb Ltd. introduced an egg-shaped continuous capsule containing an appropriate quantity of chloral: the convenience of this formulation (Noctec) has boosted the drug's popularity. The precautions and contra-indications to be observed with chloral and derivatives are essentially the same as those for barbiturates, with the obvious addition of abdominal complaints such as peptic ulcer. Interactions with other drugs have not been fully studied, but it is recognized that chloral potentiates other CNS depressant substances, may interfere with the action of warfarin and similar anticoagulants, and is dangerous in conjunction with alcohol. Chloral has often been recommended as night sedation for patients, such as the terminally ill, who must take morphine or a similar opiate: the hypnotic supposedly enhances the analgesia which they provide. This combination may be inappropriate: as chloral resembles the barbiturates in so many respects, it is not unlikely that like them it might antagonize the effectiveness of analgesics.

New-Generation Hypnotics – Methaqualone and Others

The explosion in production of psychotropic drugs, which has been going on for some 30 years, has led to the synthesis of several new compounds with soporific action. In most instances this effect is secondary to the principal applications for mood-altering drugs, and some examples have already been cited. Both in terms of cost and frequency of prescription, diazepam (Valium) and those of its derivatives which are marketed specifically as hypnotics have become the most important: nitrazepam (Remnos, Mogadon) now accounts for well over half of the prescriptions for hypnotics filled in the UK. This drug and its close relatives are described in more detail below.

Of the new-generation sedatives and hypnotics, some like nitrazepam have been found both effective and safer than most alternatives, while others have turned out to be as dangerous as the barbiturates. In the latter category methaqualone is conspicuous. Introduced to the UK in the 1960s amid much publicity and advertised in ringing tones as a safe, reliable remedy for insomnia, methaqualone preparations were freely and extensively prescribed. One product in particular, combining methaqualone with the sedative antihistamine diphenhydramine, dominated the market: this was Mandrax. All other formulations of this drug having been deleted, Mandrax enjoys the dubious distinction of being the only hypnotic (barbiturates not excepted) which is restricted under the Misuse of Drugs Act. With the benefit of hindsight, one wonders why prescribers did not more quickly discover that Mandrax was powerfully euphoriant, tolerance- and dependence-producing, possessing all the undesirable qualities of the barbiturates and none of their advantages. In the USA, where methaqualone is still not adequately controlled under the law, abuse of the three branded tablets Quaalude, Parest and Sopor has in the past few years constituted a virtual epidemic among young people, and the expression 'luding out' (on Quaalude) has become part of the rock-culture's vocabulary. In this context the drug is not taken to promote sleep: the idea, on the contrary, is to remain awake and 'stoned' after consumption of doses often far in excess of those indicated therapeutically. Despite its restriction in Britain, and its high price on the illicit market, Mandrax is today much sought after by drug abusers. Its gross effects are, to the onlooker, very like those of alcoholic excess: gait becomes unsteady, speech is slurred, inhibitions are lost, and paradoxical excitement can be observed. Despite the considerable hazard of lethal overdosage, alcohol is often taken concurrently with methaqualone to increase its euphorigenic activity. Abuse of this kind tends rapidly to the onset of tolerance (the authors have observed the ingestion of 10 or more tablets at once by some persons) and to psychic and physical habituation of the barbiturate type. Chronic intoxication and withdrawal reactions are virtually indistinguishable (see under Barbiturates, above). Until legislative control of the drug, victims of accidental overdosage with methaqualone, stuporous or comatose, were a common sight in casualty departments, and death often supervened. There is currently no legitimate indication for prescribing methaqualone except to a patient who is already known to be dependent upon it. Why Mandrax in the UK, and Quaalude in the USA, continue to be available at all is beyond the present writers' comprehension. True, it is an effective sleep-inducer, and if used as directed may not be taken abusively; but given the accessibility of so many other, less hazardous hypnotics and the fact that it cannot be therapeutically used for any other purpose, methaqualone should be deleted.

Listed in the accompanying Chart III (C) are two related compounds (piperidinediones), glutethimide (Doriden) and methylprylon (Noludar). Both are employed more in continental Europe than in the UK or America, where they are no longer heavily promoted. Methylprylon and glutethimide have been included in the Chart because some authorities consider them to be helpful in insomnia, particularly when there are good reasons for contra-indicating a barbiturate. Cases of Doriden abuse and dependency have been cited, but these seem to be uncommon. Except at very high dosages the two compounds are unlikely to provoke euphoria, and fatal overdosage (either accidental or suicidal) occurs infrequently. There is little to choose between the two: however, methylprylone may have a slightly quicker onset (20–30 minutes) and marginally longer duration of action (6–8 hours). Apart from hangover in a few subjects, adverse reactions are seldom a problem. As in the case of almost all other hypnotics, caution must be exercised the day after dosage with driving and other tasks requiring swift reflexes.

Other sleeping-preparations which have not been included in the Chart are covered, like all relevant substances, in the Alphabetical Entries for individual drugs: these comprise chlormethiazole, methylpentynol, ethinamate, ethchlorvynol, and diphenhydramine and promethazine, two sedative antihistamines.

New-Generation Hypnotics: The Benzodiazepines

The reader may feel that to leave the most frequently chosen class of hypnotic until last is capricious. However, the authors considered that these agents could best be elucidated against the background of those which preceded them. All of the soporifics described thus far have real disadvantages, and most of them serious ones. In the past decade two new drugs, nitrazepam (Mogadon, Remnos) and flurazepam (Dalmane), have almost saturated the market for sleeping-preparations, and only two years ago were the related compounds temazepam (Euhypnos, Normison) and triazolam (Halcion) added to the armamentarium.

These four drugs are members of the benzodiazepine class, which means that they are similar chemically and in effect to diazepam (Valium) and chlordiazepoxide (Librium). The latter products, together with a veritable host of close chemical analogues, were originally and are still promoted as daytime tranquillizers and relievers of anxiety and tension states: these are reviewed in more depth elsewhere (see Essay VI(A): Tranquillizers). Suffice it to state here that, as all the world must be aware, when Valium and Librium became available in the early 1960s, they were advertised as almost miraculous remedies, lacking substantial adverse effects, being almost immediately effective, having no contra-indications; and, best of all, being so safe that (as one wag has put it) the only way to kill an experimental animal with a benzodiazepine was to bury it in Valium. At last, the Swiss-based firm Hoffmann-La Roche averred, the psychotropic millennium had arrived.

That some of these benzodiazepines are now marketed as hypnotics rather than as tranquillizers is arbitrary, in the sense that all the compounds of this class produce drowsiness which is dose-related. Thus, nitrazepam (advertised as a hypnotic at doses of 5–10 mg) will do very well to alleviate anxiety, if, say, 2.5 mg is taken twice daily; and conversely, that diazepam will combat insomnia in many people given 10–20 mg at night (vs 2–5 mg twice or thrice daily as an anxiolytic).

Mutatis mutandis, any of the diazepam-derived agents recommended for use during the day can be thus taken. The only real difference between them lies in their length of perceptible action (usefully indicated by the plasma $t_{1/2}$: see above under Barbiturates). Nitrazepam and flurazepam are not generally recognized to be long-acting drugs, like diazepam. But these hypnotics are likely to exert some effect through much of the day following night-sedation with them. Temazepam has a slightly shorter duration of action, but even so hangover effects are noticed by some patients. Only with triazolam, which has a plasma $t_{1/2}$ of only just over 2 hours and a pharmacological, hypnotic activity of 4–6 hours, are insidious after-effects relatively improbable (but see also below). The problem of impaired reflexes following ingestion of almost all sleeping-preparations has been mentioned and should not be overlooked merely because the individual does not feel hungover.

The Committee on Review of Medicines (CRM), already referred to in connection with the barbiturates, was busy in 1980. In March it laid down a series of recommendations concerning benzodiazepines and systematically reviewed these compounds (*British Medical Journal* vol. II for 1980, p. 1009). Most of the body's findings are summarized elsewhere in this book (pp. 344–5). As far as the prescription for benzodiazepines to induce sleep is concerned, it advocates short-term treatment only (as it does for all hypnotics). This is partly because so many thousands of people in Western countries are repeatedly – and much of the time unnecessarily – given prescriptions for nitrazepam and its relatives. This practice can easily lead to psychological and, less rarely than is usually believed, physical habituation, which for diazepam and chlordiazepoxide is well documented.

Professor Leo Hollister, a leading authority on psychotropic drugs, gives six criteria which should apply to the 'ideal' hypnotic: (1) onset of sleep should be rapid; (2) the normal pattern of sleep (especially REM sleep) should not be impaired; (3) the drug should act for sufficiently long to avoid early waking; (4) after-effects should not persist into the daytime; (5) the drug should not produce tolerance or dependence; and (6) an overdose should not be fatal. These are not listed in order of importance, but do illustrate the goal which pharmacologists have been trying to attain. How then do the benzodiazepines measure up? Hollister considers that this class of compounds most closely approaches his (intrinsically unrealistic) requirements. Numbers (1), (3) and (6) certainly apply. Flurazepam and nitrazepam (respectively the most frequently prescribed hypnotics in the USA and the UK) do affect REM sleep, and thus dreaming, only to a small extent unless very high doses are taken (2). Criterion (4) on after-effects has been touched upon: caution in driving or operating machinery after use of nitrazepam or flurazepam should be exercised. Regarding requirement (5), tolerance to any and all benzodiazepines occurs when individuals are exposed to them on a long-term basis. Physical addiction, as attested by the onset of distinct withdrawal symptoms and signs when drug is suddenly discontinued, undoubtedly represents an additional hazard to the chronic user. Nevertheless such reactions are often not severe enough to justify administration of a substitute drug (if such existed) for humane withdrawal. These may be characterized by delirium and confusion, and convulsions are sometimes experienced. As yet the extent of physical dependency is difficult to gauge, whereas the psychological craving felt by many Valium-habitués is coming to be well recognized. The lesson is obvious: short-term or intermittent prescription only of benzodiazepine hypnotics, except in psychiatric conditions (e.g. chronic anxiety states) considered severe enough to justify regular administration.

We have remarked upon the phenomenon of cross-tolerance in relation to barbiturates: this effect, whereby any one member of a class of drugs will substitute for any other, applies equally to the benzodiazepines, which with one exception are virtually identical in chemical structure. The present practice perpetrated by an alarming number of physicians (and even psychiatrists) of prescribing two or three different diazepam-type agents concurrently is to be discouraged. In many cases it appears that practitioners are unaware that the drugs which they are giving belong to the same category. Thus we find people receiving Valium three times daily and flurazepam at night. When a daytime anxiolytic effect and a sedative action are required, either drug can be used, e.g. a single adequate dose of Valium taken at night will not only ensure sleep but alleviate anxiety through the next day.

Adverse reactions to flurazepam, nitrazepam, temazepam and triazolam vary according to dosage, idiosyncrasy and other factors. Oversedation and hangover obtain more often with the first two drugs, whose actual duration of action may be double that of temazepam and triazolam. With all, blurring of vision, unsteadiness of gait and confusion may be experienced, particularly by the elderly: dosage of benzo-diazepines should generally be halved for the over-60 patient. Disinhibi-tion – loss of normal inhibitions, leading at times to bizarre or antisocial behaviour – is often ignored as an effect of high dosage regimens. Rarer side-effects are dealt with in Essay VI(A).

The authoritative *Drug & Therapeutics Bulletin,* in which new drugs are objectively analysed, has stated: 'Triazolam may help patients who have delayed onset of sleep or marked hangover effects with other benzo-diazepines, but more data are needed' (vol. 17, 1979, p. 66). A couple of weeks after this opinion, the journal published a warning. In Holland, where triazolam is very popularly prescribed, reports had appeared of severe psychological reactions to the drug, including intense anxiety, restlessness, 'paranoia' and even depersonalization. For the time being, the supply of triazolam in the Netherlands has been suspended, pending further investigation by the manufacturers and the relevant authorities. In the UK, side-effects of any kind have been stated to be uncommon. This may be because here 0.125–0.25 mg is the accepted hypnotic dose, and tablets are produced only in these two strengths. However, the Dutch have available also 0.5 mg and 1.0 mg formulations, these higher doses being often taken for sleep. (*Drug & Therapeutics Bulletin* vol. 17, 1979, p.73.) This report is quoted here because there may be sound reasons for anticipating instances of such effects with other benzodiazepines, and because it behoves all of us to treat with utmost caution claims by pharmaceutical companies that their hypnotic (or whatever) 'is well tolerated, with few unwanted reactions', an assertion frequently made in those precise terms before large-scale assessment is possible.

Nitrazepam and its analogues are not recommended for children (except when night terrors are severe), for use in pregnancy or during lactation, or for patients who have acute respiratory ailments, or serious liver or kidney complaints. Alcohol and all other CNS depressants will potentiate (enhance) these compounds' activity. Interactions which may be significant can occur with tricyclic antidepressants, such as amitriptyline (Tryptizol, Elavil) and imipramine (Tofranil); thyroid extract (thyroxine); and the anticonvulsant phenytoin (Epanutin). Hypersensitivity reactions to one benzodiazepine will occur if any other is administered.

Dosage requirements must be judged on an individual basis on account of remarkable variability in response. The figures shown in Chart III(2) should be regarded as no more than a general guide: some patients sleep well on 5 mg of nitrazepam, while others remain awake even after 20 mg of the same drug. Dosages in excess of the latter may be considered by some practitioners to be too high, but are needed for some individuals. It is evident that the standard hospital dose of nitrazepam for night sedation (one 5 mg tablet) is quite inadequate for many patients. Given the very wide margin of safety which benzodiazepines have, we feel that some physicians are too conservative in the regimens they prescribe: both the present authors, for instance, neither of whom is habituated, have found that nitrazepam 20 mg exerts no more than a slightly calming, but not a soporific, effect. In this respect they may be unusual, but the finding suggests that greater flexibility is required in determining the correct dose for any given patient. Naturally, the lowest quantity should be given which does its job, a dictum applicable to all types of medication.

Concluding Remarks

It is accepted, even by doctors who are themselves guilty of the practice, that psychotropic drugs in general, and hypnotics in particular, are overprescribed. We have seen that no individual compound or class of compounds meets Leo Hollister's criteria in all respects: he concludes, as do most of us, that benzodiazepines are probably the least harmful of the choices available. Now, however, with a spate of popular magazine articles and television reports which have recently played up these agents' adverse effects and 'mother's-little-helper' dependency, some GPs are switching their patients off benzodiazepines (as, previously, they did with barbiturates, and then methaqualone, etc.) and on to the more sedative of the tricyclic antidepressants (see Essay I) such as dothiepin (Prothiaden). This is happening not because tricyclics are safer or more effective (they are neither) but because people do not become habituated to them. Such a move is particularly unfortunate because this type of antidepressant is cardiotoxic and for this and other reasons is dangerous in overdosage.

In choosing a hypnotic, the prescriber (especially in Britain, where the £1-per-item prescription charge is nominal) should at least consider the cost as one factor in reaching a decision. Barbiturates are extremely cheap: amylobarbitone tablets 100 mg cost about £1 per hundred on a private prescription, while for the newest benzodiazepine, triazolam (Halcion) 0.25 mg tablets × 100 a charge of nearly £10 is made. These are extreme examples: they nevertheless illustrate the enormous difference in price between barbiturates, glutethimide and a few others, and the more recently introduced compounds like flurazepam and temazepam. With the annual NHS bill for hypnotics now running at £6 million per year, and with the necessity of making savings within the Health Service, one may reasonably ask how to obtain the best value. The final choice must lie with the practitioner.

Non-pharmacologic techniques of overcoming insomnia fall outside the scope of the present work. It is a fact, though, that many people find yoga, meditation, est, bio-feedback and other approaches helpful, and there is no need for the physician to be reticent about suggesting one of these.

Suggestions for Further Reading

It is a pity that there is no detailed, accurate book-length guide to sleep and hypnotics which is not somewhat technical. The following references are worth finding, nevertheless.

Hollister, Leo E.: *Clinical Pharmacology of Psychotherapeutic Drugs.* New York, 1978. pp. 50–67.

Perhaps the most up-to-date succinct account. Hollister can be criticized because of his clear predilection for the benzodiazepines, but of these he provides an excellent survey.

Harvey, S. C.: 'Hypnotics and sedatives' in Goodman and Gilman, *op. cit.* pp. 339–75.

This author gives a searching and detailed analysis, which will, however, be useful only to readers who have a background in science and understand the terminology.

Williams, R. L. and Karagan, I. (ed.): *Pharmacology of Sleep.* New York, 1976.

For those interested in the mechanisms of action of the various natural and other substances involved in sleep, and in its detailed physiology, this book can be recommended.

Zelvelder, W. G.: *Therapeutic Evaluation of Hypnotics: an experimental study in hospitalized patients.* Assen (Holland), 1971.

For the reader interested in learning how hypnotics are tested in human beings, this work will provide a first-rate introduction.

CHART III: THE BARBITURATES AND OTHER HYPNOTIC (SLEEP-INDUCING) DRUGS

NOTE: The generic (official) names of barbiturates having not been standardized worldwide, these drugs are known slightly differently in the UK and US: e.g. amylobarbitone (UK) = amobarbital (US). In the US the suffix -al is used instead of -one as in UK. Products in which a barbiturate is combined with other drugs, e.g. simple pain-killers, which are very numerous, are not listed here. Barbiturate/amphetamine combinations are considered under Amphetamines (Essay I). SLEEPING PILLS, BARBITURATE AND OTHERWISE, SHOULD BE PRESCRIBED ONLY INTERMITTENTLY.

1: BARBITURATES

Drug name	Brand name	Nightly Dose Range
a. Intermediate-Acting		
AMYLOBARBITONE (AMOBARBITAL) AMYLO-BARBITONE SODIUM	UK;US: Amytal, Sodium Amytal	50 – 200 mg
BUTOBARBITONE (BUTETHAL)	UK: Soneryl	50 – 200 mg
CYCLOBARBITONE	UK: Phanodorm	100 – 400 mg
HEPTABARBITONE	UK: Medomin	100 – 300 mg
HEXOBARBITONE (HEXO-BARBITAL)	UK: Evidorm* US: Sombulex	125 – 500 mg
PENTOBARBITONE (PENTO-BARBITAL) PENTOBARBITONE SODIUM	UK,US: Nembutal	50 – 300 mg
QUINALBARBITONE (SECOBARBITAL) QUINALBARBITONE SODIUM	UK,US: Seconal, Seconal Sodium, Tuinal**	50 – 300 mg
SECBUTOBARBITONE (BUTABARBITAL) SODIUM	US: Butisol, Buticaps	50 – 250 mg
TALBUTAL	US: Lotusate	120 – 360 mg

*with cyclobarbitone   **with amylobarbitone sodium

b. Long-Acting		
BARBITONE (BARBITAL)	UK: unbranded	150 – 300 mg †
BARBITONE SODIUM	US: unbranded	150 – 450 mg
METHARBITONE (METHARBITAL)	US: Gemonil	50 – 100 mg †
METHYLPHENOBARBITONE (MEPHOBARBITAL)	UK: Prominal US: Mebaral	30 – 100 mg †
PHENOBARBITONE (PHENOBARBITAL) PHENOBARBITONE SODIUM	UK,US: Luminal, Luminal Sodium	50 – 200 mg † 50 – 350 mg

†twice daily doses (barbiturates given in e.g. epilepsy)

Side-Effects
Common: Hangover, oversedation, unsteady gait, dizziness, impaired reflexes
Occasional: Skin rashes, fall in blood-pressure, physical and/or psychological dependency, disinhibition (see Text)
Less common: Abdominal upsets, hypersensitivity, blood disorders, paradoxical excitement

Warnings, Contra-Indications, Interactions etc

CONTRA-INDICATED in porphyria, severe liver disorders, respiratory ailments, severe pain states, known hypersensitivity; for persons liable to drug abuse
GREAT CAUTION: kidney disease, prostate enlargement, hyperthyroidism, diabetes, severe anaemia, heart disease, raised intra-ocular pressure (e.g. in glaucoma)

BARBITURATES SHOULD NEVER BE PRESCRIBED CONTINUOUSLY FOR LONG PERIODS, AS TOLERANCE OCCURS READILY. DEVELOPMENT OF PHYSICAL DEPENDENCE MAY BE INSIDIOUS.

INTERACTIONS WITH OTHER DRUGS: Barbiturates should not be given concurrently with alcohol or, in general, with other drugs which depress the central nervous system. Particularly to be avoided or used with utmost care are: coumarin anticoagulants; corticosteroids (e.g. cortisone); the contraceptive Pill; thyroxine; phenothiazines & other antipsychotic agents; phenylbutazone (Butazolidin); griseofulvin (Grisovin); pethidine & other narcotics. Phenytoin (Epanutin) may be necessary as an adjunct to a barbiturate in control of epilepsy, but in such cases regular monitoring of the patient is recommended.

2: **BENZODIAZEPINES** (members of this group used as hypnotics: see also Chart VI A: Anxiety-relieving Tranquillizers)

Drug name	*Brand name*	*Nightly Dose Range*
FLURAZEPAM	UK,US: Dalmane	15 – 45 mg
NITRAZEPAM	UK: Mogadon, Remnos	5 – 25 mg
TEMAZEPAM	UK: Euhypnos, Normison	10 – 40 mg
TRIAZOLAM	UK: Halcion	0.125 – 0.75 mg

Side-Effects
Common: Hangover (except triazolam), oversedation, unsteady gait
Less common: Physical and/or psychological dependence, skin rashes
Rare: Blood disorders, jaundice, fall in blood-pressure (see Text)

Warnings, Contra-Indications, Interactions etc
CAUTION: severe liver or kidney disease. Great care if driving or operating machinery. Possibility of physical/psychic dependence. Avoid during pregnancy. Contra-indicated in myasthenia gravis.
DRUG INTERACTIONS: Alcohol and other drugs which depress the central nervous system should be avoided if possible (e.g. antipsychotic tranquillizers, narcotics). Caution with tricyclic antidepressants, thyroid hormone, phenytoin (Epanutin)

3: **OTHER HYPNOTIC/SEDATIVE DRUGS** (see also under individual entries in alphabetical section)

Drug name	*Brand name*	*Nightly Dose Range*
CHLORAL HYDRATE	UK: Noctec US: Noctec, Felsules	500 mg – 1.5 G
DICHLORALPHENAZONE	UK: Welldorm	650 mg – 2.0 G
TRICLOFOS (SODIUM)	UK: unbranded US: Triclos	750 mg – 2.5 G

Side-Effects
Common: Abdominal upsets, e.g. stomach irritation (more likely with chloral hydrate), hangover, oversedation

Occasional: Physical and/or psychological dependence; disinhibition; rashes
Less common: Paradoxical excitement

Warnings, Contra-Indications, Interactions etc
CONTRA-INDICATED in severe liver or kidney disease, porphyria, severe cardiac or gastro-intestinal illness. Great caution in cases of respiratory insufficiency. Watch for hypersensitivity, tolerance, possibility of dependence.
DRUG INTERACTIONS: Coumarin anticoagulants should not be given with chloral and derivatives. Alcohol is contra-indicated. Other CNS depressants should be administered cautiously, if at all.

Drug name	Brand name	Nightly Dose Range
GLUTETHIMIDE	UK,US: Doriden	250 – 750 mg
METHYLPRYLON(E)	UK,US: Noludar	200 – 600 mg

Side-Effects
Common: Hangover, unsteady gait
Occasional: Disinhibition, skin rashes, paradoxical excitement, blurred vision, physical and/or psychic dependence
Rare: Dermatitis, blood disorders

Warnings, Contra-Indications, Interactions etc
CONTRA-INDICATED: known hypersensitivity, epilepsy. Caution when driving or operating machinery. Physical dependency has been reported.
INTERACTIONS: Chlorpromazine-type tranquillizers should be avoided; likewise other CNS depressants and alcohol; care with coumarin anticoagulants

Drug name	Brand name	Nightly Dose Range
METHAQUALONE	UK: Mandrax‡	150 – 500 mg
	US: Quaalude, Parest	

Side-Effects
Common: Hangover, dizziness, oversedation, disinhibition, temporary amnesia, euphoria
Occasional: Physical/psychic dependency, euphoria, paradoxical excitement, itching, sweating, abdominal upsets
Rare: Blood disorders (anaemia), toxic psychosis (see Essay)

Warnings, Contra-Indications, Interactions etc
CONTRA-INDICATED in cases of severe liver disorders, and for individuals liable to drug abuse. Physical addiction has become common. Reflexes may be impaired.
INTERACTIONS: Concurrent administration of methaqualone and alcohol is HIGHLY DANGEROUS. Effect of other CNS depressants will be enhanced, including antihistamines. Diazepam (Valium) can be fatal in combination with methaqualone.

‡ with diphenhydramine, a sedative antihistamine

IV: Morphine and Other Potent Analgesics (Narcotics)

Pain and the Discovery of the Endorphins

The subject of pain and its relief has always proved puzzling, and even with very recent advances in our knowledge of the nervous system's physiology and biochemistry much remains obscure. This is not the place for a detailed account of the physical and psychological processes whereby pain is evoked, but a particular series of fundamental discoveries has an important bearing on our comprehension of this sensation and of the drugs used to palliate it: these are described in the following pages.

First: what is pain? A deceptively simple question. All existing definitions are unsatisfactory, except perhaps that of the great Harvard anaesthesiologist Henry Beecher, who said: 'Pain is what the patient says hurts.' Many tests are employed on laboratory animals to induce pain of a type which can be measured or at least observed. Such include electrical stimulation of areas of the brain and of isolated organs, the placing of animals on hot plates, pinching the tails of rodents and so forth. Although these sound (and are) to some extent repugnant, they are necessary for the proper preliminary evaluation of pain-relieving drugs. Only a limited number of techniques may be used on human volunteers, for ethical reasons. In man, experimentally-provoked pain – such as the induction of mild electrical shocks – can be quantified but cannot reproduce the acute and chronic agonies which may be caused by trauma, surgery, cancer and a host of other conditions. The only really useful way of assessing the analgesic potency and other attributes of a new drug involves administration of the substance to actual patients. So far as potent drugs such as morphine are concerned, the first human clinical trials are almost invariably conducted on postoperative patients, whose responses can be closely monitored. Typically, one group of such patients receives the new agent, while a control group, matched for age, sex, etc. is given a standard analgesic such as morphine or pethidine. The medications are prepared, for example in capsule form, to appear identical, and only someone not directly connected with the experiment knows which units contain which drug. At the end of such a 'double-blind' trial, the code is broken and the effects of each compared. Pain relief is often measured on a numerical scoring system. Sometimes (despite the dubious ethics of such procedures) a new analgesic is compared with placebo, an inert preparation, even among patients with severe pain.

It may be well to interpolate here an explanation of the relevant terminology. 'Analgesia' is the relief or abolition of pain, and 'analgesics' (some choose the etymologically preferable 'analgetics') are substances which serve this purpose. Analgesics are commonly divided into two groups, 'simple', e.g. aspirin, and 'potent': it is the latter, as being mood-modifying drugs, with which we are concerned. Strong pain-killers like morphine or pethidine are known as 'narcotics': this expression has been used even in the medical profession to refer to any substance which is likely to be abused. However, the strict definition, employed here, applies only to powerful analgesics, most of which have a high potential for tolerance and physical or psychic dependency. In the great majority of cases such drugs are stringently controlled by law. Synonymous with 'narcotic' is the term 'opiate' or 'opioid': the latter are strictly speaking derivatives of opium but generally opiates are held to comprise both these and synthetic drugs which act in a similar manner. It will be seen from Chart IV that the main opium alkaloids morphine and codeine and their derivatives ('manufactured' and 'semisynthetic' substances) are differentiated from analgesics which are produced entirely synthetically. The expressions 'narcotic antagonist' and 'partial antagonist' are explained below.

The feeling of pain travels along nerve cells from its point of origin to the brain as waves of electrical signals: these are converted to molecular groupings known as neurotransmitters which transmit the sensation to specialized nerve-endings. The latter are called receptors and those concerned with pain nociceptors. They are found chiefly in certain areas of the mid-brain but in other regions to a lesser extent. These receptors affect the individual's perception of pain by reacting with ('binding to') a natural brain substance or substances. For some years it had been strongly suspected that a 'natural opiate' existed which bound to pain receptors. Phenomena such as the severely wounded soldier's temporary inability to feel pain in battle conditions, and the possible mechanism of acupuncture-induced analgesia (e.g. in tooth extraction), provided indirect evidence that such a chemical or chemicals existed.

In 1975 John Hughes, working under the direction of Hans Kosterlitz at the Addiction Research Unit at Aberdeen, convinced that an 'endogenous' or internal opiate-like substance existed, conducted a simple but effective series of tests. He applied extracts of pigs' brains to animal tissues (such as the isolated small-intestine of the guinea-pig) which were known to be particularly sensitive to opiate analgesics. For instance, the isolated ileum of rodents can be made to convulse by the administration of strychnine, and these convulsions are abolished when morphine is administered. Having discovered that the brain extracts exerted a definite morphine-like activity on such tissues, Hughes and others went on to identify a number of peptides, or chains of amino-acids, which had this characteristic. Three of these sequences, which he termed enkephalins, were isolated from diverse regions of the brain, and a fourth, christened endorphin, was found embedded in the pituitary gland hormone β-lipotropin. Other such peptides were subsequently discovered. Both enkephalins and endorphins bind firmly to the opiate receptors, in man as in other mammals.

The very latest research suggests that there are at least three different types of pain receptor. Morphine, heroin, methadone and other opiate 'agonists' react chiefly with μ-receptors, while partial antagonists such as pentazocine bind to κ- and σ-receptor sites. The μ-receptors are responsible for some analgesia, as well as feelings of well-being (euphoria) and dependence capacity; κ-receptors are associated with pain relief, sedation and anaesthesia and a different form of dependency; and σ-receptors with lowering of mood (dysphoria), stimulation of respiration and dilation of the pupils. This information could go far towards explaining how dependency on pentazocine, and other compounds not previously believed to be habit-forming, may arise. (cf 'Characterization of opioid receptors in nervous tissue' in *Neuroactive Peptides,* ed. A. Burgen, H. W. Kosterlitz, & L. Iverson. Royal Society: London, 1980, pp. 113–22.)

Although we are, at the time of writing, only on the threshold of understanding exactly how these endogenous opiates (and morphine-type medicaments, whose natural activity they mimic) operate, we are now closer than before to a specific understanding of the physical processes of pain, the development of addiction to narcotic drugs, and much else. While there are many apparent paradoxes to be sorted out, the discoveries mentioned constitute a major advance. Endorphin has been injected into experimental animals and gives pain relief of a type and quality which are associated with narcotic drugs: however, for reasons that are not yet clear, tolerance to its effects develops (with cross-tolerance to morphine and its analogues) and physical dependency occurs when the natural peptides are administered repeatedly to laboratory animals.

One of the most intriguing aspects of this research concerns the possible applications of enkephalins/endorphins in psychological illness and in human opiate dependency. For instance, the individual who is habituated to a narcotic has been demonstrated to possess depleted levels of these substances. It is not known whether such levels obtained prior to the onset of addiction, but if so we may have found a relatively simple, physiological explanation for the fact that some people and not others are 'predisposed' to opiate use, and take such drugs, albeit unwittingly, to bring up their endorphin titres to the required levels. This is speculation, but it is based on convincing evidence. Avram Goldstein and others have demonstrated that persons diagnosed as 'schizophrenic' likewise have abnormally low endorphin concentrations in their brains. This finding could mark the beginning of a radically new methodology for the treatment of psychiatric illnesses. An enormous amount of work remains to be carried out in this field and this is almost certain to have profound implications.

Opium and its Derivatives: History

Opium is the dried latex or gum which is extracted from the unripe seed-capsule of *Papaver somniferum,* the opium poppy. This species, similar in appearance to the common poppy, usually has white flowers and stands 3 to 5 feet tall. Its habitat is diverse: supplies of opium, both for legitimate medical use and for the black market, come mostly from India and Turkey. The 'Golden Triangle' where the borders of Thailand, Laos and Cambodia meet has also provided the raw material for illicit traffic to Western European countries and North America. The harvesting of the latex is extremely hard work: techniques differ according to place and custom, but the farmers score the seed-heads with a special knife, later returning to scrape off the sticky brown exudate.

The principal alkaloid (as plant-derived drugs are known) of *P. somniferum* is morphine, and of the two dozen others only a few have any therapeutic value. As is shown in Table '5, the quantity of opium's medicinal ingredients varies according to the country where the plant is cultivated: the morphine content may be as low as 8% or as high as 20%. Of the other alkaloids, thebaine, like morphine, has strong analgesic and narcotic properties, and one derivative of it, thebacon, has been marketed in Germany for many years as a morphine alternative (Acedicon). Papaverine has muscle-relaxant properties, but no psychotropic or analgesic activity, and is prescribed as an antispasmodic. Noscapine (narcotine), like other opium alkaloids, possesses a useful cough-suppressant action: it is an ingredient of numerous proprietary remedies in conjunction with antihistamines and other agents. Codeine too has excellent antitussive properties, and as Codeine Phosphate Linctus is prescribed more because of these than because of its analgesic effectiveness.

Opium has been employed (and on occasion enjoyed) since prehistoric times: in Switzerland, seeds and capsules of the plant dating from the late Stone Age have been found. The ancient Egyptians and Assyrians were familiar with some at least of its attributes. Greek physicians, from Hippocrates onwards, included opium in prescriptions. A remarkably accurate account of its effects was given by Dioscorides, the author of numerous Greek medical writings in the 1st century AD. The following is from his book *On Medicaments*: 'The sap [extract] itself is still further cooled, compressed, and dried. If a quantity about the size of a pea of this concentrate is taken, it relieves pain, promotes sleep, and also helps with coughs and abdominal complaints' (c.65).

Table 5: OPIUM ALKALOIDS: DIFFERENCES IN CONCENTRATION

Percentage (%) by Weight

	India	Iran	Turkey	China/'Golden Triangle'	Variation
MORPHINE	20	8–16	12	11	3–25
CODEINE	3	4	1	4	0.3–4
THEBAINE	2	3	1.5	1	0.2–3.2
PAPAVERINE	1.5	2	1.5	1	0.8–2.7

adapted from: *Benigni, R., Capra, C. and Cattorini, P. E.: Piante medicinali: chimica farmacologia e terapia* vol. 2 (Milano, 1964) pp. 1038–40.

If one had to summarize this substance's effects in a couple of sentences, Dioscorides' description could hardly be bettered, except perhaps for a reference to its habituating nature. The use of opium in the West dates back to the 16th century and beyond, as attested by its inclusion in some of the earliest Herbals. By the following century it had assumed an extremely important place in medicine. Sir Thomas Sydenham wrote in 1680 that: 'Among the remedies which it has pleased Almighty God to give man to relieve his sufferings, none is so universal and so efficacious as opium'.

Powdered Opium retains its time-honoured niche in modern pharmacopoeias, including the British and American. This dark brown, rather coarse and granular powder is standardized by modern assay techniques to contain 10% of anhydrous morphine. Contrary to the statements of some who should know better, opium powder does not have a 'characteristic' odour, unless it is first heated. Strangely, while if a small quantity is placed on the tongue its bitterness is nauseating, when smoked opium tastes sweet, even sickly. Opium tincture, or Laudanum, is also listed in the current British Pharmaceutical Codex and (though recently there have been shortages) may be prescribed, usually in diluted form. This dark brown, alcoholic liquid contains 1% morphine, which sounds very little but in fact represents 10 milligrammes per millilitre, and a normal adult dose is only 1–2 ml. Laudanum is also present in Camphorated Opium Tincture, known in the USA as Paregoric; and whereas the former is administered to provide analgesia, Paregoric (containing only 0.05% morphine together with camphor, anise oil, etc.) is liked by some physicians for the control of diarrhoea or to stop intractable coughing. It is effective for both purposes, and the content of opiate is so low that Paregoric has not much abuse potential, except of course by those already abusing drugs. Most patients are unlikely to experience psychotropic effects at the proper dosage (5–10 ml), and the taste, not dissimilar to neat Pernod but harsher, will discourage improper use. The only other available preparation containing medicinal opium as such is Ipecacuanha and Opium Tablets BPC (Dover's Powder), which are now seldom seen. These contain equal amounts of opium and of ipecacuanha, a highly potent emetic included to prevent abuse or overdosage, and prescribed to relieve diarrhoea. To most practitioners all the above-named formulations are obsolescent.

One of the greatest milestones in the history of pharmacology was the isolation of morphine from opium. For this feat Friedrich Sertürner, an apothecary working at Eimbeck, near Hanover, was responsible in about 1814. Sertürner did not merely extract the main active principle from poppy gum but carried out experiments on himself and his colleagues with the new, pure analgesic. He was evidently aware of the greater specificity of action of morphine, of the abolition of some of crude opium's unwanted effects, and of the potential therapeutic benefits. Sertürner's most important monograph on the subject, which is still well worth reading, was published in the prestigious *Annalen der Physik* in 1817 under the title 'Über das Morphium, eine neue salzfähige Grundlage, and die Mekonsäure, als Hauptbestandtheile des Opiums' (On Morphine, a new soluble base, and meconic acid, as the most important constituents of opium). The appearance of this paper spurred others on, and was quickly followed by the identification of codeine by M. Robiquet in 1832 and of papaverine by E. Merck in 1848.

The importance of his discovery was not lost on Sertürner, and the availability of a relatively pure, soluble, concentrated drug was very quickly put to widespread therapeutic use for the control of severe pain. Further, the invention of the hypodermic syringe in about 1850 greatly augmented the medicinal advantages of morphine over crude opium extract or tincture, which had of course to be taken orally. Injection of the drug, generally by the subcutaneous route, was soon the established mode of administration, providing excellent analgesia within 10–20 minutes (vs up to 1 hour for opium). Although the early syringes were mostly opaque, silver or brass, with needles to match, and aseptic techniques were (to put it mildly) not too often used or even tried, the incidence of infections resulting in skin abscesses, hepatitis and other now very familiar hazards seemed to be low. Some practitioners were even dissolving morphine in sherry before administering it to patients. Codeine, ethylmorphine and other purified alkaloids and derivatives were given in much the same way, though the absolute analgesic effectiveness of these in comparison to morphine was overrated.

Research into and development of drugs derived from the opium alkaloids have continued through to the present day. Diamorphine (diacetylmorphine, heroin) was prepared first in 1874 by C. R. A. Wright – by the heating of morphine with acetic anhydride – but it was not until 1898 that Heinrich Dreser of Düsseldorf introduced this compound to clinical medicine, under the brand name Heroin. It was Dreser, too, whom we have to thank for the synthesis of acetylsalicylic acid, better known as aspirin, which was accomplished a year later.

By this time addiction to morphine, and even more extensively to laudanum, was widespread. It was common among the higher classes and also among the poor, who used to add laudanum to their babies' feeds in order to keep them quiet. Dreser and his colleagues claimed that not only was diamorphine an excellent remedy for severe pain and cough, but it was in addition most effective in the treatment of morphine dependency. For the latter purpose heroin was a huge success: it completely abolished withdrawal symptoms within a short space of time. Only after heroin had been on the market a few years was it realized that there existed an unfortunate snag: as we now know, the new drug proved just as addictive as morphine.

Other semisynthetic opiates, most of which could also be substituted for morphine, were prepared during the period 1881 to 1959. For many years large prizes had been offered to anyone who could produce morphine synthetically, but not until 1946, when R. Grewe accomplished the difficult task, was this possible because of the complexity of the molecule. Even now, when many drugs of plant origin (e.g. cocaine) are prepared from scratch in the laboratory, pharmaceutical companies find that it is prohibitively expensive in the case of morphine, and so importation of the raw material continues.

All the morphine and codeine derivatives which are at present marketed in the UK and/or the USA as analgesics are shown in Section 1 of Chart IV. These represent more or less slight adaptations of the basic morphine or codeine (methylmorphine) molecule, but they do differ in a number of ways as is illustrated. In terms of absolute analgesic potency, dihydrocodeine and hydrocodone do not match the others, but are useful in the mitigation of mild to moderate pain and for their antitussive action.

Immediately before the Second World War, when synthetic substitutes for the above-mentioned compounds were being most actively sought, O. Eisleb and O. Schaumann prepared a large number of agents of the phenylpiperidine series, one of which was pethidine (meperidine, Demerol). Initially noted for its antispasmodic action, this drug was seen to be a viable alternative to morphine. Present-day clinicians may (justifiably, we believe) assert that its analgesic potency is not as great as that of the original opiate, and may be inadequate to control the most severe pain, and also that its usefulness is circumscribed by its very short (2–4 hour) duration of effect. Even so, pethidine is today the most popularly used of the strong analgesics. This drug was the prototype of several other medicaments developed in the post-war period, notably alphaprodine and anileridine, which are useful in obstetrics, fentanyl and phenoperidine for anaesthesia and the special technique of neurolept-analgesia (see below), and ethoheptazine, which may be taken only by mouth and relieves mild to moderate pain.

With the onset of the Second World War, Germany was cut off from its regular source of medicinal opium, as Turkey was inaccessible. Thus stocks of morphine quickly became depleted and could not be renewed. This undoubtedly spurred the researchers on to find other strong analgesics which could be made by synthesis. By 1942 Schaumann, with his colleagues M. Bockmühl and G. Erhart, had prepared methadone from a different series of compounds from that which yielded pethidine. Methadone, it was found, compared favourably with morphine for analgesia and was longer-acting. At the time both pethidine and methadone were considered to have a low dependence potential, a view which has subsequently had to be revised. From methadone, during the 1950s, dextromoramide and dipipanone were derived: both tend to produce fewer side-effects than morphine or methadone, are potent analgesics, and are certainly addictive. A further derivative, propoxy-phene (dextropropoxyphene), was less active as a pain-killer but had considerably less abuse liability.

The aim, all along, was to produce a drug which (a) would be capable of alleviating very severe pain without serious adverse effects such as respiratory depression; (b) would not be tolerance-producing if adminis-tered regularly; and (c) would lack the characteristic abuse and addiction liability typical of the opiates. Since Grewe synthesized morphine, the specific aim was to modify the morphine molecule in such a way that its analgesic activity was retained, but without its undesirable attributes. To this end, J. Hellerbach and his associates at the multinational company Hoffman-La Roche in Basel tested more than 300 compounds of the morphinan series. Of these, only three were found to be therapeutically useful. Dextromethorphan had no analgesic effect but suppressed chronic cough, and this drug now forms an ingredient in numerous over-the-counter expectorants. Levallorphan relieved pain, but as a narcotic antagonist it provoked serious adverse reactions and is now used almost exclusively to counteract opiate overdosage. The third compound, levor-phanol, demonstrated genuine advantages over standard narcotics: it relieved even the most intractable pain and was more effective when taken orally than almost all alternatives.

Concurrently with Hellerbach's work, a group led by the distinguished pharmacologists Everette L. May and Nathan B. Eddy were examining still another class of compounds, the benzomorphans. Of these one drug, phenazocine, looked promising, and in 1960 it was introduced for prescription in the USA and the UK. Here the basic morphine 'skeleton' had been adapted still further, and phenazocine emerged as an acceptable alternative for conventional opiates. Like levorphanol it could palliate extremely severe pain and, while less effective orally than levorphanol, side-effects were shown to be few and dependence potential not high. A few years later another benzomorphan, pentazocine, was developed. A partial narcotic antagonist, this agent was a moderately successful analgesic: initial predictions that it was unlikely to be habituating, however, proved incorrect (see below).

Since the introduction of pentazocine, only one new drug with fundamental morphine-like 'agonist' activity has been put on the market: piritramide, which was made available in 1972. However, the emphasis in analgesic research had shifted towards partial narcotic antagonists, of which the first introduced to relieve pain was pentazocine. Narcotic antagonists are, as their name implies, drugs which reverse the effects of morphine-like agents, such that they are useful in treating poisoning with opiates and, if administered to individuals already dependent on morphine or one of its analogues, they will precipitate withdrawal symptoms in a dramatic and, for the patient, singularly unpleasant fashion.

The original antagonist, apomorphine, was developed early in the century. Although it does counteract the effects of opiates, it is unpredictable in this respect and side-effects described as 'psychotomimetic', i.e. hallucinations, disorientation and other bizarre states, are common. Such effects are typical of narcotic antagonists. Apomorphine is seldom prescribed today, and then almost exclusively for its powerful emetic action. Nalorphine and levallorphan, prepared in the 1950s, have a similar profile of activity (but do not always produce nausea) and were known to possess good analgesic effects. Unfortunately, at therapeutic doses psychotomimetic reactions were found to occur in an unacceptably high proportion of patients. With pentazocine such side-effects were less common, and it was reasoned that because these drugs antagonized narcotics they themselves would not be habituating. The three newest additions to the armamentarium of strong analgesics – buprenorphine, butorphanol and nalbuphine – are all partial narcotic antagonists which provide effective analgesia but do not generate many unwanted reactions (below, p. 301). The attempts, which have been made by pharmacologists for many years, to separate the pain-relieving element from the undesirable effects, have now, apparently, been to some extent successful. Experience with the three new compounds, which were made available in 1977, 1979 and 1980 respectively, is as yet too limited for definitive statements to be delivered: time will tell whether they live up to expectations.

Opium Alkaloids, Morphine and Derivatives: Actions and Uses

The opium preparations already referred to, such as laudanum, have little contemporary medical use. Nevertheless, other products which contain all the opium alkaloids in purified form are still popular: these are tablets and injections which consist of 'papaveretum', i.e. of the active ingredients 50% is morphine and 50% other substances, such as codeine, papaverine and noscapine. Under the brand names Omnopon and Pantopon, papaveretum has been used for many years, and many anaesthetists prefer it to morphine for premedication before surgery. The assertion that, unlike morphine alone, papaveretum provides 'balanced' analgesia rests on the assumption that the typical side-effects of morphine, such as gut hypermotility which causes vomiting, are negated by the addition of papaverine, which relaxes smooth muscle. On the other hand, most authorities aver that the analgesic and other actions of papaveretum are entirely due to its morphine content.

Morphine itself may be given in a variety of forms – the pharmacopoeias list injections, tablets, elixirs, solutions, suppositories and others – but in common with most strong analgesics it is considerably less active orally than by injection. A tablet, for example, takes 30–60 minutes to begin exerting noticeable pain relief, while a subcutaneous injection will provide analgesia within 10 minutes in most cases. In each case effect is sustained for between 3 and 5 hours. About twice the injected dose is required for morphine to give relief when administered orally.

After an average dose of 10–20 mg, most individuals experience some side-effects. The commonest of these are sedation, nausea (with or without vomiting), constipation and respiratory depression. Other reactions are listed in Chart IV according to their probable frequency. Like other narcotics, it does not banish pain: it alters the patient's perception of it. A characteristic observation made by patients receiving opiates is: 'Yes, I can still feel the pain, but it doesn't bother me.' This is obviously related to the mood modification which some individuals find agreeable (euphoria), the sensation which leads susceptible people to crave for narcotic drugs and to become dependent on them. However, other patients dislike their psychic effects (dysphoria). The drowsiness induced by morphine differs from that promoted by other CNS sedatives, such as barbiturates, insofar as the former may not allow of sleep: thus the patient can hover in a strange state between sleep and wakefulness, which some enjoy and others find distressing.

Diamorphine, or heroin, is preferred to morphine by many clinicians because, in spite of a shorter duration of action, it begins to work very rapidly after subcutaneous or intramuscular injection (the intravenous route is rarely used therapeutically, for although onset is quicker analgesia wears off much less slowly). Almost immediately after administration, heroin is broken down in the body to morphine and other metabolites: thus heroin itself cannot be detected by blood or urine tests, which will be positive only for morphine. It is generally agreed that, by weight, diamorphine is twice as effective as morphine (5 mg being thus equivalent to morphine 10 mg). We believe that the actual ratio is closer to 1.5:1. One of the disadvantages of diamorphine is that the drug is not stable in solution, such solutions becoming unusable within a few days: thus for many years physicians adopted the inconvenient practice of dissolving special hypodermic tablets in sterile water or saline when the drug was required. Now a major manufacturer in the UK is producing freeze-dried ampoules of different strengths: each ampoule contains what appears to be a white tablet-shaped bolus, and this is readily soluble in a small volume of liquid. This presentation has enhanced a recent upsurge of popularity, and now, whether in dealing with acute pain states such as myocardial infarction ('coronary thrombosis') or terminal ones, e.g. inoperable cancer, practitioners may choose heroin over morphine. They feel that the former is less likely to depress respiration and the functions of the CNS than morphine; also that it is no more euphoriant. Most objective studies have shown little or no difference between the two drugs in analgesic or other effects, and addicts injected with morphine or heroin on a 'blind' basis have been unable to differentiate them. The comparative incidence of the most important actions of opiates is shown graphically in Chart IV and also in Table 6.

The clinical applications of the opium alkaloids and their derivatives are numerous: they may be suitable for relieving postoperative pain, inoperable malignant disease, severe trauma, in renal and biliary colic, and for premedication. Morphine and its closest analogues are less suitable than synthetic drugs (particularly pethidine) for use during labour: because some of the drug crosses the placental barrier, the baby may be born with impaired respiration. This neonatal apnoea, as it is called, can be reversed by naloxone or one of the other narcotic antagonists, but obviously it is unfortunate to have to resort to this. The effect of opiates on respiratory function makes them undesirable where breathing difficulties already exist, for instance in bronchial asthma and chronic bronchitis. Other reasons for caution, such as raised intra-cranial pressure, as may occur after head injury, are listed in the Chart. Where severe liver or kidney disorders are present, very great care must be exercised.

Hydrocodone, hydromorphone (Dilaudid), oxycodone (Proladone) and oxymorphone (Numorphan) are in all significant respects similar to morphine: equivalent dosages are shown in Table 6. Hydrocodone (Dicodid) is less active than the others for pain relief; but its cough-suppressant properties are noteworthy. In the UK the only formulation to contain this compound is Dimotane-DC, an expectorant which, although giving only 1.8 mg per 5 ml of hydrocodone, is restricted in the same way as much more potent opiate products. The 1980 edition of *American Drug Index* lists five similar preparations, while in Canada more than 20 syrups or linctuses, usually containing hydrocodone with antihistamines and

Table 6: PHARMACOLOGY OF NARCOTIC ANALGESICS

Drug	Analgesia	Sedation	Respiratory Depression
Morphine	+ +	+ +	+ +
Diacetylmorphine (Heroin)	+ +	+ +	+ +
Ethylmorphine (Dionin)	+		+ +
Nalorphine (Nalline)		+ or 0	±
Codeine	+	+	+
Hydromorphone (Dilaudid)	+ +	+	+ +
Methyldihydromorphinone (Metopon)	+ + +	+ +	+ + +
Hydrocodone (Dicodid, etc.)	+		±
Dihydrocodeine (Paracodin, etc.)	+		+
Dihydrodesoxymorphine (Desomorphine)	+ + +		
Oxymorphone (Numorphan)	+ +		+ + +
Oxycodone (Percodan)	+	+ +	+ +
Levorphanol (Levo-Dromoran)	+ +	+ +	+ +
Racemorphan (Dromoran)	+ +	+	+ +
Levallorphan (Lorfan)		+	+
Pentazocine (Talwin)	+ +	+ + or 0	+ +
Oxilorphan (BC–2605)			
Buprenorphine (M–6029)	±		
Naloxone (Narcan)			
Naltrexone (EN–1639A)			
Methadone (Dolophine, etc.)	+ +	+	+ +
L-alpha-acetylmethadol (LAAM)		±	
Propoxyphene (Darvon)	+	+	+
Fentanyl (Sublimaze)	+ +		+
Noracymethadol	+ +	+ +	+ +
Dextromoramide (Palfium, etc.)	+ +	+	+ +
Meperidine (Demerol, etc.)	+ +	+	+ +
Alphaprodine (Nisentil)	+ +	+ +	+ +
Anileridine (Leritine)	+ +	+ +	+ +
Piminodine (Alvodine)	+ +	+	+ +
Ethoheptazine (Zactane)	±		+
Methotrimeprazine (Levoprome)	+	+ + +	+

NOTES

+ = Degree of activity from the least (±) to the greatest (+ + +) activity.
0 = Produces the opposite effect.

from: Morris, R. W. 'The use and abuse of narcotic analgesics and antagonists', in *pharm Index* vol. 19 no. 7 (1977) p. 13 (reproduced by kind permission) cf Chart IV

Emesis/Nausea	Constipation	Anti-tussive	Physical Dependence	Dose in mg
+ +	+ +	+ +	+ +	10
+	+ +	+ +	+ + +	4
		+ + +		
				C
+	+	+ + +	+	120
+	+	+ +	+ +	2
+ +	+	+ +	+	3
	?	+ + +	+	15
+		+ + +	+	60
	+		+ + +	1
+ + +	+ +	+	+ + +	1
+ +	+ +	+ + +	+ +	10
+	+ +	+ +	+ +	2
+	+	+ +	+ +	2½
+		+		C
+ +	+		+	45
			+	C
				C
				C
				C
+	+ +	+ +	+	10
	+			
+	+		±	240
				0.2
+ +			+	10
+ +	+		+	5
?	+		+ +	100
+	+		+	40
?	+	+ +	+ +	40
+	+		+ +	10
	+		±	100
				20

? = Questionable activity.
Blank space indicates that no such activity has yet been reported.
C = Used solely as narcotic antagonist and not as analgesic.

respiratory stimulants, are marketed. Oxycodone may be obtained in Britain only as suppositories: the drug is an excellent analgesic in this form and its duration of action is significantly greater than that of most analogues. In the USA oxycodone is available in tablet form, the best-known product being 'Percodan', whose analgesic effect gains little from the addition of aspirin, phenacetin and caffeine. Oxymorphone (Numorphan) is presented only in injectable form, and hydromorphone (Dilaudid) as tablets, ampoules, syrups and suppositories. Hydrocodone has an intermediate abuse potential, but the other three compounds described here are as liable as morphine to give rise to addiction. The fact that hydromorphone (Dilaudid) tablets are advertised in American medical journals to relieve 'the pain you [the physician] see every day' is quite incredible.

Codeine itself has been overrated as a pain-killer: in this respect its potency does not approach that of morphine or hydromorphone, however much is administered. It is nonetheless useful in the control of moderately severe, especially chronic, pain states. There is little if any evidence that its effectiveness is enhanced by the standard combinations with aspirin and caffeine. The stronger oral codeine tablets (30 and 60 mg) are surprisingly under-used. As an injection, the alkaloid is predictably more potent as an analgesic: it should, however, be borne in mind that codeine injections are incompatible with several other medications which may need to be given concurrently. Ethoheptazine (Zactane, Zactipar, Zactirin) and dextropropoxyphene (propoxyphene, Darvon, Doloxene, Distalgesic), mostly available in conjunction with aspirin or paracetamol, are similar to codeine in analgesic effect, while codeine has the additional advantage of being still one of the most efficacious remedies for diarrhoea and for chronic cough.

Dihydrocodeine was developed in the early years of the present century, but the introduction of DF-118 preparations about 20 years ago heralded a resurgence of interest in this drug. Today, in the UK, dihydrocodeine tablets are perhaps more frequently prescribed than any other strong analgesic. One of the principal explanations for this commercial success is undoubtedly that fact that these tablets are exempt from Misuse of Drugs regulations (although the ampoule formulation is not). In absolute terms, the pain-relieving potency of DF-118 bridges the gap between the simple analgesics and the narcotics, and is rather stronger than codeine. As it is not under special legal restriction it is difficult to estimate the extent of dependency, but on the basis of anecdotal evidence it seems that dihydrocodeine has a significant potential for habituation, and tolerance certainly develops quickly in some cases. The drug is given occasionally to suppress cough but chiefly to mitigate a wide variety of pain states. It is not always effective in controlling the symptoms of inoperable cancer and other extremely severe types of pain where morphine would usually be employed.

Synthetic Narcotics: Agonists

Pethidine (meperidine, Demerol) has become a standard drug, having outstripped morphine in the quantity given in emergencies and in the numbers of prescriptions written annually. Its apparent tendency to produce less respiratory depression than other opiates has made it the compound of choice in handling labour pains, although it has many other applications and may be used in place of morphine in many clinical situations. As is usual with strong analgesics, pethidine has a slow onset of action when taken by mouth, while injection produces very rapid relief. Whatever route of administration is chosen, however, the drug has an appreciably shorter duration of effect than most other comparable analgesics. Its newer analogues alphaprodine (Nisentil) and anileridine (Leritine) share this disadvantage, and provide pain relief for a maximum of about 4 hours, often less. The capacity of these compounds for abuse and addiction is slightly less than that of morphine, but pethidine dependency is, relatively, not uncommon: for reasons which are obscure it is the drug most often chosen by physician addicts.

Fentanyl (Sublimaze) and phenoperidine (Operidine), which are pethidine derivatives, have a highly specialized application. This is in the technique of neuroleptanalgesia: fentanyl in combination with the major tranquillizer (neuroleptic) droperidol is administered to induce a state of anxiety-free analgesia (thus neurolept-analgesia), whereby the patient may be operated upon while conscious and can co-operate with the surgeon. The two compounds are given intravenously to produce respiratory depression in operations where assisted ventilation is necessary. This mode of injection gives fentanyl and phenoperidine a duration of action of only ½–1 hour, but lately, administered by the intramuscular route, the former has been used to alleviate pain postoperatively and may then be effective for a much longer period than had been supposed. Side-effects of pethidine and its analogues bear close relation to those of morphine but, while qualitatively similar, they tend to be milder at the doses normally prescribed.

From the shortest-acting of the narcotics, we now turn to one which may provide pain-relief for up to 6 hours and other effects for more than 8: this is methadone (Physeptone, Dolophine), which as has been stated was devised in wartime Germany as a synthetic alternative to morphine. It is slightly more potent, weight for weight, and is prescribed in the same range of clinical situations. Adverse effects are almost identical to those of morphine, and addiction liability is high. Methadone's derivatives dextromoramide (Palfium) and dipipanone (Diconal) show the same profile of activity as the parent drug and both have become popular among opiate users in the UK during recent years: over the past decade a steep increase in the number of notified addicts to dipipanone (Diconal) has been observed. Methadone is used widely in the treatment of heroin addiction (see below, p. 307).

The three last-named compounds listed in Section 2 of Chart IV each belong to separate chemical categories but they all possess some morphine-like characteristics and are administered in situations where conventional opiates would normally be given. Because clinical experience with it is relatively limited, piritramide (Dipidolor) is so far recommended only for use following surgery, when patients' responses can be carefully watched. At the time of writing, the authors are not aware of any particular benefits which piritramide, introduced in 1972, can confer which other analgesics cannot. Published studies indicate that side-effects are basically similar to those of morphine, say, or pethidine, and importantly that the drug produces at least as much respiratory depression as agents of comparable analgesic potency. Theoretically piritramide is considered a substance which can be abused in the same way as other opiates: however, given the very high cost of the drug and its limited clinical applications, it is not surprising that so far there have been few reported cases of addiction.

While the chemical resemblance of levorphanol (Dromoran, Levo-Dromoran) to morphine is more apparent than that of other strong synthetic analgesics, this drug does show some degree of separation of the mandatory pain-relieving from the undesirable actions which has been so long sought. Whereas most morphine analogues are poorly absorbed from the gut, levorphanol is often successful in alleviating very intractable pain if it is administered in the form of tablets. The assertion of its manufacturers, Hoffman-La Roche, that the compound is almost as effective by weight by the oral route as by injection is an exaggeration: the ratio is probably about 1 to 2 or 2.5, which is still higher than for many opioids. Adverse reactions from levorphanol tend to be mild, with little or no euphoria normally felt at therapeutic doses. Dependency on this compound is not common.

Most of the statements made in the foregoing paragraph apply equally to phenazocine (Narphen): it is a very potent pain-killer, with rather few side-effects, it is not normally euphorigenic, and addiction is even rarer than for levorphanol. Clearly in both cases the fact that mood changes, when they occur at all, are slight would render them unpopular with opiate abusers, although phenazocine and levorphanol are restricted under the Misuse of Drugs Act. Phenazocine is now available only in tablet form and nowhere but in the UK: this is unfortunate because as an injection it is an excellent analgesic, and its oral potency is reckoned to be about only a quarter of its strength when given parenterally.

In the case of each analgesic described, we have noted what is considered to be the potential for misuse and addiction, relative to well-known 'drugs of abuse' such as morphine, diamorphine and pethidine. It should be understood, however, that precise estimates cannot in most cases be made, particularly where completely illegal use is concerned. For some years now there have existed a number of protocols for determining the physical dependence capacity (PDC) of any new analgesic. One of the most important tests which are carried out before the drug is marketed has been developed by H. F. Fraser, Harris Isbell, and latterly by Donald R. Jasinski and his colleagues at the Federal Addiction Research Center at Lexington, Ky. Since experiments on laboratory animals are for various reasons unsatisfactory, volunteers are used in this institution who are generally ex-addicts. In one test a group of such patients are maintained on morphine for a given period and then the drug under trial is given instead: whether or to what extent the new compound abolishes the withdrawal syndrome which would normally arise is established. Thus, if this completely suppresses the abstinence reactions of morphine, it must have a comparable PDC. Under another protocol the subjects are allowed to take the new drug as often and in as high a dosage as they wish, perhaps for a period of several weeks. At a certain point they are given what is euphemistically termed a 'naloxone challenge': naloxone is a very pure and potent narcotic antagonist, so that if the compound being tested is significantly morphine-like the administration of naloxone induces almost immediate withdrawal effects. During the earlier part of the trial the patients are monitored for physical signs and asked a series of questions about a substance's psychological effects, e.g. whether it makes them 'high'. Experiments of this sort are carried out under 'blind', and usually controlled, conditions, to eliminate observer bias and other problems. Nevertheless the set-up is inevitably artificial and may ultimately bear little comparison to the PDC as this might be seen, for instance, in a group of cancer sufferers, or even in the circumstances of the illicit drug market. Sadly, it appears that the Lexington protocols provide the least unreliable predictive assessments of new analgesics which it is possible to devise. Their limitations, however, are not sufficiently realized.

Partial Antagonists and Pure Narcotic Antagonists

The expression 'narcotic antagonist' has been referred to briefly in connection with apomorphine, nalorphine (Lethidrone, Nalline), levallorphan, (Lorfan), pentazocine (Fortral, Talwin) and other drugs. For convenience the strong analgesics may be divided into the 'agonists', such as morphine, which are antagonized by all the above-mentioned compounds; and 'partial antagonists', e.g. pentazocine, which are prescribed for pain relief but which partially reverse the effects of narcotics (see above, p. 290, and Chart IV). A third category consists of pure antagonists, of which the only example yet available is naloxone (Narcan): this has no analgesic activity but in recent years has proved far superior to the partial antagonists (nalorphine, levallorphan) in the treatment of opiate overdosage. To make matters yet more complicated, the partial antagonists are in most cases themselves antagonized by 'pure' drugs such as naloxone. It will be recalled that apomorphine, nalorphine, and levallorphan, despite having some analgesic efficacy, were found to be unusable clinically because of the high incidence of weird and distressing adverse reactions, notably hallucinations, depersonalization and other symptoms more usually associated with psychotic states (hence the adjective psychotomimetic).

In the half-dozen years since its introduction, naloxone (Narcan) has proved to be a remarkably safe and effective remedy for poisoning with morphine and its analogues: it has a short duration of action (½–1 hour) but because of its low toxicity repeated doses can be given. Naloxone is spectacularly good at reversing narcotic-induced respiratory difficulties, not only in the overdosed adult patient but in newborn babies whose mothers have received pethidine to relieve labour pains. Unlike the vast majority of new drugs, which have been developed by the multinational pharmaceutical companies or large organizations such as the US National Institutes of Health, naloxone was synthesized by Mozes Lewenstein in his private laboratory. While this compound itself has become an essential part of the therapeutic armoury, some of its derivatives and analogues are being evaluated for various possible applications.

The development of pentazocine in the early 1960s has been seen as important, because here at last was a partial narcotic antagonist which gave a reasonable level of analgesia without, evidently, also provoking psychotomimetic side-effects. Early testing of this benzomorphan compound suggested a favourable comparison with morphine and pethidine: apparently, it appeared to lack PDC almost entirely. Pentazocine (Fortral, Talwin) was first marketed amidst much fanfare and is still heavily promoted by advertisements in medical journals. Apart from the claim that Fortral is as powerful for analgesia as pethidine, the fact that the product is not restricted under the Misuse of Drugs Act is stressed. Partly on account of this physicians are prescribing the various formulations of pentazocine increasingly, and for conditions – e.g. chronic pain states in illness that is not immediately life-threatening – when opiates would seldom be given. So far as the most severe pain is concerned, many have found the drug disappointing, for it may not only be ineffective but its adverse reactions have been understated. Psychotomimetic states can follow administration of pentazocine, more often when it is injected than when taken orally, and a variety of other unpleasant reactions may occur whatever route is chosen: nausea, dizziness, sedation and dysphoria are not uncommon. Additionally, several papers in the medical literature have documented abuse of the compound and in some cases habituation, chiefly but not exclusively among persons who had previously abused narcotics. Some authors in the UK have lately recommended that pentazocine be placed under the same legal control as the agonist opiates, and in France this has been done.

So, after all, the fact that an analgesic happens to be a partial narcotic antagonist gives no guarantee that it will not be liable to abuse. Recent research in the field has continued to centre on drugs of this category, as is evidenced by the appearance in rapid succession of three new partial antagonist analgesics: buprenorphine (Temgesic, UK 1977), butorphanol (Stadol, US 1979, UK 1980) and nalbuphine (Nubain, US 1980). All three are unquestionably strong pain-relievers, and appear comparable with morphine and pethidine in this respect. Side-effects tend to differ slightly from those commonly associated with opiates, as indicated (Chart IV, Section 3), and seem in most cases to be mild and transient. According to the Lexington protocols already described, these new analgesics are predicted to have a low potential for abuse, development of tolerance, and dependency. But until further studies have been carried out, in general practice as well as in the hospital environment, it is not possible to declare with certainty that they are unlikely to be misused – and, given experience with pentazocine, all claims should be examined critically. Buprenorphine, of the three, has one particular advantage and one disadvantage: respectively, its long duration of action (6–8 hours), and the fact that it is not antagonized by naloxone. A most important point concerning all antagonists, partial or otherwise is that if pentazocine, buprenorphine, butorphanol or nalbuphine are administered to patients who have been receiving morphine or other agonists (and who may therefore have become dependent), withdrawal reactions may be very rapidly provoked. Contra-indications for partial antagonists are similar to those for conventional opiates (see Chart), and in addition, until further clinical experience is gained, these should not be given during pregnancy. Interactions with other drugs (apart from agonists) have not as yet been documented.

Research in an entirely different direction is being actively pursued at the present time. Hitherto all the potent analgesics which have become available have been, by virtue of their chemistry and/or their pharmacology, narcotic agonists or partial Pantagonists. The American-based pharmaceutical company Pfizer is responsible for the development of a quite new type of pain-killer. The compound on which studies are continuing is nantradol (levonantradol), an extremely complex chemical structure which has been modified from $\triangle^9$-tetrahydrocannabinol (THC), one of the active alkaloids of cannabis (q.v.). Tests with laboratory animals and with a limited number of human volunteers show that nantradol has strong pain-relieving activity, without any opiate-like effects (it does not bind to opiate receptors and is not antagonized by naloxone), although immediate plans involve its use in clinical trials as an anti-emetic. In this respect the drug's potency has been established, but it could, if preliminary findings are confirmed by experiments with sufferers from severe acute or chronic pain, represent a remarkable breakthrough in analgesic research. Nantradol appears to be active both orally and by injection, and to give pain relief lasting from 3 to 6 hours. It has not yet been revealed whether, or to what extent, the compound's psychological effects are cannabis-like. Even if this should prove to be the case, it would not necessarily detract from nantradol's clinical usefulness.

The role which opiates play in the prevention and control of intractable pain states, such as may occur in terminal cancer, can hardly be overemphasized. It is as yet unclear whether partial antagonists which are said to be very potent analgesics will be satisfactory in this kind of situation. The hospice movement, pioneered by Dame Cicely Saunders, has fully understood the need to keep cancer patients not only free from pain but from anxiety that it will recur: this can be achieved in most cases by a 3- or 4-hour regimen of a suitable drug (morphine is one of several alternatives), by whatever route is necessary. A syrup may be preferable to tablets for some patients, and others may need injections or suppositories for greater or more long-lasting effect. The quantity of drug required varies considerably: 10–20 mg of morphine may be adequate for the majority of patients, 4-hourly, but others may need 100 mg. This may sound a lot, but the authoritative *Drug & Therapeutics Bulletin* (18: 70, 1980) regards it as 'quite acceptable'. Many practitioners still balk at prescribing at such levels: however, when intense, insupportable pain is present, it is wholly inappropriate to play the numbers game. Some doctors worry about the prospect of addiction, but in terminal cases this is irrational.

According to a recent study by Murray Parkes (*Journal of the Royal College of GPs* 28: 19–30, 1978), whose findings have been confirmed by Robert Twycross and other specialists in terminal care, more than one-half of terminally ill patients continued to suffer severe pain up to the time of their death. This is an appalling reflection on GPs and others, who could in virtually every case provide substantial relief of symptoms by proper prescribing of strong analgesics, and in certain cases other drugs concomitantly. Evidence from the hospices shows that this goal can be achieved, and that many sufferers can be maintained on a stable dose regimen for months or even longer. The present authors have known many instances in which patients with inoperable cancer have been denied opiates altogether, or have been prescribed ludicrously ineffective doses at far too long intervals.

It sometimes happens that an individual, old or young, is afflicted with a chronic or intermittent severely painful illness for which only palliative treatment is available: trigeminal neuralgia is one example (though surgery helps in some cases), and herpes zoster (shingles) another. While neither ailment is lethal, intense suffering may arise which only the most powerful of analgesics will mitigate. It is arguably unreasonable, even if such a complaint is not immediately life-threatening, for the practitioner to withhold suitable medication. It is truly remarkable how willing doctors are to prescribe pentazocine (Fortral) or dihydrocodeine (DF–118) to alleviate almost any type of pain. This has less to do with these compounds' analgesic effectiveness (which is limited) than with the fact that neither is subject to the Misuse of Drugs Act. This although both drugs are probably more likely, *ceteris paribus*, to produce dependence if taken repeatedly than certain other strong analgesics – e.g. levorphanol (Dromoran) and phenazocine (Narphen) – which are thus restricted. A kind of phobia obtains in Anglo-Saxon countries in respect to this and similar statutes among many practitioners. While obviously we are not advocating the indiscriminate prescribing of narcotics, we do believe that one of the physician's paramount responsibilities is to relieve pain, by whatever means may be appropriate in individual cases. Naturally the doctor should take care to titrate dosage accordingly and to watch for signs of tolerance and habituation in patients suffering from very severe but not necessarily terminal pain states.

In the Federal Republic of Germany, recent (1978) amendments to the relevant legislation have set maximum daily doses for opiate analgesics: the drugs and quantities concerned are described in Annex 3 of this book. These could serve as a general guide to acceptable doses in the higher range, which may be required for some patients (e.g. terminal cancer sufferers with bone metastases), bearing in mind the possibility of tolerance developing over time and, possibly more importantly, of the variation – which may be great – in individual response.

Still popular as a preparation for use in terminal cancer is the 'Brompton Cocktail', which contains a mixture of diamorphine and cocaine in equal quantities. The addition of cocaine is intended to decrease the risk of respiratory depression and perhaps to induce a greater euphoria. So far as the cocktail's analgesic effectiveness is concerned, Ronald Melzack and his colleagues have found it to be indistinguishable from that provided by morphine elixir alone (*Canadian Medical Association Journal* 120: 435, 1979). It does seem likely, nonetheless, that the mixture enhances a feeling of well-being: this is why opiate addicts, in the days when heroin and cocaine were prescribed for them concurrently, enjoyed the combination more than the opiate alone.

Opiate Addiction – Myth and Fact

The World Health Organization has laid down three main criteria for addiction, which are now generally accepted: (1) the individual has an overpowering desire or craving for repeated administration of the drug;

(2) tolerance to the drug's effects develops readily with repeated use; and (3) a clearly defined withdrawal syndrome sets on when the drug is suddenly discontinued. All the opiate agonists, and maybe the partial antagonists, possess these characteristics in different degrees. It is commonly supposed that if any individual takes morphine or another narcotic analgesic (even therapeutically, to alleviate pain) for a period of weeks or months, addiction will occur. This has been demonstrated to be false: for example, some, not all, patients discharged from hospices after unexpected remissions of inoperable cancer, who may have been receiving quite large doses of opiates for considerable periods, may evidently be withdrawn from morphine without the appearance of withdrawal symptoms. Likewise, experience in the hospice movement indicates that terminally ill patients may need no increase in the dose of narcotic prescribed, even over a period of months. And in most of these patients craving for drug does not occur, provided obviously that sufficient doses are given in the first place to attenuate pain and to forestall the apprehension that it will recur. It has already been observed that a proportion (perhaps even a majority) of patients do not find the opiates' mood-modifying effects agreeable.

When such drugs are taken non-medically, however, the matter is different; but even in these circumstances the WHO criteria do not necessarily apply. Individual response to this class of compounds is extremely variable, in terms of the time taken for tolerance to occur and of frank dependency to begin. The popular image of 'one-shot-and-you're-hooked' is absurd. While many so-called authorities write of unstable young people drifting into opiate addiction, who as it were become addicted by accident, a much more frequent phenomenon (as the present writers believe) is the knowing, even purposeful, development of a narcotic 'habit'. To illustrate: heroin (or morphine, or any opiate) must be taken daily for a period of at minimum several weeks before severe withdrawal reactions are felt on abrupt discontinuation. Some would claim that the required time is longer still. It is perfectly true that addicts can eventually tolerate many times the therapeutic dose of their chosen drug; but even persons habituated for many years may be 'maintained' on dose levels which hardly exceed those normally used in medicine. The speed with which abstinence reactions follow the last dose varies according to the narcotic used: with pethidine, one of the shortest-acting, these symptoms may begin in less than 8 hours; with heroin or morphine, in 8–16; and with long-acting methadone they may not be apparent for 24 hours or more. If the withdrawal syndrome is left to run its course, and the addict kicks 'cold turkey', this may last 2–4 days in the case of heroin and about 7 days with methadone.

The severity of abstinence reactions will also vary according to the length of time that the individual has been dependent and the previous daily dose, as well as the addict's own idiosyncrasy. How serious these may be also depends on the drug or drugs used: at one end of the scale, it appears that heroin and methadone withdrawal is extremely painful and debilitating, while on the other dihydrocodeine and levorphanol may provoke reactions which are not much more than uncomfortable. But it is impossible to generalize on the subject: the treatment of withdrawal symptoms must be empirical, depending on all the factors mentioned. Graphic descriptions of abstinence phenomena have been provided by William Burroughs in such works as *Junky* and *The Naked Lunch*, the latter an inspired, surrealistic account of the processes of opiate addiction: the reader will learn more about the field from these works than from many of the available medical texts.

What then are the principal features of the withdrawal state? The patient's pupils will be dilated (or will respond to light), and he may experience trembling, diarrhoea, profuse sweating, nausea and vomiting, stomach cramps, profound depression and a phenomenon which Burroughs has called the 'cold burn' (a kind of fever). Apprehension may play a role in eliciting any or all of these effects, which may begin early on account of auto-suggestion if the habitué can reasonably predict that he will not obtain his next dose. Cross-tolerance is an important element, i.e. virtually any opiate agonist will substitute for any other. Thus, if heroin becomes unavailable, pethidine, methadone and several other compounds will stave off withdrawal symptoms completely, while the milder opiates (codeine, dihydrocodeine) will do so partially. Techniques of humane withdrawal from narcotics are various: often, methadone is substituted for heroin during the acute phase. Another method involves administration of diphenoxylate (Lomotil) and chlormethiazole (Heminevrin) tablets to mitigate the worst reactions. Diphenoxylate is technically an opiate because of its chemical structure (it is related to pethidine), but it has no analgesic activity and is prescribed almost exclusively as a remedy for diarrhoea. Chlormethiazole is a sedative and anticonvulsant which has been found useful in treating alcoholic delirium tremens.

The popular image of the heroinist as an emaciated, ill person who is dirty, unkempt, dishonest and unstable undoubtedly applies to many of the street addicts seen in London, New York and other Western cities: to such individuals their drug is the most important thing in life and all else may be subordinated to buying ('scoring'), selling and taking it. It is often not realized, however, that the appearance and attitude of the 'junkie' are not necessarily due to the direct effects of heroin (or any analogous drug). For example, because opiates decrease appetite, some chronic users do not eat properly: hence, resistance to illness and infection are lowered. This may be further undermined by unsterile injection techniques. Street heroin ('Chinese H') is obviously not sterile and is commonly adulterated, or 'cut', with lactose and other substances which bulk it out. If such powders are dissolved in ordinary water, aspirated into an unclean syringe, and injected via a dirty hypodermic needle, the likely effects on the organism are obvious: abscesses and cellulitides at the site of injection, and the real hazards of septicaemia (blood-poisoning) and hepatitis, a viral infection of which a virulent, dangerous new strain ('B: Australia antigen' type) has appeared in recent years. In these circumstances, it is remarkable that fatalities do not occur more often.

Most of the phenomena described are a function of opiate use which is illicit, although some of them may arise even when an addict is receiving his drugs on prescription. Social attitudes may drive the habitué into a *demi-monde* of outcasts and criminals: something that Thomas Szasz has aptly described as the 'ritual persecution of addicts'. In previous eras, when no stigma was attached to the taking of opiates, it was perhaps easier for the user to live a near-normal life. It should be remembered that many famous and highly talented people – De Quincey, Coleridge, Elizabeth Barrett Browning, J. M. W. Turner, and in our own time Billie Holliday, Lenny Bruce, Jimi Hendrix – have relied on opium and its derivatives, their creativity not necessarily impaired. The present authors have known a number of individuals, including physicians, whose dependency on narcotics in no way precluded their making a valuable contribution to society, whose health was evidently not impaired, and whose secret (for such today it must be) would not be detectable. We are not seeking to condone addiction, but neither must we condemn opiate use without applying the most stringent ethical standards. On the one hand, the West allows and even encourages the use of alcohol, with all its sequels, while opium and its derivatives, which objectively can hardly be described as more dangerous, are outlawed.

Most people would quite properly condemn the organizations involved in smuggling and selling hard drugs. The poor populations of the Golden Triangle can, though, hardly be blamed for continuing to grow a cash crop, opium, which they have done for centuries and whose use in the local community (like alcohol in the West) is institutionalized. Harvesting the poppy gum is back-breaking labour, for which the farmer in Laos or Burma may receive less than $50 per kilo (200 man-hours). By the time this opium is converted to 80% pure heroin it is worth $4,000 a kilo: the process, carried out increasingly in the country of origin but also in European countries such as France and Italy, is simple, requiring no more skill than a chemistry graduate can provide. This process was graphically shown in the two *French Connection* movies. By the time the heroin reaches its ultimate and most profitable destination, the USA, its value has jumped to $20,000, paid by the wholesaler, and to more than $400,000 when, adulterated to a purity of 3–6%, the street 'pusher' obtains it.

All kinds of measures have been adopted by governments to try to stop this traffic. Law-enforcement agencies in all Western countries have been reinforced and today the US government spends $20 billion annually to combat the trade in various ways: the attempts to persuade the Thai farmer to grow alternative crops, the breaking of the 'French connection' (which has now re-formed), increased facilities for treating users, the persuasion of Turkey to cease opium production for a large sum in dollars (which failed), recruitment of more and better-trained police and customs-officials, training of dope-sniffing dogs . . . Yet still enough heroin gets through to supply the requirements of the estimated 600,000 American addicts and the growing number of opiate habitués in Britain and the continent of Europe. The Vietnam war provided extraordinary opportunities for smuggling via the US military postal service, and the thousands of veterans who returned, addicted to heroin, shocked the American government anew. With this channel closed, alternative smuggling systems were devised, via Mexico and South America, to meet the ever-expanding demand.

In the UK, before 1970 the quantity of black-market heroin was negligible, for reasons which we shall discuss. Since then, according to Home Office records, 3.3 kilogrammes of the drug were seized in 1973, rising to 20.2 in 1976 and 60.8 kg by 1978. At the time of writing (1980) there exists in London, partly due to the Iranian revolution, more illicit heroin than there are individuals who require it, and the price has dropped from £120 per gramme in 1978 to £60 or less now. It is assumed that only a small fraction of the total quantity imported is intercepted.

The British System and Methadone Maintenance

For several decades in the UK a system operated which obviated the kind of situation which obtained in New York and other American cities, where the only way an addict could receive heroin was through the black market and at prices which forced him to crime in order to pay for his habit. Prior to 1967, any British physician could prescribe opiates, whether morphine, heroin, or whatever was chosen, for persons who were addicted: under a voluntary scheme, such addicts were notified to the Home Office. Up to the 1960s less than five hundred people were thus 'registered', whether because they had begun opiate use non-medically or because they had become dependent in the course of medical treatment. There was no social problem. Then, by about 1964, it became known that a few practitioners (literally no more than a dozen) were overprescribing heroin and cocaine to a considerable extent, in the case of the worst offenders simply for ready money. There was thus available a surplus of legally prescribed drugs which proved sufficient to introduce many novices to opiate addiction. Addicts often obtained large prescriptions, a portion of which would be sold to cover the doctor's and pharmacist's charges. The philosophy was then that if a person was opiate-dependent, he should be encouraged by his doctor to 'kick the habit', but that otherwise the humane course of action was to prescribe as the individual practitioner deemed appropriate.

In 1962 about 500 opiate users were registered, but by 1966 the total had risen to 1,349 and by 1967 to 1,729. Partly on account of this increase, especially among the young, and partly because of the sensational treatment by the press of two or three irresponsible prescribers, in 1968 there were hastily established Drug Dependency Clinics (DDCs). These were attached to the psychiatric departments of a number of hospitals, mostly in London. Henceforth, only specially licensed practitioners, who ran these clinics, most of whom had no previous experience of treating narcotics users, were permitted to prescribe heroin or cocaine to addicts. (These drugs could continue to be given by other doctors in cases of organic illness or injury.)

Many practitioners resented this curtailment of their prescribing rights, at least in principle. One of the ironies of the new arrangement was that some of the very few physicians who had any knowledge of opiate addiction were not among those licensed to prescribe in these circumstances, while others without practical experience were permitted to do so. Formerly, scripts for heroin and cocaine (the most popular combination) 300 mg of each daily were not uncommon. Under the DDC system the prescription of cocaine, which enhances the narcotic 'high', was virtually abolished, the psychiatrists in charge having belatedly realized that this stimulant was not, strictly speaking, addictive. True, craving for cocaine could be great, but the absence of a well-defined withdrawal syndrome on its discontinuation precludes 'addiction' in the WHO sense (see further under Cocaine). For a time, methylamphetamine (Methedrine) was substituted, but both the acute and chronic ill-effects of this drug proved almost as bad as those of cocaine itself.

Opiate habitués did not much care for the DDCs, either: first, prescriptions had to be dispensed only a day's supply at a time, having been stamped and signed on special pink forms which were sent to a local pharmacy. This obviated the possibility of forgery, but many chemists were unwilling to carry out the chore of daily dispensing. More important, the quantities of drugs considered appropriate fell far below most addicts' expectations. The DDCs have since their inception drastically reduced administration of heroin and of other injectable narcotics, now almost uniformly giving methadone syrup instead.

The idea of 'methadone maintenance', whereby if an addict cannot or will not accept cessation of opiate supply he is 'maintained' on a single, oral dose of methadone which should last the day and keep withdrawal symptoms at bay, began in the USA. Vincent Dole and Marie Nyswander in the early 1960s realized that most of the patients who had been arrested for possession of heroin (which is illegal in any form in America) would, very soon after detoxification, become recidivists, i.e. would resume their illegal and preposterously expensive habit. To discourage this, a programme was established in which former heroinists attended the hospital daily and consumed a dose of Kool-Aid-flavoured methadone. By this means it was hoped that formerly (almost by definition) criminal and asocial people could be rehabilitated, obtain jobs, and otherwise be 'useful' to society.

It was indeed found that a certain proportion of patients could be assisted in this way: the incidence of criminal behaviour, including 'scoring' heroin, dropped, while a few well-motivated people managed to withdraw from opiates entirely. Methadone programmes were soon sprouting all over the USA, and the idea of maintenance with this drug, failing the ideal of an opiate-free patient, found favour with the British DHSS and the staff of the Clinics.

The UK statistics relating to registered opiate addicts for 1979 have just become available: currently, of 2,809 users, more than 2,000 are receiving methadone alone, while fewer than 200 get heroin. For the past several years the number of notified addicts has continued to increase, but it is fairly sure that fewer than one-quarter of persons addicted to narcotics are thus registered: a proportion of these, and the remainder, obtain black-market heroin and/or other drugs. One obvious explanation for the apparent reluctance of many heroinists to become notified is the present difficulty, partly due to staff shortages, of obtaining a prescription for an opiate. In virtually all new cases, oral methadone, at a rather conservative dose of 50–150 mg per day, is all that is offered, heroin being given again only in small quantities, and only to those who have a long history of dependency and might be called 'incurable'. Methadone syrup is often rejected, because at the dose regimens used it is unlikely to promote euphoria, and also because for many users the rapidly-acting 'high' following an injection of heroin is the principal desideratum.

It has been argued, often forcefully, that with methadone maintenance persons who previously were considered irredeemable have been enabled to get back their self-respect, to hold down employment, to desist from criminal activity, and much else. However, it has to be recognized that methadone is a highly addictive drug, whether taken by mouth or by any other means: some claim, on good evidence, that it is just as dependence-producing as heroin. Therefore, according to one school of thought, practitioners are merely substituting one addiction for another. Also, there is scant indication that patients maintained on methadone fare better than those for whom heroin is prescribed. On the contrary, it seems that DDC patients who receive only methadone feel in many cases compelled to supplement their legal regimen with black-market heroin. There exists now a vast body of medical publications concerning the technique of methadone maintenance, most authors favouring the continuation of these programmes. In the treatment of opiate dependency, moral support, psychotherapy and sustained striving towards the patient's rehabilitation have been signalized as important elements, which nobody would dispute. Ideally, methadone is employed for a very short period. But in practice, the drug is, as we have said, itself highly addictive, and withdrawal from it may be more difficult than that from heroin: abstinence reactions are certainly more prolonged, and, according to some who have experienced both, more severe.

So far, surprisingly, there is only one detailed comparison of groups of patients prescribed oral methadone on the one hand and of those receiving injectable heroin on the other. Martin Mitcheson, with R. L. Hartnoll and colleagues, has undertaken an evaluation of this kind: their results have now been published in *Archives of General Psychiatry* and were kindly made available to us before publication. The workers randomly assigned to patients who were treated at University College Hospital, London, doses of (injectable) heroin and methadone syrup respectively, each dispensed on a daily basis. The two groups of subjects were monitored for a period of 12 months. Independent observers assessed such factors as illicit drug use, frequency of injection (in both groups), total opiate consumption, crime as a source of income, and frequency of arrests during the study period. The findings of these workers have been summarized as follows:

> Heroin can be seen as maintaining the status quo with the majority continuing to inject heroin regularly, and to supplement their maintenance prescription from other sources; it was associated with a continuing intermediate level of involvement with the drug subculture and criminal activity. Refusal to prescribe heroin while offering oral methadone constituted a more confrontational response and resulted in a higher abstinence rate; but also a greater dependence on illegal sources of drugs for those who continued to inject. Those offered oral methadone tended to polarise towards high or low categories of illegal drug use and involvement with the drug subculture, and were more likely to be arrested during the 12 month follow-up. *There was no difference between the two groups in terms of employment, health, or consumption of non-opiate drugs.* Refusal to prescribe heroin resulted in a significantly greater drop out from regular treatment. (*Archives of General Psychiatry* vol. 37 (1980) pp. 877–84; our italics.)

These results may lead some concerned with the problem of opiate use to judge that the prescription of heroin, as the majority of addicts want, has no worse a prognosis in important respects than that of oral methadone, which heroinists often reject. It is arguable that the provision of reasonable doses of heroin by legal means is preferable to the 'scoring' of impure, illicit drug.

At present there are some 3,000 notified opiate addicts in the UK, chiefly concentrated in London, most of whom are being prescribed methadone and many supplementing their prescriptions with illicit heroin. The knowledge that only oral methadone is likely to be offered to a person coming to a Drug Dependency Clinic has evidently proved a deterrent: the total number of narcotics users is estimated to be approximately 10,000 throughout the UK, not counting those individuals who have become dependent in the course of medical treatment (therapeutic addicts). Meanwhile, the number of Home Office notifications continues to rise year by year.

It is noteworthy that prior to the introduction of the clinics in 1968 virtually no illegal, imported heroin was available for sale; but since then the drug has been smuggled into Britain – formerly just an entrepôt for the USA – for domestic consumption at a level which escalates annually, as the statistics for Customs and other seizures indicate. We believe we are justified in asking whether this would have been the case had the old system of unfettered prescription been maintained. Of course there must be facilities accessible for withdrawal, rehabilitation, help with housing and employment; and there are already adequate mechanisms for dealing with irresponsible prescribers. But perhaps prescribing trends during the past decade have become so conservative that many habitués who want a legal source of opiate are discouraged even from trying to obtain treatment at the DDCs. A more flexible approach is called for, not just domestically, but in the USA and other countries as well, where the social problems caused by illicit drug use are more widespread.

Suggestions for Further Reading

Parkhouse, J., Pleuvry, B. J. and Rees, J. M. H.: *Analgesic Drugs.* Oxford, 1979.
    A useful, up-to-date account of the properties of pain-killing drugs, with some details of recent research into the endorphins and enkephalins.

Gordon, Maxwell (ed.): *Psychopharmacological Agents* vol. 4. New York, 1976, containing:
    Eddy, N. B., 'Drug abuse and drug dependence' pp. 1–11
    Gordon, M., 'Perspectives in drug abuse' pp. 13–34
    May, E. L., 'Research toward nonabusive analgetics' pp. 35–58
    Gearing, F. R., 'Treatment of opiate abuse by methadone maintenance' pp. 147–64
    This volume of a technical series in medicinal chemistry offers a number of contributions which will be useful to the non-specialist. However, the chapter on methadone maintenance is heavily biased in favour of this method.

Jaffe, J. H. and Martin, W. R., 'Opioid analgesics and antagonists' in Goodman and Gilman, *op. cit.* pp. 494–534.
A concise overview of the field.

Glatt, M. M.: *A Guide to Addiction and its Treatment.* Lancaster, 1974.
Of the available guides to the subject, this is adequate and written in reasonably non-technical style. Not everyone will agree with Glatt's opinions, however, or his approach to the treatment of opiate users.

Judson, H. F.: *Heroin Addiction in Britain.* New York, 1974.
A breezy, but thorough, account by a journalist from the American perspective of the history of opiate addiction in the UK and its treatment. Recommended.

Burroughs, William S.: *Junky.* repr. Harmondsworth, 1977.
This novel, by the 'master addict', provides insights which only those who have been through the experience can give.

Zekert, O.: *Opiologia: ein Beitrag zur Geschichte des Opiums und seiner Wirkstoffe.* Wien, 1957 (HMW Jahrbücher).
A fascinating account, replete with quotations, of the history of opium use. For anyone who is able to locate a copy, this is well worth reading.

Pachter, I. J., 'Can We Make It Useful? the novel therapeutic approach' in Clarke, F. H. (ed.): *How Modern Medicines Are Developed.* Mount Kisco, NY, 1977, pp. 75–84.
Recent advances, particularly in the use of opiate antagonists as analgesics, are reviewed here. Useful for those who have some knowledge of chemistry.

Chart IV: Morphine and Other Potent
Analgesics (Narcotics): *overleaf*

CHART IV: MORPHINE AND OTHER POTENT ANALGESICS (NARCOTICS)

Drug Name	Brand Name(s)	Dependence Liability	Average Dose (Oral) mg	Average Dose (Injected) mg	Duration of Action (hrs)
1: Natural and Semisynthetic Drugs					
*PAPAVERETUM (OPIUM ALKALOIDS)	UK: Nepenthe, Omnopon US: Pantopon	+++	10–30	20–40	4–5
*MORPHINE	UK,US: unbranded UK: Cyclimorph†, Duromorph, MST-1	+++	5–20	5–20	4–5
*DIAMORPHINE (HEROIN)	UK: unbranded	+++	(5–20)	5–15	3–4
*HYDROMORPHONE	US: Dilaudid	+++	1–3	2–4	4–6
*OXYMORPHONE	US: Numorphan	+++	–	1–2	4–6
‡CODEINE	UK,US: many branded preparations	+(+)	10–60	(30–60)	3–4
‡DIHYDROCODEINE	UK: DF-118	++	30–90	50–100	3–4
*HYDROCODONE	UK: Dimotane-DC (syrup)† US: Dicodid	++	5–15	5–10	3–4
*OXYCODONE	UK: Proladone (suppositories) US: Percodan†	+++	5–15	–	5–8
2: Synthetic Compounds					
*PETHIDINE (MEPERIDINE)	UK: unbranded, Pamergan† US: Demerol	++(+)	25–100	50–150	2–4
*ALPHAPRODINE	US: Nisentil	++(+)	–	40–120	2–3
*ANILERIDINE	US: Leritine	++(+)	25–50	25–75	2–4
ETHOHEPTAZINE	UK: Zactipar† US: Zactane†	+	75–225	–	4–6
*FENTANYL	UK,US: Sublimaze	++(+)	–	0.1–0.6	2
*PHENOPERIDINE	UK: Operidine	++(+)	–	0.5–5.0	1
*METHADONE	UK: Physeptone US: Dolophine	+++	5–10	5–10	4–6

314

NOTE: For an account of the distinction between narcotic 'agonists' and partial 'antagonists', refer to accompanying Essay. Physical dependence liability (addictiveness) is rated: + = slight, ++ = moderate, and +++ = high: brackets indicate intermediate degrees of this hazard. Injectable doses generally refer to intramuscular route: when any of the following drugs is given intravenously, lower dosages are used and duration of action is shorter. * indicates that a compound is restricted by the Misuse of Drugs Act or corresponding US legislation.

Uses	Adverse Effects	Contra-Indications (all drugs in
Severe pain, e.g. postoperative, inoperable cancer, trauma, spasm (renal & biliary colic), myocardial infarction; as premedication; for intractable cough	*(excluding withdrawal reactions)* *Common:* Sedation, constipation, nausea, vomiting, respiratory depression, euphoria/dysphoria *Less common:* Confusion, itching, allergic reactions, sweating, urinary retention, hyperexcitability, mental depression *Uncommon:* Tremors, insomnia, convulsions, hallucinations, cardiac irregularity	Sections 1 and 2 except codeine, ethoheptazine and dextropropoxyphene): Conditions of respiratory insufficiency (e.g. bronchial asthma), severe head injury (raised intracranial pressure), urethral stricture, acute alcoholism, delirium tremens, Addison's disease, pregnancy (except labour), convulsive states *Maximum Caution* in severe liver and kidney disorders,
as for morphine	as for morphine	hypothyroidism, myxoedema, known hypersensitivity to opiates; children, the elderly and debilitated.
as for morphine	as for morphine	
Moderately severe pain; persistent cough; diarrhoea	Dizziness, restlessness, excitement after high doses, seldom euphoria; constipation	Codeine, ethoheptazine & dextropropoxyphene: caution in liver or kidney ailments, known hypersensitivity
Moderate to severe acute & chronic pain; inadequate for most severe pain	as for codeine but more frequent; flushing of face, euphoria may follow injection	
Moderate to severe pain; intractable cough	generally as for morphine but much less severe	TOLERANCE & PSYCHOLOGICAL/PHYSICAL DEPENDENCE HAZARD SHOULD BE CONSIDERED.
Postoperative and other very intense pain states	as for morphine	
Obstetrics (labour pains), premedication, other acute & chronically painful conditions as for pethidine	similar to morphine but somewhat less severe; hyperexcitability more common and euphoria probably less as for pethidine	*Interactions with Other Drugs:* Morphine-type agents should not be used within 14 days of a MAOI antidepressant (see Chart II). Great care if other CNS depressant drugs (e.g. tranquillizers) are prescribed concurrently, as effects such as
Obstetrics, premedication; unsuitable otherwise because of short action	as for pethidine	respiratory depression are enhanced. Avoid alcohol. Barbiturates counteract or diminish the effectiveness of opiates.
Moderate acute & chronic pain	nausea, vomiting, dizziness, gastro-intestinal upsets after high doses as for morphine; muscle rigidity	
Neuroleptanalgesia (see Essay), anaesthesia, postoperative pain as for fentanyl	as for morphine	CONCURRENT ADMINISTRATION OF ANY DRUGS IN GROUPS (1) and (2)
as for morphine (except premedication); maintenance of opiate addicts (v Essay)	as for morphine; euphoria no less likely at equivalent doses	i.e. AGONISTS WITH

Drug Name	Brand Name(s)	Dependence Liability	Average Dose (Oral) mg	Average Dose (Injected) mg	Duration of Action (hrs)
*DEXTROMORAMIDE	UK: Palfium	+++	5–10	5–10	4 – 5
DEXTRO-PROPOXYPHENE (PROPOXYPHENE)	UK: Doloxene US: Darvon	+	65–200	–	3 – 5
*DIPIPANONE	UK: Diconal†	+++	10–20	–	4 – 5
*LEVORPHANOL	UK: Dromoran US: Levo-Dromoran	+ +	1.5–3	2–4	4 – 6
*PHENAZOCINE	UK: Narphen	+ +	5–10	–	4 – 6
*PIRITRAMIDE	UK: Dipidolor	+ +(+)?	–	15–30	5 – 6

3: **Partial Narcotic Antagonists** N.B. None of the drugs in this group should be given to patients who are prescribed any morphine-like compound (groups 1 and 2 of this Chart) on a regular basis: the latter are antagonized by the former, withdrawal symptoms may be provoked.

PENTAZOCINE	UK: Fortral US: Talwin	+ +	25–100	20–60	3 – 4
BUPRENORPHINE	UK: Temgesic	+?	–	0.3–0.6	6 – 8
BUTORPHANOL	UK,US: Stadol	+?	–	1–4	3 – 4
NALBUPHINE	US: Nubain	+?	–	10–20	3 – 6

†denotes that the product contains an additional ingredient, e.g. an anti-emetic

‡In the USA, all pure codeine preparations are restricted. In UK, only injectable dihydrocodeine is controlled.

'Technical' opiates (i.e. compounds chemically related to these) which are used other than for analgesia (dextromethorphan, diphenoxylate) are described in the Alphabetical Entries, likewise narcotic antagonists (naloxone, nalorphine, levallorphan, apomorphine).

Uses	Adverse Effects (excluding withdrawal reactions)	Contra-Indications
severe acute & chronic pain states	as for morphine but possibly less severe	NARCOTIC ANTAGONISTS (NALOXONE) AND WITH COMPOUNDS IN GROUP 3 (PARTIAL ANTAGONISTS) CAN BE DANGEROUS because they may provoke withdrawal symptoms in patients habituated to morphine and other opiate agonists.
Moderate pain, acute & chronic	as for ethoheptazine, following high doses; incompatible with orphenadrine (Disipal)	
as for morphine	as for morphine but rather less severe (Diconal contains cyclizine as anti-emetic)	
as for morphine	as for morphine but rather less severe	
as for morphine	as for morphine but much less severe (seldom euphoriant)	
Postoperative pain	as for morphine	

Uses	Adverse Effects (excluding withdrawal reactions)	Contra-Indications
Moderate to severe pain; premedication; obstetrics	Nausea, vomiting, dizziness, sedation, headache; less commonly euphoria/dysphoria, tremor, excitement, psychotomimetic effects (e.g. hallucinations); ulceration at site of injection, convulsions (rare)	Contra-indicated in head injury (raised intracranial pressure), respiratory depression; caution – impaired liver or kidney function; narcotic-dependent patients; serious interactions with agonists, MAOIs & perhaps nicotine (cigarettes)
Moderate to severe pain	Drowsiness, mood changes, nausea, dizziness, sweating, respiratory depression following high doses; headache, dry mouth, bizarre psychological states in some cases	Should be avoided in cases of impaired liver or respiratory function; MAOIs & agonists must not be given concurrently; drug not antagonized by opiate antagonists (e.g. naloxone); contra-indicated in pregnancy
Moderate to severe pain	similar to buprenorphine	Contra-indicated in respiratory insufficiency & during pregnancy, myocardial infarction; not recommended in cases of severe liver or kidney disorders; with MAOI antidepressants & opiate agonists
Moderate to severe pain; premedication; obstetrics	similar to buprenorphine	as for butorphanol

V: Lysergide (LSD) and Other Psychedelics

The non-medical use of LSD and other chemicals which produce altered states of consciousness has, for the past decade at least, become so widespread as to be probably ineradicable. Certainly this is true with respect to cannabis (q.v.). And the taking of lysergide (LSD) is inextricably linked in the public mind, though not in fact, with the more irresponsible elements in the counter-culture, or 'alternative society'. Because the subject of this and kindred substances' psychological effects is so complex, and because of the highly emotive overtones of 'psychedelic states', this Essay has a more discursive character than the others in this volume. It is difficult for even the most impartial observer to describe accurately a class of drugs about which such hysterical claims, and counter-claims, have been made. Indeed the pitch has been reached when, chiefly on account of lurid stories in the yellow press and even in medical journals, even researchers with the most impeccable credentials have immense difficulty in obtaining LSD for legitimate studies. Alexander Shulgin, one of the foremost scholars in the field, has remarked sadly:

> In this area of research, as in many others that have become charged with social and political overtones, there is an unfortunate enthusiasm with some researchers to search only for negative findings, to emphasize hazards out of context in the hope that such statements might dissuade the potential drug user from exploration with these chemicals ('Psychotomimetic Drugs' in *Psychopharmacological Agents,* ed. Maxwell Gordon vol.4. New York, 1976, p.133).

The psychedelics (as listed in Chart V), together with cannabis and its derivatives, have the dubious distinction of having been assigned, in the USA, the UK and elsewhere, a special schedule among restricted drugs, whereby they are far more rigorously controlled than all others. Under the British Misuse of Drugs Act 1971 and the corresponding American legislation, lysergide, mescaline, and several other so-called 'hallucinogens' may not be prescribed by physicians, and are regarded as having no (or very few) therapeutic indications together with a supposedly strong abuse liability. In effect this means that any researcher who wishes to study the effects of LSD on humans must obtain a special licence from the Home Secretary (in the USA, the Drug Enforcement Administration) in order to get supplies of drug legally: such licences are seldom granted in the USA and hardly at all (even for cannabis) in the UK. The administrative difficulties involved have, to borrow Shulgin's apt term, a chilling effect on research into an area of considerable interest and potential importance. It is noteworthy, and symptomatic of public attitudes to this class of drug, that a number of people (including a chemist and two physicians) concerned with illegal production of lysergide, who were arrested in the course of 'Operation Julie', received harsher sentences than large-scale traffickers in heroin. The judge in this case showed a quite remarkable degree of ignorance and prejudice, evidently believing that LSD was, among other evil attributes, addictive: this is inaccurate and misleading.

The majority of reference works refer to this category of substances as 'psychotomimetics', a term which the reader will perhaps already have encountered in connection with the side-effects of amphetamines and narcotic antagonists, and which means 'mimicking' a psychotic state. This label has been applied to lysergide because persons under its influence are regarded by some psychiatrists as suffering from a temporary form of psychosis. The expression 'hallucinogen' has similar connotations and is inadequate, insofar as persons under the influence of lysergide often do not hallucinate but do nevertheless experience profound perceptual distortions. There are certain elements in common between mental states provoked by the drug and those which occur spontaneously in schizophrenia, but the differences are more significant. In this book we have adopted the etymologically unsound but more accurate term 'psychedelic', which is derived from the Greek *psyche* ('mind') and *dēloō* ('show') and indicates 'mind-revelation'. Many who have experienced LSD or mescaline report, as one of the most profound phenomena, that these agents enable the subject to gain surprising insights into his own consciousness. Indeed it is because of this faculty, and the ability to gain access to the subconscious mind, that lysergide has been used in psychiatry. The present authors have coined the noun 'psychedelosis' to refer to this kind of insight.

For many centuries, 'primitive' peoples, particularly the Indians of Central and South America, have employed decoctions of plants containing psychedelic alkaloids. Most of the compounds shown in Chart V are derived from vegetable sources: mescaline from the cactus *Lophophora williamsii*, psilocin and psilocybin from several species of *Psilocybe* mushrooms, harmine and harmaline from *Banisteriopsis caapi*. In fact, a number of plants yield several distinct compounds with psychedelic activity, and some of these compounds are found in two or more generically different plants. Many groups in Latin America take psychedelic plant extracts as part of a religious ritual, in order to achieve a transcendental or mystical state. Carlos Castaneda, in several books (e.g. *The Teachings of Don Juan),* vividly illustrates how seriously the use of these substances is taken, for instance among Mexican shamans.

There exists in nature an extraordinary variety and number of plants whose active principles yield effects analogous to those of lysergide: only a tiny percentage of these compounds have been studied in any detail. The interested reader will find an enormous amount of fascinating material on numerous little-known botanical psychedelics in *The Botany and Chemistry of Hallucinogens,* by Richard Evans Schultes and A. Hofmann (Springfield, Ill., 1973).

It was an accidental discovery of Albert Hofmann's which was to lead directly to current non-medical use of psychedelics. In 1938 Hofmann was working in the laboratories of the multinational drug company Sandoz in Basel. He began to prepare a series of chemical modifications of ergometrine. This compound and its congener ergotamine are used medicinally to stop bleeding from the womb after delivery and to constrict bloodvessels, which has the effect of relieving migraine for many sufferers. These agents were derived from the micro-fungus ergot (*Claviceps purpurea*) which grows on rye.

As so often in the history of therapeutics, a serendipitous thing happened. In 1943, while studying the ergotamine derivative lysergic acid diethylamide (lysergide, LSD), Hofmann accidentally ingested a minute quantity of this substance. (It is likely that he either breathed some in or that a quantity of the drug was absorbed through the skin of his fingers.) While journeying home from work he fell off his bicycle and underwent an extraordinary series of sensations: his state of consciousness was completely altered. As he later described what came to be known as the 'psychedelic experience':

Experience of the environment, its forms and colours, as well as a person's own mental and corporeal personality are altered . . . Not only space, however, but also time, the other fundamental category of our existence, is experienced . . . otherwise than in the normal state. Frequently the sense of time seems altogether to have vanished. Yet all these changes in perspective are experienced with undiminished awareness. Fully conscious, the subject is transported into other worlds, dream worlds as it were, but worlds which are experienced quite realistically, generally in fact more realistically, intensely and meaningfully than the normal everyday world. The senses, especially the sense of sight, are abnormally sensitized; objects appear to be in greater relief, colours more lustrous. With rather high doses this stimulation of the senses is apt to produce visions and hallucinations. It would appear that the control mechanisms in the nervous system, which normally exercise a limiting function, are inactivated and that consequently from the external world the entire store of cosmic experience, and from within, from the subconscious, a vast flow of sensations, images and recollections penetrate the conscious mind. It is not surprising that in its intensity, vehemence, and unfamiliarity this experience [is] frequently interpreted as a religious revelation. (A. Hofmann, 'Psychotomimetic Substances' *Indian Journal of Pharmacy* vol. 25, 1963, p.246)

There are many more poetic and graphic accounts, but that of Hofmann has been quoted because (a) he has taken lysergide himself, and (b) he is a highly trained professional pharmacologist. There are rather few individuals who fulfil both criteria: indeed, it might be argued that any medically qualified person who presumes to make judgments about LSD should first take the drug himself. The difference which this might make to his understanding of the psychedelics could be considerable.

One of the most astonishing facts about lysergide, as Hofmann discovered, is that it provokes the kind of reactions he describes at a minute dose – between 100 and 300 μg – a quantity not visible to the naked eye. The pure drug, which occurs as a highly soluble powder or fine crystals, is also colourless, tasteless and odourless. Hofmann's discovery triggered an enormous increase in research into psychedelics, and his laboratory at Sandoz subsequently synthesized a range of other compounds with LSD-like activity. In particular, the pharmaceutical firm was interested in the potential applications of lysergide in the treatment of mental illnesses. Also, it was felt, 'model psychoses' could be induced by administration of the compound to healthy volunteers: this would maybe provide clues to the biochemical changes which are believed to be the basis of schizophrenia and other severe psychoses as these occur spontaneously.

Although the latter goal has not been achieved, there is no doubt that understanding of mental states regarded by the medical profession as 'abnormal' has been enhanced by the study of psychedelics. During the 1950s and early 1960s many psychiatric studies were published which indicated that the administration of lysergide or psilocybin could unlock the 'doors of perception' (Aldous Huxley's expressive phrase), for example by unearthing a traumatic experience buried in the patient's subconscious mind which may have been the cause of the present malady. Huxley's accounts of psychedelic experiences, *The Doors of Perception* and *Heaven and Hell,* are recommended as an introduction to this extraordinary field.

The celebrated experiments by Timothy Leary and his colleagues at Harvard, in which healthy subjects were given psilocybin, were followed, in the late 1950s and early 1960s, by a colossal demand for psychedelics among members of the counter-culture. Many of these people had glimpsed 'consciousness-expansion' with cannabis, some of whose effects are qualitatively similar (though far less intense) to those of lysergide. Leary himself was sacked from his post at Harvard for advocating the unrestricted use of psychedelics, and his advice to 'turn on, tune in, and drop out' became a *Leitmotiv* for the hippie community. He was convinced, as Huxley had been, that a genuinely important, transcendental (or 'mystical') experience could be obtained on a lysergide-impregnated sugar-cube. Unlike Huxley, however, who appreciated the need for intellectual honesty and extreme caution, Leary wanted to turn on the world.

In the context which prevailed within the American counter-culture, people other than thrill-seekers were drawn to experiment. Here in Britain, during the period 1963-5, there was very little knowledge of or interest in psychedelics. One of the present writers, having first taken lysergide under careful conditions, was responsible for some pilot experiments with the compound in Oxford at that time. It was then possible for qualified individuals to obtain lysergide without difficulty: the psychedelics were not yet under legal restriction. Pure lysergide, at an average dose of 250 μg, was used. Only intelligent, healthy subjects with a genuine interest in altered states of consciousness participated. The criteria which we laid down at this period are still applicable. One should not even contemplate taking lysergide or any other psychedelic substance *unless*: (1) the individual concerned has a stable personality; (2) an accurately measured dose of pure drug is available; (3) a fairly relaxed environment, free from interruption, can be found; (4) there is expert, sympathetic and preferably medically qualified supervision; and (5) antidotes (see below) are to hand.

This may seem like a counsel of perfection, but the above are sensible precautions. At Oxford, a number of persons who very much wished to participate in the trials were refused on the grounds of psychological instability or a poorly-defined sense of identity. Of the 30 subjects studied, all but one felt that the experience was worthwhile, and the great majority asserted that profound insights into their personality had been gained. Although episodes of fear occurred in some cases, in only one instance did it prove impossible to overcome such states by means of verbal reassurance and/or physical contact. Suggestibility is greatly enhanced during a lysergide 'trip', and the presence of a trusted friend who has personal experience of psychedelics can be an important factor. In no case did we find a desire for repeated administration of the drug, though some persons subsequently took additional doses, at intervals of at least 2–3 weeks. More regular consumption was uncommon, in spite of the ease with which LSD could be obtained a short time after our pilot study. More than half of the subjects decided that, although they believed the experience to have been valuable, they did not want to take the chemical again. 'Flashbacks', or after-effects hours or days following lysergide administration, were reported in a few instances but did not cause concern. In no case did any psychotic state or other severe mental disturbance arise following dosage: in part this may have been due to careful screening beforehand. Unfortunately, chiefly on account of legal sanctions and administrative problems, this research had to be discontinued at a relatively early stage.

One of the most noteworthy features of several studies of psychedelics, including our own, involved a heightened aesthetic sense as reported by subjects: poets, musicians, painters and others have fervently asserted that their experiences with lysergide or mescaline added a new dimension to their creative work, both during sessions of psychedelosis and long afterwards. The feeling of many individuals, especially practitioners of various art forms, that they had achieved a real transcendental experience was, and is, extremely strong.

By about 1960 a number of clinicians were convinced that psychedelic compounds had proven efficacy in the treatment of mental illness, especially when such drugs were given to severely disturbed patients who had failed to respond to other forms of therapy and whose prognosis was poor: chronic alcoholics, criminal psychopaths, sexual deviants, and narcotic addicts, among others, were apparently helped. When the distinguished Czech researcher Stanislav Grof arrived in America in 1965, he was astonished at how the climate had changed and how controversial the medical use of psychedelics was regarded. In his native country lysergide was listed on the official pharmacopoeia as a therapeutic agent, and Grof had never experienced any problem in either obtaining or administering it. But by this time the compound had been placed under stringent legal control in the USA, and the manufacturer of lysergide, Sandoz, had recalled most supplies, so that it was available only, in effect, on application to the government. Grof noted that the earlier claims for the drug's success in psychiatry were being vociferously challenged, and practically all clinical trials with psychedelics had been abandoned. At this point LSD was seen by most people, including physicians, as a highly dangerous drug, more likely to provoke psychotic states than to mitigate them. Horror stories abounded: tales of individuals under the influence of lysergide believing they could fly or walk on water, and consequently meeting an untimely end, made – and still occasionally make – excellent copy, although attempts to follow up such accounts proved consistently unsuccessful. A real threat to society was seen: but hippie talk of revolution was misconstrued. What the beats and their followers sought was an *inner* metamorphosis. Several detailed accounts of LSD synthesis having been published in academic journals, counter-culture chemists began to make their own. Given the minute quantities required, a single illicit laboratory could supply an entire country, as the Operation Julie story demonstrated. And demand was always ahead of supply. The synthesis of lysergide, from ergotamine base, is a complex operation, and manufacturers have shown a remarkable degree of sophistication: the purity of drug produced in Wales during the 1970s was said to be greater than that of Sandoz, the only company in legal production.

Given the large-scale availability of cheap (£1 per dose or less) and often impure LSD, it is hardly suprising that there have been some casualties. What is much more astonishing is that there have been so few. Undoubtedly, persons described as having a pre-psychotic personality, if they take a psychedelic, may then exhibit florid schizophrenic signs. Also, the belief that these compounds will produce a 'high' has led to much incautious and irresponsible use. For such individuals psychedelic experience is apt to be very frightening. On the question of the toxicity of lysergide much nonsense has been written: the lethal dose in experimental animals is many many times higher than any human would take, and, during the last year for which figures are available, no accidental or deliberate cases of lethal poisoning were reported in England and Wales from lysergide or any other psychedelic. Physical addiction to these drugs does not occur, and psychological dependency is, at least, uncommon.

The reader who has not himself taken a psychedelic substance may be puzzled by descriptions of its effects, including that of Hofmann quoted above. Many attempts to translate the experience into words have been published, some of them articulate and vivid. Yet none can provide more than an impressionistic picture, and a blurred one at that. Simply stated, the problem is that the events or effects triggered by psychedelics are intrinsically indescribable. Whether or not one agrees that a lysergide 'trip' constitutes a mystical experience or revelation, by its very nature it can be described only allusively, metaphorically, allegorically, poetically – but not literally.

Physical reactions to the psychedelics are easily summarized: dilatation of the pupils is characteristic. Tachycardia, or fast heartbeat, nausea, trembling, muscular weakness, numbness and elevated temperature may occur, but for some subjects these effects are transient or absent. As we have already stated, physical dependency does not arise with this class of drugs. The question of tolerance is more problematic, but the weight of evidence suggests 'reverse tolerance' among those who use psychedelics regularly. This is similar to the phenomenon found among habitual smokers of cannabis (q.v.), in that the more experienced one is with the drug the less of it is required to achieve the desired state. It is extremely difficult to find out about the incidence of 'regular' lysergide consumption, as few of those involved may come to the attention of the authorities, and even then evidence can be misconstrued. Given the almost incredible intensity of a lysergide-induced state, it is probable that only a very small proportion of those who have taken one 'trip' will repeat the experience within, at least, a week. Anecdotal data suggest an average frequency of far less than one psychedelic session per month.

The first perceptible effects of lysergide (to which we principally refer, since its availability is greater than other psychedelics') may be apparent within 30 to 90 minutes after administration. At the outset one may feel a tingling in the extremities. Nausea is not uncommon at this point, and does not often lead to vomiting: this tends to be transient. Little by little, one's surroundings seem to change, subtly at first. One's attention may be held arbitrarily by a particular object, for example a painting on the wall. The images within the picture may appear to move, change colour, alter in shape, become three-dimensional. An examination of one's hand may reveal the musculature, the blood-vessels, the bones, as if it had become transparent. By this juncture, the process of 'sensory overload' may commence: thoughts, feelings, all the data normally filtered through the senses, crowd in on one vertiginously. Synaesthesia – an odd phenomenon whereby the faculties are jumbled – may find one hearing the painting, tasting the music, smelling the voices. Time seems to stop or to slow down: the other referent of space may be perceived in an entirely different manner. Weird shapes scurry past one's peripheral vision.

Rational thinking may by this stage have become hard. A classic observation is that: 'It's too much. Everything's flooding in on me . . . I must try to control it.' The novice may not be able to control it, however, although the more experienced user finds he can to a degree. Concurrently with the synaesthesia, one's sense of identity begins apparently to disintegrate. An inner battle may be fought to try to ward off this process. This, indeed, may be the most critical phase of the session, since fighting against this seeming loss of identity may be frightening. But when one has eventually 'let go', subject and object fuse into one. The paradoxical situation arises in which there undoubtedly is perception, only without a percipient. This phenomenon has been described by psychiatrists, aptly for once, as 'depersonalization'; and it is principally because of this aspect of psychedelic experience that some practitioners associate it with schizophrenia and other psychotic states, and term lysergide a 'psychotomimetic' agent. Yet whereas these conditions of grave mental illness are involuntary and may persist over long periods, psychedelosis is both voluntary and self-limiting. This is not to say that parallels do not exist nor that comparisons should not be made.

Ironically, it is this very state of depersonalization which, according to Huxley, Laing and others, the Zen Buddhist strives to attain by meditation: oneness with the previously perceived world, predicated on dissolution of the 'self'. Hofmann's description, it will be recalled, concentrates on alterations in perception such as visions or heightened colours, and does not specifically mention depersonalization. This is understandable because those schooled in Western ways of thought, unlike practitioners of yoga, assume that the 'self' exists in an absolute sense, with the necessary corollary that there is always a duality between the percipient and that which is perceived. The psychedelics help to break down this apparent duality, and therein lies their possible significance for certain serious-minded and intelligent individuals, to whom the sensory distortions ('hallucinations') are only peripheral to the main object of the exercise. It should not surprise anyone that responsible and careful use of psychedelics may lead to profound insights and be regarded as a quasi-mystical experience. Neither LSD nor any other chemical will provide a 'quickie nirvana', but arguably it could help set the neophyte on the right road.

The so-called 'bad trip' appears to arise when some or all of the criteria which we have set down above have not been met, for example if impure drug is taken, or if set and setting are not relaxed and reassuring. Worried friends and relatives, observing an inexperienced and young person who is in a state of panic and whose words make no sense, may think that the subject has gone mad. Certainly, if a psychedelic is taken with the intention of 'getting a kick', the probability of a negative experience is increased. The best way of handling such a situation is to give strong reassurance to the affected person that the state will pass, and perhaps to clasp the hand as a gesture of moral support and affection: the subject will probably be very suggestible to such actions and can usually, with care, be 'talked down'. Should such tactics fail, a number of remedies have been suggested, e.g. giving large quantities of sugar. This will have no more than a placebo effect but may be sufficient if the individual believes it will work. Conventional medical practice in such cases is to take the tripper to a local hospital casualty department, there to be injected with a substantial dose of a potent antipsychotic drug such as haloperidol (Haldol, Serenace). This may restore the patient to a semblance of normality fairly quickly, but with the risk that severe depression can arise or, if already present, be enhanced. Also, the blocking action of antipsychotic tranquillizers is temporary, so that after discharge from hospital psychedelic-type effects may recur ('flashbacks') in even more distressing form. The present writers have found, after some experience of handling 'bad trips', that when a talk-down does not achieve the intended result an unproven but effective measure can be taken: this is the intramuscular injection of 2,000-3,000 µg of hydroxocobalamin (vitamin B_{12b}, 'Neo-Cytamen'). The risks involved are negligible and the patient can often be thus restored to rationality within 20 minutes or less. Occasionally this may be ineffective, and then a moderate dose of a minor tranquilliser such as diazepam (Valium, 10–30mg IM) is likely to do the trick without adverse sequelae.

The various substances listed in Chart V, whether they be of plant origin or whether synthetic, have similar *qualitative* psychological effects. The differences are hard to explain: some say that mescaline is more likely than lysergide to provoke wonderful visual phenomena, or that harmine (also known as telepathine) is more apt to induce states of apparent thought-transference. At least, in dealing with quantifiable distinctions, we are on firmer ground. Duration of action of psychedelic drugs varies from ½–1 hour in the case of the tryptamines (DMT and DET) to 24 hours or even longer for DOM (2,5-dimethoxy-4-methylamphetamine). The active dosage levels given in the Chart have been reasonably well established for lysergide, mescaline and psilocybin/psilocin. In the case of other compounds, such as lysergamide and DMT/DET, a number of clinical studies have been carried out, so dosage can be estimated approximately. With bufotenine and ibogaine, however, practically no research involving human subjects has been published. In the improbable event of either compound becoming available even to practitioners, the quantities required to elicit psychedelic effects are a matter of guesswork. Although neither iboga alkaloids nor bufotenine are obtainable legally, and they have not appeared on the illicit market, both are under exactly the same legislative restriction as lysergide and mescaline. In clinical experiments, workers have tended, for reasons quite unfathomable to these authors, to administer psychedelics by intravenous injection. This route is quite unsuitable even for compounds which are inactive by mouth, because its use will provoke virtually all the most intense psychic effects almost immediately. This might be calculated to freak subjects out.

The appropriate mode of administration is different for a number of psychedelics. Most can be taken orally, but some are inactivated by the stomach acids and therefore some other technique must be employed. It is possible to smoke cigarettes impregnated with DMT/DET and harmaline/harmine (and theoretically phencyclidine – but see below), as these are fairly well absorbed via the mucous membranes. Subcutaneous or intramuscular injection is a more reliable means of delivering them to the system: if this is the route chosen, dosage must be calibrated with particular care and, obviously, aseptic procedures must be followed. DMT and harmine are not stable in solution, so they should be freshly dissolved in sterile water or isotonic saline. It goes without saying that all the other specified precautions should be taken.

An extra set of precautions may be needed for harmaline and harmine, because these are (albeit to a slight extent) inhibitors of the enzyme monoamine oxidase (MAO-inhibitors). In this respect they resemble a certain type of antidepressant (e.g. iproniazid, Marsilid and tranylcypromine, Parnate). The various warnings and contra-indications obtaining with this group of drugs are shown in Chart II (Antidepressants): importantly, alcohol should be avoided, and certain foods such as concentrated meat or yeast extracts, in addition to a formidable list of other medicaments (above, p. 250 under Antidepressants) may be dangerous concurrently.

Two substances which have been included in Chart V because of their illicit availability are nevertheless absolutely contra-indicated: these are DOM (STP) and phencyclidine (Sernylan, 'angel dust'). Phencyclidine is manufactured legally as a veterinary anaesthetic, but most of the angel dust which reaches the black market in the form of tablets, crystals or powder is 'home-produced' and often sold as Δ^9-tetrahydrocannabinol (THC), one of the active constituents of cannabis: the latter promotes quite profound mood-altering states. At the time of this writing there is a craze for angel dust in the USA. Phencyclidine is extremely dangerous, the margin between active and toxic doses in the human being narrow, and large doses cause confusion, aggressiveness, hypertensive crises, convulsions and coma: death may then supervene. As there is no specific antidote, and phencyclidine overdosage is not uncommon, its treatment must be entirely symptomatic. Thus the inherent risk of experimenting with this compound is unacceptably high.

The same is true of DOM, an amphetamine derivative which produces effects stronger than, but qualitatively similar to, those of the conventional amphetamines (see Essay I). Like these, it has a potent central stimulant action, which is however much more protracted. The psychological effects of DOM resemble those of methylamphetamine (Methedrine, Desoxyn) more closely than those of the true psychedelics. DOM and phencyclidine are included here only because at high doses they may provoke hallucinations and possibly depersonalization, and because their illicit use is quite widespread and likely to become more so. Chronic DOM administration leads to a state indistinguishable from 'amphetamine psychosis'. Like angel dust, DOM should not be taken under any circumstances.

Repeated use of any psychedelic, even under the conditions laid down, is to be avoided. This will not be difficult for the great majority of individuals, for whom a single dose of lysergide may take weeks or months to 'digest'. But of course abuse is possible and does occur: whether psychedelics precipitate permanent psychotic states which would not otherwise have occurred is an open question. Similarly, reports that lysergide produces chromosomal (genetic) damage if taken regularly, and thus could be dangerous if taken during pregnancy, have not been substantiated in human beings: laboratory animals exposed to enormous doses have apparently undergone such damage in some cases. Certainly we would contra-indicate the use of any psychedelic substance during pregnancy, as we would the taking of virtually any other psychotropic drug. In general, the utmost caution must be observed by every person, however apparently stable, intelligent or sophisticated, who may consider experimentation with these chemicals. If such substances are capable of showing you heaven, then they are also capable of demonstrating hell.

While illicit use of lysergide and other psychedelics continues, hardly
checked by all the efforts and sanctions which have been brought to bear,

conl. a few researchers specializing in psychological medicine are again wondering about the possible therapeutic applications of these drugs. For most the numerous administrative hurdles and difficulties involved in obtaining approval to prescribe psychedelics have proved too great a hassle, as doubtless has been the intention on the part of the authorities. But the field of LSD psychotherapy is gradually opening up again and new areas of research have begun. Stanislav Grof, for instance, has been administering lysergide to terminally ill patients: he has found that the substance not only abolishes the pain of advanced cancer, but that it induces a state of dignified serenity immediately preceding these patients' death. Aldous Huxley himself, moribund and unable to speak, had his wife administer a dose of LSD to help him pass on in the way that he wished.

It is to be hoped that research into this fascinating group of compounds be encouraged, rather than discouraged as at present. For the layperson, one can only advise extreme caution if a psychedelic experience is being contemplated and point to what one believes are the proper criteria (see above) in that event. If you are seeking a new kind of thrill or 'kick', the psychedelics will do you more harm than good. Only if you are philosophically interested in the mysteries of existence and genuinely seeking to follow the great dictum 'know thyself' should you even consider taking such a step.

Suggestions for Further Reading

The literature on psychedelic drugs is voluminous: most of it is highly technical, while only a few of the popular suveys of the subject even approach adequacy. The following should be found of interest:

Aaronson, B. and Osmond, H. (ed.): *Psychedelics: the uses and implications of hallucinogenic drugs.* London, 1971.
  This anthology, which includes first-hand accounts, will provide an easy way in to the field. While non-technical, the work is sensible and eclectic.

Masters, R. E. L. and Houston, J.: *The Varieties of Psychedelic Experience.* New York, 1966 repr. London, 1973.
  A very good account of subjective experiences with psychedelic drugs, collated and interpreted intelligently.

Cohen, S.: *Drugs of Hallucination.* London, 1965 repr. London, 1972.
  This work is useful in terms of the facts which it provides, although it is coloured by the author's conventional medical bias against non-medical use of psychedelics.

Grof, S: *Realms of the Human Unconscious: observations from LSD research.* New York, 1975 repr. London, 1979.

This is the first of a projected series of works in which not only are the medical applications of lysergide and its analogues considered but also an entire theory of the unconscious is being formulated. A fascinating work by this pioneer in the field.

Lewin, L.: *Phantastica: narcotic and stimulating drugs,* trans. P. H. A. Wirth, ed.3. London, 1931 repr. London, 1960 etc.

Although the book's English title is misleading, arising from difficulty in exactly translating the original German, it provides an interesting series of descriptions of ritual use of hallucinogens, e.g. that of mescaline among Mexican Indians.

Shulgin, A.T.: 'Psychotomimetic Agents' in *Psychopharmacological Agents,* ed. M. Gordon vol.4. New York, 1976. pp. 59-146.

For the reader with some scientific or medical knowledge, this is a first rate overview of the many different types of psychedelic substances, by one of the foremost researchers in the field.

CHART V: PSYCHEDELICS: LYSERGIDE (LSD) AND OTHER PSYCHEDELICS

N.B. (None of the following drugs is available for prescription)

Drug	Other Names	Source (Plant)	Habitat	Active Human Dose*	Approximate Duration of Action
MESCALINE	peyotl	Lophophora williamsii Trichocereus pachanoi	Central America Peru	300–750 mg PO	6–8 hours
PSILOCIN PSILOCYBIN	teonanacatl	Psilocybe mexicana Psilocybe spp Stropharia cubensis	Mexico Worldwide Cuba	4–8 mg PO,SL	3–4 hours
DIETHYLTRYPTAMINE DIMETHYLTRYPTAMINE	DET DMT	Piptadenia peregrina Piptadenia macrocarpa Virola theiodora	Central America Central & South America Brazil, Colombia	50–100 mg IM or smoked	½–1 hour
BUFOTENINE	parika. cohoba. mappine	Anadenanthera peregrina Virola peruviana (the toad Bufo marinus)	Central America Peru Worldwide	70–140 mg PO ?	1–2 hours
IBOGAINE	–	Tabernanthe ibóga	West Africa. Zaire	300 mg PO ? 100 mg IM ?	3–4 hours
LYSERGAMIDE	ololiuqui. ergine	Rivea corymbosa Ipomoea violacea	Mexico Mexico	1–5 mg PO	3–5 hours
HARMALINE HARMINE	yage. telepathine	Banisteriopsis caapi Peganum harmala	South America Asian steppes	100–300 mg IM	3–5 hours
LYSERGIDE	LSD. acid	synthetic	–	100–300 µg PO	6–8 hours
†2,5-DIMETHOXY-4-METHYL- AMPHETAMINE	DOM.STP	synthetic	–	3–5 mg PO	12–24 hours
†PHENCYCLIDINE	Sernylan. angel dust	synthetic	–	3–10 mg PO or smoked	4–6 hours

*Mode of administration: PO = by mouth; SL = sublingually; IM = intramuscularly (injected). For many compounds the 'active' dosage level has not been properly established. Always err on the side of caution if psychedelics are to be used.

IMPORTANT NOTE: None of the above-listed drugs should ever be taken except under expert medical supervision. In the event of a 'bad trip', contemporary hospital practice is to give large doses of antipsychotic tranquillizers (e.g. haloperidol, Haldol, Serenace): this may trigger delayed reactions and is seldom necessary (see Text). Harmaline and Harmine are MAO-inhibitors: like certain antidepressants, these should not on any account be taken with a range of other drugs nor with certain foods, such as meat and yeast extracts (see Chart IIB: ANTIDEPRESSANTS – MAO INHIBITORS)

†ABSOLUTELY CONTRA-INDICATED

VI: Tranquillizers

Introductory

This Essay is concerned with two distinct types of medication, both of which are commonly referred to as 'tranquillizers'. It may seem capricious to include both 'minor' and 'major' tranquillizing agents under the same heading. Those designated as 'minor' comprise the drugs prescribed to alleviate anxiety and tension, while 'major' tranquillizers are chiefly given to control the symptoms of schizophrenia and other severe forms of mental illness. Both types of drug tend to exert a calming, often sedative effect: otherwise they could hardly be more dissimilar. However, because both are still referred to as tranquillizers by most practitioners and in many reference texts, they are dealt with here. The reader is directed to section A of Chart VI (pp. 368–9) for comparative information on anxiety-relieving agents, and to section B (pp. 370–2) for data on antipsychotic preparations.

The former group consists mostly of the chemically related benzo-diazepine compounds, of which chlordiazepoxide (Librium) and diazepam (Valium) are the most familiar and most frequently prescribed. Drugs of this kind are also known as anti-anxiety (anxiolytic) agents or 'ataractics', from the Greek *ataraxia*, which indicates a state of profound harmonious quietude to which the philosopher aspired.

'Major' tranquillizers, as represented by chlorpromazine (Largactil, Thorazine) and its derivatives and analogues, are more appropriately termed 'antipsychotics', since this is the purpose for which they are principally prescribed. These are described with increasing popularity as 'neuroleptics' (see below, p. 349). The important chemical groupings to which most such drugs belong are the phenothiazines, the buty-rophenones, and the thioxanthenes: when authorities refer to phenothiazines, they may indicate members of any of the three principal categories, which are pharmacologically very similar.

Like depression, anxiety and tension are practically ubiquitous in Western society. It was reported that in 1978 no fewer than 44.5 million prescriptions for diazepam (Valium) alone were filled in the USA. It has been further estimated that some 18% to 20% of British women – and rather less than half that number of men – are currently under treatment with one psychotropic drug or another. Sophisticated rating scales have been devised to test for depression, anxiety and other symptoms (see Table 2 above, under Antidepressants). But, in the main, prescription of a minor tranquillizer follows a quick and informal assessment by the practitioner. Like depression, states of undue tension or stress may be superficial symptoms of a more profound physical or psychological illness. Anxiety itself clearly has a proper role in an individual's makeup, as an element in the 'fight or flight' reflex. This may be an appropriate defence mechanism when the feeling can be followed up by positive action: all sorts of potentially dangerous situations provoke this state. It is when the anxiety serves no useful purpose – i.e. is considered an inappropriate response to a given set of circumstances – that it comes to be regarded as pathological, the province of the physician.

Almost any phenomenon – bereavement, loss of job, difficulties involving a spouse or partner – can trigger sensations of tension and anxiety. And in a society where, increasingly, people are unwilling to make use of their own resources and will not tolerate disagreeable mood changes for long, the doctor is expected to provide chemical remedies. Depending on the type and severity of symptoms, other types of treatment may be more suitable: if anxiety is secondary to an illness accompanied by severe physical pain, then the original ailment should be treated, if not curatively, then palliatively. Or a patient presenting apparently because he is anxious may in fact be suffering from an underlying neurosis or even psychosis. The desirability of careful history-taking in these circumstances is evident. One should also distinguish between what may be termed constitutional and reactive anxiety: i.e. the person who is over-anxious 'by nature', irrespective of other factors, and the one whose tension is precipitated by a specific event or situation. Whatever the cause of the condition, it is handled ever more commonly by the prescribing of a tranquillizer.

A: ANXIETY-RELIEVING TRANQUILLIZERS

Historical

For many decades prior to the late 1950s and the 1960s, when a vast armamentarium of new psychotropic drugs was made available, virtually the only chemical remedy for tension or anxiety was one of the old-fashioned soporifics, taken at lower dosage than that required for sleep. Pre-eminent among these were the barbiturates, notably the long-acting phenobarbitone, which certainly 'calmed the nerves'. A surprising number of proprietary preparations which contain small amounts of this or other barbituric acid derivatives, alone or in conjunction with bromides, are to this day marketed in the USA. There and in Britain some physicians still prescribe amylobarbitone or one of its analogues to quell anxiety, directing the patient to take a dose (anything from 15 to 100 mg) two or three times daily: the amount given as a single daytime dosage is half or a third of that required to promote sleep. This is quite inappropriate today, because so many modern drugs may be given which have a more selective action and do not damp down the faculties to the extent that barbiturates do. The longer-acting barbiturates in particular, barbitone and phenobarbitone, are unsuitable as anxiolytics for many reasons: immediate side-effects such as confusion and oversedation may be expected; repeated use causes the drug to accumulate in the tissues, which can be dangerous; tolerance sets in quickly for many people; psychological and physical dependency are real risks; and barbiturates have an almost unequalled potential for suicidal use (see further Essay III). Ability to drive or perform other skilled tasks may be impaired at almost any dosage level. As Malcolm Lader has written: 'The more complex the human psychological function, the more it is impaired by barbiturates. Tasks requiring intricate and dexterous manipulations, for example handwriting, are also markedly affected.' ('Drugs for Anxiety', *Practitioner* 215: 469, 1975). Almost the only advantage which barbiturates offered was their cheapness: 100 tablets of phenobarbitone 60 mg are priced at less than £1, while a prescription for a newer tranquillizer may cost five times as much, or even more (see Table 7).

The first drug specifically promoted as an anxiety-reliever, meprobamate, became available in the USA in 1951. Originally proposed as a muscle-relaxant, it was soon realized that this compound had tremendous sales potential as an alternative to barbiturates for inducing a state of tranquillity. Under the trade-name Miltown – the name of the place where it was manufactured – meprobamate proved immensely successful. Indeed, up to about 1962, when Valium was introduced, this was the most frequently prescribed drug in America. Miltown was also the first psychotropic agent to be named a tranquillizer: the term was coined to obviate the slightly pejorative overtones of 'sedative'. During the 1950s two other compounds, related to each other but not to meprobamate, became popular as barbiturate surrogates for inducing sleep and for their calmative effects: glutethimide (Doriden) and methylprylon (Noludar) may still be prescribed, although neither is really suitable for daytime use (see Chart IIIC).

Meprobamate, known in the UK as Equanil, proved after careful comparative studies to possess effects almost identical to those of the barbiturates. Its acute toxicity is said to be relatively less, however, so that among patients who might be suicide-prone the compound is not so hazardous. Still, it is dangerous in overdosage, and withdrawal symptoms in persons addicted to meprobamate match those of the barbiturates both in type and severity. The tranquillizer and its chemical cousin tybamate

(Tybatran), which is also prescribed as a muscle-relaxant, are significantly shorter-acting than even the supposedly 'short-acting' barbiturates such as pentobarbitone. This necessitates a three- or four-times-daily regimen of doses. Even when taken in modest quantities (the strength of the standard tablet is 400 mg) meprobamate may slow reflexes and decrease short-term memory. Adverse effects and interactions with other drugs are similar to those of the barbiturates. Despite its continued favour with a few practitioners (and more than a few patients), meprobamate should be regarded as obsolete in the treatment of anxiety and tension states.

The Benzodiazepines: Valium and its Kin

Chemicals of a particular class, known as benzodiazepines, were synthesized as early as 1933, but nobody considered them to be of any importance until the mid 1950s. It was then that Lowell O. Randall and his colleagues noticed that one of these drugs – chlordiazepoxide – produced a remarkable taming action when administered to aggressive monkeys and, what is more, did so at a lower dosage than that required to send them to sleep. Profound muscle-relaxant and anticonvulsant properties were also observed at this time.

The potential implications of this research were not lost on workers at Hoffmann-La Roche, one of the largest of the multinational drug companies, which is based in Switzerland. Chlordiazepoxide was extensively tested in human beings and, in addition to relaxation of the smooth muscles and the abolition of seizures, as in epilepsy, the compound demonstrated a hitherto unmatched capacity for mitigating anxiety and tension: excessive sedation occurred only when much larger doses were given. Chlordiazepoxide came on to the market in 1960 with the now universally familiar trade-name Librium. A similar, but more potent, drug belonging to the same chemical group, diazepam (Valium), appeared amidst much fanfare a couple of years later. Compounds of this benzodiazepine class were shown to act selectively at certain sites in the midbrain, whereas the barbiturates and meprobamate have a much more generalized effect in depressing the central nervous system. They also turned out to be far safer than any of the previously used anxiety-relieving drugs. The margin between effective and toxic doses is wider for Valium and its kin than for any other type of mood-modifying agent.

Precisely how these compounds quell anxiety is still unclear, since they influence a number of the neurotransmitters which conduct nerve impulses to the brain. In particular diazepam and its analogues enhance the activity of γ-aminobutyric acid, or GABA, which is known to be associated with anticonvulsant effect and improved mood. Other factors are involved and research is proceeding apace with the aim of discovering precise mechanisms of action. On the basis of studies being conducted at the time of this writing, it appears that the benzodiazepines 'bind' to receptor-sites in the brain which are specific for these drugs alone, and that a 'natural tranquillizer' is produced in the human brain, perhaps analogous to the 'natural opiates' or endorphins to whose receptor-sites molecules of morphine and similar pain-killers specifically bind (see Essay IV). The actual molecule has not so far been discovered, but there seems little doubt of its existence.

Whatever the means whereby Librium and Valium exert their effects, these two drugs soon supplanted the earlier anxiolytic agents. Roche and other companies are still promoting these and other benzodiazepines vigorously. Diazepam, whether dispensed as an unbranded ('generic') preparation or under the Valium tradename, now accounts for over 70% of all prescriptions for tranquillizers written in the UK. And, according to evidence submitted to a US Senate Commission in 1979, American physicians issued almost 45 million prescriptions for Valium alone. Thus it is by far the most extensively used of all psychotropic drugs: Valium and analogues are now taken by 14% of the population in Britain, 17% in France and Belgium, 15% in Denmark, 14% in Germany, 10% in Italy and Spain, and 10% in the USA. Ten years ago the British Monopolies Commission established that prescriptions for Librium and Valium cost the National Health Service £6.8 million, from which at least £4 million was made by Roche as a clear profit. The cost of these and other benzodiazepines will be referred to below, in connection with the introduction of newer compounds of the same chemical class.

While diazepam and chlordiazepoxide remain more heavily used than all other anti-anxiety agents, a large number of other benzodiazepines have been introduced since 1963. Those currently available for prescription in the UK and/or the USA are displayed in Chart VI(A) and also in Chart III(B): most are recommended by their respective manufacturers to quell tension and anxiety, while others are promoted as remedies for insomnia. In fact both are very close analogues of the original compounds, having essentially similar ranges of activity and side-effects. Those benzodiazepines which are marketed and advertised as hypnotics – flurazepam (Dalmane), nitrazepam (Mogadon), among others – could equally well be taken during the daytime at correspondingly lower doses. Conversely, the ones commonly prescribed as tranquillizers – e.g. medazepam (Nobrium), clorazepate (Tranxene, Azene) and prazepam (Verstran) – will, if taken at night in a single dose equivalent to or slightly larger than the total indicated for the day, not only help the patient to sleep but, in most cases, go on with their anxiolytic action through most, if not all, the following day. Dosages for and other information on 'hypnotic' benzodiazepines will be found in Chart III(B), and data on the remainder in Chart VI(A), which accompanies this Essay.

Most benzodiazepines in fact are broken down to other discrete substances which continue to affect the individual. Diazepam, flurazepam, nitrazepam and others are converted in the body to *N*-desmethyldiazepam (which is also the active element in clorazepate). All of them are offered to the prescriber as single-entity drugs, under various proprietary names. In only one important respect do the benzodiazepines differ (see Table 7): some have a longer duration of action than others. Chlordiazepoxide and diazepam are among the longest-acting, while oxazepam (Serenid, Serax) and lorazepam (Activan) may need to be taken more than once daily for tranquillizing purposes. For some patients, even these can be useful as a single daily dose, which is what we would advocate for the majority of drugs of this type. In a technical paper which reviews the biochemical changes wrought in the body by benzodiazepines, S. H. Curry and R. Whelpton tell us: 'In anxiety, combining a brief sedative effect with a prolonged anxiolytic effect in a bedtime dose may be particularly appropriate and diazepam is clearly the best drug for doing this' ('Pharmacokinetics of closely related benzodiazepines' *British Journal of Clinical Pharmacology* 8: 20S, 1979). Diazepam and chlordiazepoxide were found, on the basis of a survey conducted in 1973, to be the first and third drugs most often prescribed by US practitioners. Reviewing these agents and their alternatives, Barry Blackwell observes, with a hint of irony: 'It remains unclear as to why diazepam is so much preferred . . . [to other anxiolytics]. There is no convincing evidence of realistic differences apart from the anticonvulsant effects of diazepam parenterally. It would be tempting to assume that marketing influences alone are responsible, but it is equally possible that physicians and their patients know something that the scientist as yet does not' ('Psychotropic drugs in use today' *Journal of the American Medical Association* 225: 1640, 1973). Blackwell draws our attention to a ban on benzodiazepines imposed in South Carolina (because of budgetary considerations), for prescription under the Medicaid programme, which came into force shortly before he wrote his paper. Only 35% of anxiolytic drug use was replaced by prescriptions for antidepressants and major (antipsychotic) tranquillizers, while 65% of anti-anxiety drug use was unaccounted for. Although the author is careful to qualify his judgment, the conclusion – namely, that benzodiazepines were being heavily overprescribed – is surely evident.

During the past year alone, two more benzodiazepines have appeared in Britain: clobazam (Frisium) and ketazolam (Anxon). It is extremely doubtful whether either offers any advantages whatever over diazepam, and it is hard to see the justification – other than financial, in terms of profits for the drug companies – for the addition of still more 'me-too' compounds in an already crowded field. Peter Tyrer, an expert on psychopharmacology, entitled one of his articles 'The Benzodiazepine Bonanza'. That was published in 1974, and several other analogues have become available in Germany, France and elsewhere since then. Tyrer

Table 7: THE METABOLISM OF DIAZEPAM (VALIUM) AND RELATED DRUGS

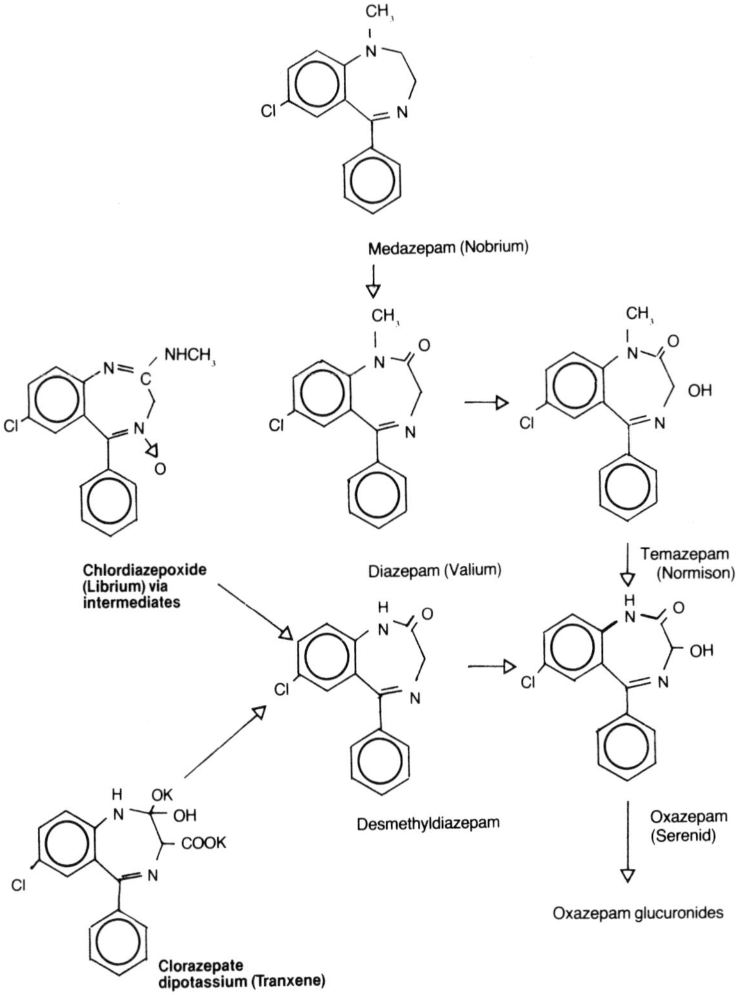

Medazepam (Nobrium)

Chlordiazepoxide (Librium) via intermediates

Diazepam (Valium)

Temazepam (Normison)

Desmethyldiazepam

Oxazepam (Serenid)

Clorazepate dipotassium (Tranxene)

Oxazepam glucuronides

adapted from: S. H. Curry and R. Whelpton, 'Pharmacokinetics of related benzodiazepines' *British Journal of Clinical Pharmacology* vol. 8 (1979) p. 16S

admits that the production of chlordiazepoxide and diazepam represented 'a development of the first magnitude – both clinically and commercially. [They] were introduced into a market in which the demand was immense and in which there were few competitors', and that 'no other class of drugs has shown the versatility and relative safety' of these drugs (*Lancet* II: 709, 1974). However, he and many other clinicians have questioned the desirability or need for such a plethora of alternatives, each more expensive than the last. This is shown by Table 8, in which the wholesale costs of equivalent dose forms of the available anxiolytics are compared: it will be seen, for instance, that the price for 100 tablets of diazepam 5 mg (unbranded) is £0.58, compared with £1.44 for the Valium brand produced by Roche and £6.56 for ketazolam 15mg capsules. In the UK, of course, the real cost of prescription under the NHS bears no relation to the still nominal prescription charges. GPs and patients alike have their own preferences for particular benzodiazepines, and it is clear that these are not always based on the results of objective studies.

Table 8: COMPARATIVE COST OF ANXIETY-RELIEVING DRUGS

Drug Name (Official)	Brand	Strength	Cost per 100 Tablets/ Capsules
Drugs prescribed as tranquillizers (Other than benzodiazepines)			
phenobarbitone	unbranded	30 mg tablet	£0.30
phenobarbitone	Luminal	30 mg tablet	£0.67
meprobamate	unbranded	400 mg tablet	£0.42
meprobamate	Miltown	400 mg tablet	£1.08
propranolol	unbranded	40 mg tablet	£2.80
propranolol	Inderal	40 mg tablet	£3.50
hydroxyzine	Atarax	10 mg tablet	£2.73
chlormethiazole	Heminevrin	500 mg capsule	£4.22
Benzodiazepines (those promoted as daytime tranquillizers)			
chlordiazepoxide	unbranded	10 mg tablet	£0.77
chlordiazepoxide	Librium	10 mg tablet	£1.35
diazepam	unbranded	5 mg capsule	£0.58
diazepam	Valium	5 mg capsule	£1.44
oxazepam	Serenid-D	15 mg tablet	£1.50
medazepam	Nobrium	10 mg capsule	£2.24
lorazepam	Ativan	1 mg tablet	£1.85
clorazepate	Tranxene	15 mg capsule	£5.21
clobazam	Frisium	10 mg capsule	£5.00
ketazolam	Anxon	15 mg capsule	£6.56
Benzodiazepines (those promoted to induce sleep)			
nitrazepam	unbranded	5 mg tablet	£1.00
nitrazepam	Mogadon	5 mg tablet	£1.40
flurazepam	Dalmane	15 mg capsule	£5.09
temazepam	Normison	10 mg capsule	£5.00
triazolam	Halcion	0.125 mg tablet	£4.44

Note: Each drug formulation is of approximately comparable therapeutic potency (daytime benzodiazepines and others); and doses of 'hypnotic' benzodiazepines are also comparable. Cost of 100 units is wholesale. Sources: *Chemist & Druggist Price List* vol. 21 (1980); *MIMS* vol. 22 etc. (1980).

A number of recommendations regarding diazepam-type tranquillizers have been promulgated by a committee of the American Medical Association. These criteria are worth mentioning and are paraphrased as follows:

1 Benzodiazepines should be used to relieve severe symptoms, not for minor complaints;
2 The underlying disorder should be diagnosed and, if possible, treated before accepting superficial relief of symptoms by prescribing these drugs;
3 Valium and its analogues should not normally be prescribed for people who have a history of drug abuse;
4 The patient should not be given an excessive dose, i.e. one that will make him sleepy or confused, or significantly impair reflexes;
5 The physician should be familiar with the type of withdrawal symptoms which can develop in cases of long-term drug overuse or abuse;
6 When it is considered appropriate to prescribe a benzodiazepine to a patient on a long-term basis, the doctor should watch for signs of tolerance and physical or psychological dependency;
7 The number of tablets or capsules prescribed at any one time should not exceed that required between visits to the physician's surgery (i.e. telephoned requests for repeat prescriptions should be discouraged);
8 Patients should be warned that the action of Valium and similar compounds is enhanced by alcohol and by other drugs which depress the central nervous system (e.g. other tranquillizers, barbiturates, opiate analgesics);
9 Patients should be clearly instructed that the drug is for their use only and should be kept out of the reach of children;
10 The doctor should convey an attitude that suggests that his prescribing of drugs is only part of the overall management of the patient's problem.

(*Journal of the American Medical Association* 230: 1440f, 1974)

The above seem to the present writers to be sensible suggestions, though they are a counsel of perfection. In a perfect world, such criteria should be met in respect of all psychotropic medicaments. The risk of taking Valium or other benzodiazepines would appear to some, on the basis of the AMA's recommendations, to be overstated: and undoubtedly these hazards are fewer than for barbiturates and for certain other mood-altering drugs. However, caution should always be the watchword.

As has already been pointed out, diazepam and its congeners have excellent muscle-relaxant properties, and so the more potent of them are given to treat tetanus (lockjaw), muscular spasm arising from cerebral palsy, and other conditions in which such an effect is needed. By intravenous injection, diazepam has been shown a successful treatment of status epilepticus, which is characterized by repeated and uncontrolled seizures, and as premedication before surgical operations, including dental procedures. Benzodiazepines are also often effective in alleviating alcoholic withdrawal reactions such as delirium tremens. Diazepam has more recently been suggested as a short-term remedy for somnambulism (sleepwalking) and night terrors in children.

Injectable formulations are available of chlordiazepoxide (Librium), diazepam (Valium), and in the UK lorazepam (Ativan). Perhaps curiously, diazepam is not more effective on a weight-for-weight basis by intramuscular than by oral administration. But if it is given by injection into a vein, great care needs to be taken. The manufacturers recommend that the vein in the bend of the elbow (the antecubital fossa) be used. We believe that this advice is inappropriate, because the antecubital vein tends to lie close to its corresponding artery, and inadvertent intra-arterial injection can be most dangerous. In any event the injection should be delivered very slowly. This is because diazepam, like most of its kin, is impossible to dissolve in water: a somewhat viscous solvent, propylene glycol, is therefore used (but see Addenda, p. 455). Too rapid or too frequent intravenous use of diazepam may collapse the superficial veins, and if any of the solution is extravasated (i.e. spills into the surrounding tissues), fibrosis of the area may occur. Still, as the benzodiazepines are very well absorbed when taken by mouth, administration by other means is suitable only in special circumstances such as those described, e.g. where rapid effect is necessary.

The usual range of doses for each of these tranquillizers is shown in Chart VI(A). In some instances patients may require less than the stated minimum, or in excess of the maximum, quantity. As for other psychotropic agents, but perhaps to a greater extent, individual requirements are enormously variable. The only way a physician can tell which dosage suits a particular patient is empirically. So the procedure would be to begin with a standard dose unit and then, according to response, to decrease or increase the daily (or nightly) regimen. Because the principal side-effects, such as impairment of reflexes, tend to be more apparent during the first phase of these drugs' action, a single bedtime dose is often the best way of achieving the desired result, as Curry and Whelpton concluded in their study of the pharmacokinetics (metabolism) of these tranquillizers. The patient could be instructed to take a single dose at bedtime of, say, diazepam or clorazepate (Tranxene), and then be asked whether any hangover effects – sleepiness, confusion, lethargy – were experienced the following morning. Shorter-acting compounds like oxazepam (Serenid,

Serax), we remind the reader, may be given 12-hourly, at breakfast and at night. There is seldom if ever any need for conventional three-times-daily or more frequent routines.

In introducing the reader to these anxiolytics, mention has been made of their low toxicity, and hence the relative rarity of successful suicide with them. There is on record one celebrated case: a depressed man took 40 × 5 mg nitrazepam (Mogadon) tablets for this purpose. On admission to hospital the patient required no supportive measures or antidotes and indeed woke up spontaneously some 10 hours subsequently feeling quite normal. Data on lethal doses of drugs are usually derived from experiments on laboratory animals, although in some cases clinical experience gives us a reasonable indication of likely fatal dosages. The LD_{50} doses are often quoted: these refer to the quantity of drug needed to kill 50% of a given number of Wistar rats or other experimental animals. The LD_{50}s for benzodiazepines are almost incredibly high, and some pharmacologists have said whimsically that the only way to kill a guinea-pig with Valium is to bury the unfortunate animal in the drug. While that is plainly an exaggeration, it must be pointed out that there have been some fatalities in which benzodiazepines were implicated, and that, though the low toxicity of these compounds is a facet to be borne in mind, this fact alone should not encourage physicians to prescribe them in excessive quanities, as some are wont to do.

The degree to which repeated use of diazepam-like drugs leads to tolerance and to frank dependency is a matter which is currently the subject of heated debate. Leo Hollister and his colleagues recounted withdrawal reactions on the abrupt cessation of treatment with Librium: trembling, fever and even convulsions were described. Interestingly, his account was published as early as 1961, long before the explosion of tranquillizer use, and this concerned patients who had been on very high doses over long periods (L. E. Hollister, F. P. Motzenbecker, and R. O. Degan, *Psychopharmacologia* 2: 63-8, 1961). There is no question that some tolerance – diminution in the effectiveness of constant dosage – develops in some patients quite quickly, necessitating higher doses to achieve the required therapeutic result. On the other hand, many who have taken benzodiazepines for months or longer have been adequately maintained at the original levels. The extent of psychological, and of physical, dependency is difficult to establish, in large measure because these drugs are so freely prescribed. Still, in a recent article David Greenblatt and Richard Shader, who are notable authorities on the subject, reviewed the relevant clinical literature. And they observe that the 'barrage of irresponsible and sensationalistic journalism by popular newspapers, periodicals and television' have made it 'almost impossible . . . to gain a rational clinical perspective of this problem'. These authors conclude that the dangers both of physical addiction and of psychological habituation have been greatly overstated. They make the important point that what some practitioners assume to be withdrawal reactions – e.g. tenseness, hyperagitation – simply represent the recrudescence of the symptoms for which the drug was originally prescribed. ('Dependence, tolerance, and addiction to benzodiazepines: clinical and pharmacokinetic considerations' *Drug Metabolism Reviews* 8: 13-28, 1978) The British Committee on Review of Medicines, which reported on benzodiazepines in 1980, acknowledged the possibility but hedged their bets as to the likelihood of dependency: this body advocates only short-term or intermittent, rather than continuous, treatment with these tranquillizers, with slow, stepwise withdrawal at the end of such therapy. The CRM report that abstinence reactions may set on 3 to 10 days after discontinuation of longer-acting, and within 24 hours in the case of shorter-acting, drugs of this class ('Systematic Review of the Benzodiazepines' *British Medical Journal* II: 1,009, 1980).

According to the authoritative *Drug and Therapeutics Bulletin*:

> The Committee has to some extent fudged the issue of benzodiazepine dependence. It attaches considerable importance to withdrawal symptoms after prolonged use, yet states that on the published evidence the risk of dependence with [these drugs] seems low. If withdrawal symptoms are common and occasionally severe (e.g. fits or psychosis) after long-term therapy, and if they lead to patients seeking supplies of the drug, this suggests true dependence, although it may be milder than with opiates and barbiturates. If the CRM believes that benzodiazepines produce dependence, it should have said so more clearly. More studies are urgently needed, especially of withdrawal after long-term use.
>
> The CRM ducks the problem of the many chronically anxious patients who obtain continuing symptomatic relief and often function better while taking [diazepam] for anxiety. Many doctors lack the time and skill to manage such patients without drugs: some patients do not accept non-drug therapy. (18: 98, 1980)

Malcolm Lader, reporting verbally on studies still in progress, has found that regular use of large doses of drug of this class can certainly lead to physical as well as psychological dependency. In a series of admittedly self-selected patients who were repeated users, he has shown that abrupt discontinuation of diazepam and analogues provoked abstinence signs and symptoms which were qualitatively similar to those known to occur in barbiturate withdrawal (Lader, personal communication, 1980).

Chart VI(A) indicates a variety of side-effects which may be expected with diazepam and its analogues. Usually these are mild and are seldom so troublesome as to necessitate stopping treatment with such agents. It has evidently escaped the notice of many practitioners that, if a patient reports adverse effects from one benzodiazepine, he will almost certainly do so if another is substituted (cross-sensitivity). Commonest among unwanted reactions are oversedation, unsteadiness of gait (ataxia), drowsiness and blurred vision: the elderly are particularly susceptible to these and other symptoms. Patients should, as the AMA recommends, be warned about possible impairment of reflexes, when driving or performing skilled tasks that require manual dexterity. This applies to the very 'new' benzodiazepines clobazam (Frisium) and ketazolam (Anxon), for despite their manufacturers' claims that they cause negligible sedation this effect is characteristic of the class as a whole, and is dose-dependent. Less frequently, other undesirable effects may arise: loss of libido and sexual potency do not seem to be as rare as is generally supposed. Skin rashes, urinary retention, headache, vertigo, hypotension (rapid fall in blood-pressure), jaundice and blood disorders have been reported sufficiently often to be worth mentioning: probably fewer than one patient in ten will experience any of these particular problems. But the phenomenon of disinhibition, to which reference has been made in connection with the barbiturates (see Essay III), is definitely under-reported. Like alcohol, diazepines may remove some or all of the conscious and unconscious inhibitions which ordinary consciousness imposes on us and which are socially necessary. As a result, 'paradoxical' effects, like excitement, over-agitation and even aggressiveness, are beginning to be recognized, especially when high doses have been taken. Depression, sometimes of a very profound kind, is sometimes intensified or provoked by these tranquillizers.

There are few absolute contra-indications to the use of Valium and its chemical relations. These compounds should not be taken by patients suffering from myasthenia gravis, acute respiratory problems, in cases of known hypersensitivity, by children (except diazepam, for night terrors or sleepwalking), and, unless the reasons are compelling, during pregnancy and lactation. Care should be exercised if it is proposed to prescribe benzodiazepines for patients with impaired liver or kidney function.

These agents enhance the CNS-depressant action of other drugs, including alcohol in any form. This does not mean that the patient should stop drinking altogether, but rather that extra care should be taken and the quantity of liquor consumed reduced. The combination will affect reflexes adversely. Cigarette smoking appears to reduce the effectiveness of usual doses of diazepines, and this is a factor which the practitioner should take into account when assessing dosage schedules. These tranquillizers increase the action of thyroxine (thyroid hormone) and decrease that of the anti-epileptic drug phenytoin (Epanutin). Dose levels of digitalis (digoxin, Lanoxin) and coumarin anticoagulants (e.g. warfarin,

Marevan), as used in heart disease, may have to be adjusted if a diazepam-type compound is being prescribed. Diazepam seems to lengthen the effect of injectable muscle-relaxants used during surgery (gallamine, suxamethonium). Concurrent administration of one of these tranquillizers with an antidepressant – such as amitriptyline (Tryptizol, Elavil) and imipramine (Tofranil) – may cause some of the latters' unwanted effects to be magnified (see Essay II: Antidepressants and Tranquillizer/Antidepressant combinations).

So far as the abuse potential of benzodiazepines is concerned, the authors of one thorough review state: 'Based on the experimental and clinical results available . . . there is an extremely low incidence of people who spontaneously increase the doses of these drugs' (Greenblatt and Shader, *op.cit.*). On the question of physical addiction and withdrawal effects, they note 'striking differences between [barbiturates and diazepines] with regard to type, severity, development, duration [of], and recovery [from] the syndrome'. G. Reggiani also reminds us that 'the so-called benzodiazepine withdrawal symptoms can be simulated by rebound effects of the underlying disease', that it is virtually impossible to commit suicide with these agents, and that they 'have been prescribed for many patients with a tendency towards excessive drug-taking, with little evidence of abuse' ('Abuse potential: discussion summary' in *The Benzodiazepines*, ed. S. Garattini, E. Mussini and L. O. Randall. Milan/New York, 1973, pp.627–9). These statements contrast with the more recent findings of Lader and others.

Reggiani, we feel, exaggerates the case for prescribing tranquillizers. Only the most blinkered of practitioners would now say that Valium and analogous drugs have 'negligible' abuse potential. On the other hand, given the extra hazards of habituation to and abuse of other psychotropic agents, such as barbiturates, and the fact that some patients' demands for chemically induced tranquillity are irresistible, perhaps the benzodiazepines are the least of several alternative evils. The American Medical Association's criteria should represent a goal, which cannot always be attained, but which should always be in view.

Other Anti-Anxiety Drugs

A novel approach to the treatment of anxiety, which has been tried for a few years now, is the use of β-adrenergic blocking agents (beta-blockers), drugs normally prescribed in hypertension, to control blood-pressure, and in heart disease. One of these, propranolol (Inderal) is at present being promoted by its manufacturers also as an anxiolytic. Certainly beta-blockers reduce the physical manifestations of tension, such as fast heart-rate, excessive sweating, and cold in the extremities – symptoms indicative of sympathetic nervous system overactivity. Propranolol does appear to relieve stress: in a celebrated study a similar drug, oxprenolol, was given to a group of musicians shortly before they were due to play at a concert. According to two professional judges, their playing was improved. Subjectively, it seems that the subjects were less nervous than usual.

There remain doubts about propranolol's efficacy, although it has become popular to prescribe it as an alternative to Valium. Part of the beta-blockers' current fashionability stems from the fact that they apparently have no abuse liability and are not tolerance-producing. One researcher, J. R. Hawkings, has tested oxprenolol as an anxiolytic with less than excellent results. As he explains: 'My excuse would be that I am protecting these patients from benzodiazepines, which I think are much more of a public danger; indeed one could say that the main success of the trial is that patients have been protected from being on benzodiazepine drugs long enough for them to get better' ('Beta-blockers in the treatment of anxiety' in *The Cardiovascular, Metabolic and Psychological Interface,* ed. R. W. Elsdon-Dew *et al.* London, 1979. Royal Society of Medicine International . . . Symposium Series no. 14, p. 79).

It is believed that beta-blockers are less likely than diazepam and its relations to affect reflexes, but clear evidence on this point is lacking. Propranolol is more likely than alternatives to provoke unwanted effects, and some serious interactions with other drugs should be, though often are not, considered. For example, beta-blockers are incompatible with MAO-inhibitor antidepressants; they may enhance the bradycardia (slowed heart-rate) produced by digitalis; and they should not be taken concurrently with the cardiac drugs verapamil (Cordilox) and clonidine (Catapres, Dixarit), and the anti-parkinsonian agent levodopa (Larodopa).

Drugs of this type are contra-indicated in heart block, cases of very poor cardiac reserve, diabetes, bronchospasm (e.g. in asthma), in pregnancy and after prolonged fasting. The studies published so far on the role of beta-blockers in the treatment of anxiety are conflicting, some indicating that they are effective, some that they may be so, and some again that they have no more than a placebo effect.

Among the compounds whose anxiolytic activity is not in question, hydroxyzine (Atarax, Vistaril) has been available for some years. This drug has antihistamine, antispasmodic and antinauseant effects, and has proved successful in relieving conditions of emotional stress, tension and agitation. It has been shown to be useful even in some psychotic states. An injectable formulation of hydroxyzine marketed in the USA has been recommended for severe acute anxiety, in alcoholic delirium tremens, and as pre- or post-operative sedation, either on its own or in conjunction with a narcotic analgesic such as pethidine (meperidine). The drug is well tolerated by most patients, though very high doses may provoke parkinsonian reactions, confusion, tremor and rarely even convulsions. The compound considerably increases the central depressant actions of other drugs. If it is to be administered concurrently with an opiate, for example, the dosage of the latter should be reduced by at least 50%. The only absolute contra-indications to use of hydroxyzine are pregnancy and known hypersensitivity. Like virtually all tranquillizers this one may slow down reflexes, an effect which is dose-related. Some cases of hydroxyzine dependency have been recorded, but this is not common. For some unknown reason this drug has never been popular in the UK.

One other substance which can be classified as a 'minor' tranquillizer has been included in Chart VI(A). This is chlormethiazole (Heminevrin), which is widely used in Europe but unobtainable in the USA. It is prescribed for night sedation, particularly to elderly patients, as its hypnotic action is mild and its toxicity relatively low. Chlormethiazole is also given to control anxiety, in withdrawal from alcohol or opiates, and its anticonvulsant activity makes it an appropriate treatment for some cases of alcoholic delirium, toxaemia of pregnancy and other conditions requiring such an effect. It should be given strictly on a short-term basis, as a fairly high proportion of patients find it euphoriant and, given the opportunity, some become dependent upon it. Principal side-effects are a strange tingling sensation in the nose, oversedation, and confusion. Chlormethiazole should be avoided in patients with severe liver disorders. As with other tranquillizers, its effects are potentiated by alcohol, barbiturates, and other depressants, and it is likely to impair reflexes. The drug has a short duration of action.

Among other obsolescent or less popular compounds which are sometimes prescribed as tranquillizers, mephenesin (Myanesin), and tybamate (Tybatran) are considered individually in the Alphabetical Entries of this book. Recently (1979) deleted in the UK has been methylpentynol (Oblivon, Oblivon-C), which chemically is a higher alcohol. This is regrettable because the compound is extremely effective in quelling situational anxiety. The present writers have found 250-750 mg of methylpentynol an excellent remedy in a variety of situations: for instance, given ½–1 hour before a visit to the dental surgery, the drug will abolish the anxious fear which so many feel at such times. It has very few and transient side-effects and an extremely short (2–4 hour) duration of action. Oblivon remains available in Germany, France and elsewhere, and it is hoped that it will be re-introduced for prescription in the UK.

B: ANTIPSYCHOTIC ('MAJOR') TRANQUILLIZERS

The thirty or so drugs described under this rubric are tranquillizers, but in many important respects they could not be more different from the benzodiazepines and other anxiety-relieving agents just discussed. Some clinicians dislike the term 'tranquillizer' for these much more potent compounds, which should be prescribed, with few exceptions, to control symptoms of profound mental disorders. It is felt that the expression is misleading, so many prefer the adjectival nouns 'antipsychotic' or 'neuroleptic' (the latter from *neuron* = nerve, and *leptos* = subtle, or fine). Neuroleptic might be translated as 'mind-tuning', to indicate the intention of producing an alteration in the chemical processes of the brain, which in schizophrenia and other 'psychotic' states are disturbed. *MIMS*, a monthly publication listing all proprietary drugs available to British prescribers, lists both Valium-type tranquillizers and antipsychotic medicaments together as 'sedatives and tranquillizers'. This fact has, we believe, been partly responsible for the practice of prescribing neuroleptics in relatively trivial conditions, the undesirability of which is considered later.

Unlike the illnesses which manifest with 'physical' signs and symptoms, the definitions of conditions classed as psychoses and neuroses are, at best, imprecise, and the label 'schizophrenia' covers a multitude of sins. There exists no definition of these terms which all psychiatrists will find acceptable. Some actually hold the conviction that, in an absolute sense, 'psychosis' does not exist or is a misnomer: Thomas Szasz and Ronald Laing, who believe the idea of 'mental illness' to be more of a myth than a reality, have written eloquently on the subject and latterly have gained a small but articulate following among younger practitioners. But to the majority of psychiatrists their views are anathema: in the UK and elsewhere the prevailing philosophy which underlies treatment techniques in psychological 'disorders' is behaviourism. This school of thought, founded by J. B. Watson and elaborated by Burrhus F. Skinner, regards normal and abnormal behaviour as the result of conditioned reflexes which are not under the control of the will. Generally, behaviouristic practitioners place more emphasis on controlling the symptoms, rather than seeking out the root causes, of the states which are defined as 'abnormal'. Hence they tend to make far wider use of neuroleptic and other psychotropic drugs than do psychoanalysts, who avoid them whenever possible. Freud still casts a long shadow over psychiatry as practised in the USA and to a lesser extent in the UK. This is not the place for a comparative critique of behaviourist versus analytic types of therapy, although it is appropriate to question commonly made assumptions which may not be valid.

All classifications of 'psychosis', and especially of those classical psychotic states known as schizophrenia, are to an extent arbitrary. According to epidemiological records, schizophrenia is a commoner ailment in the USA than in the UK. It has now been established that American psychiatrists diagnose the condition more often than their colleagues here. Most are agreed that schizophrenic states are a biological disorder or disorders, i.e. that the hormones and other substances in the brain which control and regulate mood and behaviour are disturbed. Physical injury to the cerebral cortex is not often implicated. Schizoid conditions may be acute or chronic, and occur in young or old, male or female. Opinions differ on the relative importance of a genetic predisposition to the illness and that of environmental factors. Whatever the root or proximate causes, the condition is manifested by an inability to think logically or behave rationally. The signs and symptoms are many and various. Some psychiatrists still classify schizophrenias according to the categories defined by Emil Kraepelin early in the century. Kraepelin found there to be four types: *simplex*, or simple, schizophrenia, in which the patient becomes emotionally blunted and apathetic, loses his drive, and tends to withdraw into his own inner world: in spite of these traits he may remain fairly rational. Then there is the *hebephrenic* group, characterized by hallucinations or delusions, hysteria, anomalies in speech, 'silly' and 'childish' behaviour, which suggests that the patient has 'regressed' to some point in childhood. In the *catatonic* type there seems to be a split personality, with the person apparently normal one moment and irrational the next: a feeling of being irrevocably cut off from everyone and everything ('adrift in space') may be overwhelming. Lastly, *paranoid* schizophrenics have hallucinations, sense that they are being watched, spied on or persecuted, and sometimes have delusions of grandeur ('I am Jesus Christ' etc.). Interestingly, these same types are described in the latest edition of one of the most authoritative medical dictionaries, published in 1975 (Taber's *Cyclopedic Medical Dictionary*, ed C. L. Thomas. Philadelphia, 1975, p. 517[s]).

The brilliant and iconoclastic Thomas Szasz has a different approach. According to him, schizophrenia is a sacred symbol in psychiatry. 'The largest grab-bag of all the misbehaviours which psychiatrists, coerced by "society" or convinced by their own zeal, are now ready to diagnose, prognose, and therapize', is how he refers to the condition(s) concerned. He then goes on to quote four 'inclusion criteria' regarded by the authors of a recent World Health Organization study as diagnostic of schizophrenia: (1) delusions; (2) definitely inappropriate or unusual behaviour; (3) hallucinations and (4) gross [mental or physical] over- or under-activity. The presence of these signs and symptoms, according to the WHO report, automatically qualify a patient as schizophrenic, 'regardless of the severity of the symptomatology'.

Szasz then proceeds easily to demolish all four. 'Delusions' may include a belief that one belongs to a Chosen Race; 'inappropriate or unusual behaviour' may be having long hair, short hair or no hair; 'hallucinations' could be subsumed under (believed) communication with a God or gods or with dead people; and 'over- and under-activity' – well, an example of this might be 'travelling halfway across the world to attend a psychiatric meeting and falling asleep while listening to the presentation of the papers'. *Schizophrenia: the sacred symbol of psychiatry*. Oxford, 1979, pp. 18f.)

Although the schizophrenias are the principal indication (in the view of most psychiatrists) for use of neuroleptic drugs, other conditions described as psychotic are treated with these agents. Mania, as in the manic-depressive syndrome, with its wild mood-swings which range from the most energetic euphoria to the most immobilizing depression, is one such instance: for this ailment in particular lithium carbonate is a specific therapy (see below, p. 363). Other severely disabling conditions are handled more conventionally with major tranquillizers of the chlor-promazine (Largactil, Thorazine) type. These include so-called 'acute brain syndromes', which refer to sudden (and often self-limiting) serious after-effects of amphetamines and certain other drugs (see Essay I); Alzheimer's disease, the most common form of dementia associated with old age; Gilles de la Tourette syndrome, a rare complaint manifesting with spontaneous outbursts of obscene language and a strange, barking tic; and certain forms of continuous, profound depression. Not all of these respond to antipsychotic medication, and in some conditions (e.g. the chronic depressions) such drugs are generally contra-indicated.

So far as schizophrenia especially is concerned, people tend not to fit neatly into the convenient pigeon-holes set out by Kraepelin (or indeed by more modern authorities). The point of describing certain sets of symptoms is partly to indicate the basis on which neuroleptics are often prescribed and partly to indicate the extraordinary diversity of phenomena for which the blanket term 'psychosis' is employed. This catch-all expression is thus explained in the medical glossary already referred to. Psychosis refers to 'those disturbances of such magnitude that there is personality disintegration and loss of contact with reality. [The psychotic patient] fails to mirror reality as it is, reacts erroneously to it, and builds up false concepts regarding it. His behaviour responses are peculiar, abnormal, inefficient, or definitely antiso-cial' (*op. cit.* pp. 167f.). Pragmatically, one could differentiate 'psychotic' from 'neurotic' and other conditions quite simply: if the so-called disorder is so crippling that the individual is unable to look after himself and to undertake basic tasks (washing, eating) unaided, then one may term it psychosis. On the other hand, persons with neuroses – which may still present serious problems – are at least able to cope with such tasks and remain in touch with 'reality'.

It is plain that definitions and explanations like those quoted from Taber beg many questions: who is to say what is 'normal' behaviour? And if you ask a philosopher what 'reality' is, you are likely to be told that your own existence is hypothetical. Concepts of reality are not in any sense absolute: they are culturally conditioned. Hence aberrations or deviations from an accepted norm differ according to the society in which one lives. Behaviour which in Western cultures would be regarded as bizarre or 'psychotic' may not merely be tolerated, but respected, in other societies. To give a concrete example: among the Yakut of Siberia, a particular member of the community as a youth begins to 'hear voices', to withdraw into himself, to experience what most of us would call 'hallucinations'. Such characteristics are taken to mean that this individual is a *shaman*, with healing and perhaps prophetic powers. Similar phenomena are found in African societies and elsewhere, and the interested reader will with profit read any of the works of the great anthropologist Mircea Eliade (e.g. *Shamanism*. London, 1965).

A growing number of intelligent persons in the West have come to recognize the relativistic nature of reality, some by study of Zen Buddhism, meditation, or experimental use of psychedelic drugs (see Essay V). Even if we do accept conventional Western attitudes, it is salutary to mention, in connection with schizophrenia, a brave experiment which D. L. Rosenhan and his colleagues in the USA conducted. These pseudopatients, including practising psychiatrists, assumed false identities, attended different mental hospitals in the USA and complained, fictitiously, that they 'heard voices', i.e. had auditory hallucinations. On this basis alone all but one of the eight members of Rosenhan's team were diagnosed as schizophrenic and hospitalized. Interestingly, they were completely able to deceive the doctors and nurses who were 'treating' them, but the other patients were not fooled (D. L. Rosenhan *et al*., 'On being sane in insane places' *Science* 179: 250-58, 1973).

The moral of this story surely does not need to be spelled out. One wonders how many other 'sane' people are at this moment incarcerated in mental hospitals, assumed to be psychotic. It is not irrelevant to notice that this is often the fate of dissidents in the Soviet Union: having been classified as insane, they are tranquillized into docility with haloperidol, one of the most popular Western drugs given to control schizophrenic symptoms. In the course of this book, we are describing drugs and their effects within the terms of reference of contemporary Western medical practice. In discussing antipsychotic medicaments – numerically the largest single group of psychotropic agents – we follow commonly accepted criteria for their use. However, we feel that it is right and proper to raise questions about the desirability and rationality with which such drugs are prescribed, particularly when potent neuroleptics are given to patients without informed consent and, as happens in prisons and some other institutions, quite involuntarily. The present authors' experience with 'psychological illness' spans the spectrum from the 'schizophrenic' who is violent, deluded, and has other signs and symptoms of a florid kind, to the somewhat overanxious or depressed person who to all appearances is quite normal and may need no more than reassurance. The prime criterion which one could helpfully use is: does this individual's condition cause him (or his family) unreasonable suffering? And further, whatever his concept of reality, is he able at least to dissemble sufficiently in order to cope with the realities imposed on him by society? Or can he be helped to do so with appropriate therapy, including or excluding psychotropic medication?

The current view of schizophrenia is that it results from overactivity of the neurotransmitter dopamine, and perhaps also disturbances of other chemicals such as γ-aminobutyric acid (GABA), 5-hydroxytryptamine (serotonin), or noradrenaline (norepinephrine). On present evidence it seems that at least two of these substances are implicated in severe mental disorders. And it is hopefully to restore the balance of the relevant chemicals, and not merely to improve symptoms, that antipsychotic tranquillizers are used today. Whether and to what extent these drugs are curative, rather than simply providing superficial palliation of symptoms, is a matter for debate. Conan Kornetsky has had the courage to write: 'One of the major problems in treating the mentally ill is that we do not know the nature of the illness we are treating. In fact it could be said that drug therapy in the treatment of the mentally ill is the treatment of diseases of unknown etiology [cause] by drugs of unknown actions' (*Pharmacology: drugs affecting behavior*. New York, 1976, p. 82). Nevertheless, an attempt must be made to modify this view.

Drug Treatment of Psychoses: Phenothiazines and their Analogues

Drug treatment of psychiatric conditions may be said to have begun in the West with the introduction of reserpine in the early 1950s. Reserpine is one of several alkaloids of *Rauwolfia serpentina*, an Indian plant, decoctions of which have been used for centuries in the Ayurvedic system of traditional medicine, as a remedy for insomnia and a variety of psychological complaints. Reserpine (Serpasil) will be familiar to some readers as a frequently prescribed treatment for hypertension. Although the drug had a beneficial effect on certain psychiatric patients, its use in psychiatry has been largely abandoned. At the required doses, side-effects – e.g. nausea, diarrhoea, parkinsonism and even convulsions – were unacceptably severe. And within a few years chlorpromazine, the prototype of the phenothiazine antipsychotics, had been made available.

Phenothiazine itself had been used in veterinary medicine for many years as an anthelmintic, that is to kill parasitic worms. A derivative, chlorpromazine, was synthesized by G. Charpentier in 1950. Originally this compound, which had been shown to possess sedative and antihistamine properties, was administered as premedication before surgery by Jean Delay and his colleagues in France. In 1952 Delay and Deniker tried chlorpromazine on a group of hyperagitated psychotic patients, and found that the drug afforded them remarkable relief. These workers' enthusiasm about the applications of the substance in psychiatric medicine very quickly spread, and soon chlorpromazine was marketed everywhere. In Britain and France it has the brand name Largactil, to suggest its large range of actions; in the USA it is called Thorazine; and in Germany and some other continental countries Megaphen.

The impact that this one compound had in the treatment of psychiatric inpatients was dramatic. The number of such patients in America, for example, increased steadily up to about 1956 but fell sharply thereafter. This was attributed to the success of chlorpromazine in large measure: many persons who would otherwise have been hospitalized, it was considered, could now have their psychotic symptoms controlled while still in the community. The drug's ability to restore coherent thought and behaviour was noteworthy even in long-stay psychiatric inpatients, to the point where some could be discharged. Undoubtedly, the introduction of chlorpromazine to mental hospitals proved a great boon to their staff, too: previously violent or hyperagitated patients, and those with 'antisocial' propensities, were rendered tranquil, calm, and, possibly best of all from the administrative point of view, malleable and docile. Institutions which were formerly in effect prisons, and their staff warders, did tend to become more humanized as the use of chlorpromazine became entrenched. One would not argue *post hoc, ergo propter hoc*, neither would one dismiss the fact that at some psychiatric hospitals barbarities are still practised. Not a few former patients, as well as psychiatrists, contend that the physical straitjacket has been replaced by a chemical one: the padded cell has given place to the long-acting neuroleptic injection. This view is too facile. One of the objects of this book is to arm patients with knowledge about the medicaments they are taking or will be offered; and in the absence of absolute facts about certain properties of antipsychotic drugs the reader may decide the extent to which the above assertions really obtain.

The question of whether phenothiazines and their analogues just control symptoms in psychoses or whether they are genuinely curative is much discussed. Nobody is sure, and the evidence (e.g. the number of 'remissions' or cures following treatment with these agents) can be manipulated to support both points of view. For instance, the annually falling rates of admission to mental hospitals may suggest that a greater proportion of patients are effectively treated on an outpatient basis (usually with neuroleptics), or alternatively that social attitudes towards psychological disturbances have changed. Some schizophrenics apparently get better anyway, with or without psychotropic drugs. Whatever the truth of the matter, in the two decades following the introduction of chlorpromazine, more than a hundred different compounds have been made available for prescription in Western countries, of which about 30 are in current clinical use in the UK and/or the USA. The majority of these are, like chlorpromazine, phenothiazine derivatives; of the remainder, all but a couple belong to the butyrophenone, diphenylbutyl-piperidine or thioxanthene series of drugs. Members of each class of compounds seem to act in similar fashion and to provoke the same sorts of adverse reactions. The differences are described below. (See also Chart VI(B) for comparisons.)

It is generally recognized that there are too many antipsychotic drugs available, and that this makes rational prescribing difficult. Some of the phenothiazines, for example, seem to suit individual patients better than others. But it is not possible to state that, say, thioridazine is more effective than triflupromazine for control of a specific condition. The phenothiazines all have sedative, anti-allergic, anti-emetic and a degree of pain-relieving potency. Promethazine (Phenergan) and prochlorperazine (Stemetil, Vertigon, Compazine) are given, in the main, to prevent or suppress vomiting and nausea and to enhance the action of narcotic analgesics. Since the latter often produce nausea, promethazine is often administered concurrently with pethidine (meperidine) as a premedication injection, and preparations containing both drugs are marketed (Pamergan, Mepergan). Trimeprazine (Vallergan, Temaril) and methotrimeprazine (Veractil, Levoprome) are chosen for their powerful anti-histaminic effect, in allergic conditions and to stop chronic itching. Like promethazine, these phenothiazines potentiate the pain-killing activity of opiates and may be administered with them, either in oral or injectable form. None of the above-mentioned compounds has a significant antipsychotic action.

Most drugs of the phenothiazine class demonstrate the antipsychotic effects characteristic of chlorpromazine (Largactil, Thorazine). Among the more potent chlorpromazine analogues are acetophenazine (Tindal), butaperazine (Repoise), carphenazine (Proketazine), piperacetazine (Quide), triflupromazine (Vesprin), and especially fluphenazine (Moditen, Permitil). All these have a profound effect on the consciousness, damping it down forcefully. These particular compounds should be reserved for treatment of the most severely disturbed psychotic states, partly because of the severity of their unwanted effects and partly because, if they are prescribed for other than psychotic patients, they may actually provoke mental disturbance. The specific indications for prescription of phenothiazines have been left deliberately somewhat vague, given the difficulty of defining 'psychoses' and the controversy surrounding their administration.

As the reader will see from Chart VI(B), there are three chemical sub-types of the phenothiazine class. It has been frequently, and incorrectly, stated that the aliphatic and piperidine drugs are of low potency and the piperazines of higher antipsychotic effectiveness. That this is not the case is indicated by the fact that triflupromazine, acetophenazine and piperacetazine – one member from each sub-group – are indicated only in such seriously disabling illnesses as chronic schizophrenia. However, certain adverse reactions do seem to occur more often in one sub-type than another, though the differences may not be as great as is sometimes believed.

The most frequently reported early adverse effects of chlorpromazine-like drugs are postural hypotension (rapid fall in blood-pressure on standing) and sedation: to these tolerance develops within a few weeks. 'Normal' volunteers have found that phenothiazines give them an irresistible urge to sleep. This is said to be less marked in schizophrenics, who after a short time may again be able to concentrate. These compounds act particularly on the reticular formation of the brain, which in normal people provides a 'filtering' effect on sensory stimuli. In certain psychotic states, including schizophrenia, this system is evidently overloaded, flooding the patients' consciousness with a mass of unassimilable data. To this extent the experience has resemblances to the psychedelic state (see Essay V) as this may be provoked by use of LSD, a drug whose actions are supposed to mimic spontaneously occurring psychoses. The sensory overload is in any case curtailed by antipsychotic agents. Other common side-effects of neuroleptics are of the anticholinergic type, as manifested by blurred vision, constipation, dry mouth, and urinary hesitancy or retention. Light sensitivity, allergic skin rashes, jaundice, fluctuations in body temperature and disorders of the blood picture are less regular unwanted reactions: the likelihood of one or more of these occurring seems to be related to the chemical sub-type, and this is why such reactions are listed in Chart VI(B) under three headings for the phenothiazine class of drugs as being frequent, less common, or rare.

Patients on antipsychotic medication, especially inpatients who are receiving high doses, are often seen to be docile, apathetic, and lacking in motivation. It is interesting that such traits may be a reason for antipsychotic therapy in the first place. Certainly the capacity of chlorpromazine and its congeners to control hyperagitation, violent outbursts, and other manifestations of aggression is marked, and these compounds do diminish the intensity of hallucinations and delusions. More accurately, they do not cause these symptoms to disappear. As Max Hamilton has aptly observed: 'Hallucinations and delusions continue to be present . . . What the drugs do is to diminish the disrupting effect of the symptoms. Typically, patients will say that they continue to hear the voices, but take no notice of them' ('Clinical basis of trials of neuroleptic drugs' in *Neuroleptics and Schizophrenia: Proceedings of an International Symposium*. Luton, 1979, p.56).

Mental depression, if present already, can be enhanced by phenothiazines, and may be provoked by them. The present authors are in process of collating a series of cases of suicide and attempted suicide following administration of fluphenazine, one of the most formidably potent neuroleptics. Statements that psychotic patients have, with these drugs, been returned to near-normality notwithstanding, it is quite clear that in a substantial number of patients pre-existing depressive symptoms are intensified. This is the case with phenothiazines and butyrophenones, but evidently not with members of the thioxanthene class of neuroleptics, such as thiothixene (Navane) and chlorprothixene (Taractan).

Common to all antipsychotics is their tendency to produce what are known as extra-pyramidal reactions (EPRs). These occur most often when piperazine-phenothiazines (the most numerous group) are administered: perphenazine (Fentazin), trifluoperazine (Stelazine) and fluphenazine (Moditen, Permitil) are examples. These effects are essentially a chemically-induced form of Parkinson's disease. A wide variety of signs and symptoms, all of them exceedingly unpleasant and distressing, are classified as EPRs. Characteristically, there are some loss of motor and muscular co-ordination, disturbances in gait (dyskinesia), rigidity of limbs, uncontrolled salivation, tremors, involuntary eye-movements (oculogyric crises), facial distortions and motor restlessness (akathisia, or in current US cant the 'Prolixin stomp'). Usually two or more of these phenomena occur: the degree of severity differs according to individual idiosyncrasy and the dose of the drug being administered. Because EPRs happen so often, it is some physicians' practice to give an anti-parkinsonian agent concurrently with the neuroleptic, preferably to prevent these effects from arising rather than to control them when they do so. For this purpose several drugs are available: the most effective is probably orphenadrine (Disipal), although benzhexol (trihexyphenidyl, Artane) or procyclidine (Kemadrin) may suit some patients better.

Leo Hollister believes that the appearance of EPRs is a useful diagnostic sign, which he says indicates that the antipsychotic being used is achieving its proper psychological effect. This might well be so. However, it may be regarded as unethical to expose patients who are already suffering in different ways to unnecessary, usually preventable and always alarming effects. Hence the practice of many psychiatrists of prescribing orphenadrine right at the beginning of treatment with phenothiazines.

Donald N. Franz, writing in what is arguably the most prestigious pharmacology textbook, in the course of his account of anti-parkinsonian medications, has underscored the following sentence: 'Such therapy is valid only for [the] rapid control [of EPRs] and not to prevent their possible occurrence or to mask their actual occurrence' ('Drugs for Parkinson's disease' in L. S. Goodman and A. Gilman, ed. *The Pharmacological Basis of Therapeutics*, ed.5. New York, 1975 p. 239). He contends that the development of a permanent, severe syndrome called tardive dyskinesia is 'sometimes a disastrous result of antipsychotic medication'; therefore that EPRs must be recognized early, which he says is not possible if routine anti-parkinsonian drugs are given. Tardive dyskinesia is a form of parkinsonism which occurs in patients (the proportion has not been accurately ascertained) who have been receiving high doses of antipsychotics for long periods, chiefly psychiatric inpatients. This complaint is characterized by involuntary movements of the lips, tongue and jaw, and purposeless, uncontrolled gyrations of the limbs or trunk. Autopsies of patients who have suffered from this condition show that brain damage occurs. One estimate is that between 20% and 50% of chronic schizophrenic inpatients on continuous treatment with neuroleptic drugs are likely to be affected with tardive dyskinesia. Sometimes this can be treated by lowering the dose of antipsychotic, though not by any of the available anti-parkinsonian agents. In most cases the syndrome appears to be irreversible. This problem leaves the practitioner in a dilemma: whether he should wait for symptoms to arise and have orphenadrine or a similar drug in readiness, i.e. whether he should run the risk of exposing his patients to such reactions, or whether he ought to prescribe anti-parkinsonian medicaments as prophylaxis against them. One solution might be to discontinue orphenadrine after about 6 months, when EPRs would in most cases have subsided without such treatment, and to re-institute it subsequently if there were a recrudescence of such side-effects. It should be added that anti-parkinson drugs have adverse effects of their own, particularly of the anticholinergic type, which could be intensified by phenothiazines at high dosages. There is no easy answer to these difficulties.

The American Medical Association's Department of Drugs has concluded that, because there are no less hazardous drugs in the treatment of psychotic conditions, there will inevitably be some risk of tardive dyskinesia developing in a proportion of patients. The AMA recommends that (1) neuroleptic drugs should be prescribed only when their use is unavoidable, and only one such compound at a time; (2) the smallest dose which relieves symptoms should be given; (3) orphenadrine and its analogues should be avoided until EPRs actually develop; and (4) the Committee believes that drug 'holidays' – periods, however brief, when chronic use of antipsychotics is discontinued – should be instituted whenever possible, on the grounds that this will unmask early symptoms of tardive dyskinesia and so make diagnosis of the condition easier (AMA Department of Drugs: *Drug Evaluations*, ed.3. Littleton, Mass., 1977, p. 433).

Other severe adverse effects of chronic administration of neuroleptics have been mentioned briefly. Sexuality may be impaired either by greatly diminishing the patient's libido or, perhaps, by inhibiting ejaculation. Obstructive liver disease, manifesting as jaundice, occurs in some individuals. Alterations in the blood picture, such as a massive decrease in white blood-cells (agranulocytosis), have occasionally been fatal. The lens of the eye may become opaque, so that vision is impaired. The skin may be affected by abnormal pigmentation or urticaria (itching). Epileptiform fits have been recorded. These very grave consequences of neuroleptic treatment are relatively uncommon, but large doses of any phenothiazine or butyrophenone compound given on a long-term basis make their appearance more likely. Some side-effects are associated with particular drugs – e.g. thioridazine (Melleril, Mellaril) is associated with cardiac ill-effects in a few patients – but, given the close chemical similarities between many antipsychotics, such hazards are unlikely to be specific for individual phenothiazines. On the question of cardio-toxicity, there is no doubt that this is a factor in lethal overdosage with these drugs.

The two other chemical classes shown in Chart VI(B), the butyro-phenones and the thioxanthenes, do not differ greatly from the pheno-thiazines: similar ranges of side-effects, contra-indications and other attributes obtain. The butyrophenones, of which the most widely used is haloperidol (Serenace, Haldol), are among the most potent of neurolep-tics, and their use should be confined to control of very severe psychotic states. An exception is droperidol (Droleptan), which is used in anaesthetics in conjunction with the narcotic fentanyl. One of the most recently marketed of this group of compounds is benperidol (Anquil), whose manufacturers recommend its prescription in cases of antisocial sexual behaviour, such as paedophilia and compulsive exhibitionism ('flashing'). We can find no evidence that this drug is specifically antiaphrodisiacal, and it is more probable that benperidol lessens sexual drive as an element in more general central nervous system depression.

Two other compounds of recent introduction, listed in the Chart with the butyrophenones, are pimozide (Orap) and fluspirilene (Redeptin). Technically these are diphenylbutylpiperidines, but their applications are similar to those of haloperidol, being used almost exclusively in schizo-phrenia. The third class, the thioxanthenes, are represented in the USA only by thiothixene (Navane) and in the UK by chlorprothixene (Tarac-tan) and two new additions, flupenthixol (Depixol, Fluanxol) and *cis*-clopenthixol (Clopixol). Again the principal use is in the control of schizophrenia. It has been demonstrated that thioxanthenes are less likely than other antipsychotics to produce or enhance mental depression, and that low doses of flupenthixol (Fluanxol) may in fact have antidepressant as well as anxiety-relieving properties.

According to Leo Hollister, the plethora of antipsychotic drugs, each one of which has undergone several clinical trials, constitutes 'the most massive scientific overkill in all clinical pharmacology' (*op.cit.* p. 153). So: which drug to choose, and in what form? Individual psychiatrists have their own favourites, but the selection is somewhat arbitrary. It is reckoned that we could easily do without all but perhaps half a dozen neuroleptic agents. In a way the choice has been made simpler during the past decade by the introduction of very long-acting (depôt) injectable preparations. With one exception, these are products in which the active drug is esterified in a vegetable oil base, so that following deep intramuscular injection a single dose will exert antipsychotic activity over a period of weeks. The most frequently prescribed such injection is fluphenazine decanoate (Modecate), one shot of which has a duration of 5 to 8 weeks. Because of the problem of non-compliance among disturbed patients, who find it difficult to take one or more tablets once or twice daily, the depôt preparations are extremely convenient. For hospital inpatients, management is easier, and all the outpatient must do is turn up at the psychiatric clinic at the requisite intervals to receive his injection. There are dangers, too, in that outpatients may not be monitored as closely as they should if they are seen only every two months; in this situation even quite serious adverse effects may go unreported. Alternatives to fluphenazine decanoate and the rather shorter-acting enanthate (Moditen) are the two thioxanthenes flupenthixol decanoate (Depixol) and *cis*-clopenthixol decanoate (Clopixol). A single dose of either of these will be effective for 2-4 weeks. The diphenylbutylpiperidine drug fluspirilene (Redeptin) is an aqueous suspension and is recommended for administration at weekly intervals. All depôt formulations mentioned are indicated to control schizophrenic symptoms and those of other psychic disorders of comparable severity. There has been a disturbing tendency, almost since the introduction of long-acting neuroleptics, for them to be prescribed in minor emotional/psychological disturbances: this is inappropriate and potentially very hazardous. T. R. E. Barnes and P. K. Bridges wisely warn: 'Because of the ease with which a monthly injection can be given, these preparations run the risk of being used for an undesirably wide range of psychiatric conditions. For example, they are not an appropriate means of alleviating chronic anxiety and tension. Their indications are confined to the psychoses, most often schizophrenia and sometimes mania' ('Advances in drug treatment in psychiatry' *Practitioner* 221: 515, 1978).

Whichever antipsychotic tranquillizer is prescribed, appropriate dosage regimens can be established only by trial and error: as the Chart indicates, the range of doses used is enormous. How much drug is given will depend on the severity of the condition, the patient's therapeutic response, the extent to which untoward reactions are provoked, and on individual idiosyncrasy. We have attempted to show in Chart VI(B) the order of dosages which specialists regard as acceptable, for outpatients and inpatients respectively. The higher dose levels correspond with current medical practice and, in general, with manufacturers' recommendations. With schedules for patients in hospital there can be greater latitude, as adverse effects will be more quickly noticed and also because inpatients are likely to suffer from more severe disturbances, which may require very large quantities of neuroleptic to control. When phenothiazine and similar drugs are administered orally, a once-daily routine is often sufficient. If taken at bedtime, their soporific action can be put to good use, and they may obviate the need for other night sedation. In the event that an additional hypnotic is required, chloral hydrate mixture can be given together with elixir of chlorpromazine or another antipsychotic which is presented in liquid form.

How long drug treatment should last is not settled, particularly as not all psychiatrists believe that neuroleptics are 'curative' and for various other reasons, such as the risk of tardive dyskinesia. Some favour continuous, others intermittent, therapy. Malcolm Lader has written: 'In the chronic schizophrenic, some symptoms are helped but in general overarousal is not such that a tranquillizing effect is useful. Nor is there any evidence that the natural history of schizophrenia has been materially altered by the major tranquillizers. More patients live in the community, but they still tend to relapse. Readmission, by removing them from an over-arousing environment, is itself therapeutic . . . Nonetheless, patients still become chronic although the social and personal consequences of repeated relapse may be ameliorated' ('The clinical actions of major tranquillizers' in *Schizophrenia: Dopaminergic Mechanisms, Aetiology and Therapeutics* – Proceedings of the Royal Society of Medicine 70: 24, 1977, Supplement 10).

Contra-indications, which apply to the great majority of antipsychotics, are summarized in the accompanying Chart. Phenothiazine-type tranquillizers should not be prescribed for patients with impaired liver, or seriously impaired, kidney function. If such drugs are given following hepatitis, this viral infection is likely to recur. Serious respiratory problems and cardiac ailments, e.g. advanced atherosclerosis (hardening of the arteries), would normally preclude the use of neuroleptics: the reader is reminded of the cardio-toxicity of thioridazine (Melleril) and very possibly of related compounds. Patients with Parkinson's disease, suspected brain damage, bone marrow depression, blood disorders, phaeochromocytoma (tumours of the adrenal system) and other conditions which give rise to severe hypertension, are additional contra-indications. Hypersensitivity to one phenothiazine, as manifested by an allergic reaction, will be found if any other member of this class is prescribed (cross-sensitivity): this may extend to the butyrophenones and perhaps to other antipsychotic medicaments. Neuroleptics should be avoided during pregnancy, and for children, unless the circumstances are exceptional. Because the elderly are very susceptible to major tranquillizers, dosage for this group of patients should be lower than for younger persons. An important warning: phenothiazine-type drugs can mask the symptoms of acute abdominal illness and certain feverish conditions.

The potential use of antipsychotic drugs for the purpose of committing suicide should be considered by the prescriber. James J. Brophy has reviewed the subject and concluded that the ratio of daily or weekly doses of neuroleptics to their probable lethal doses can and should be estimated before these agents are prescribed. In part because major tranquillizers are neither physically nor psychologically dependence-producing, practitioners may order an unacceptably large number of tablets or capsules. He therefore warns about such over-prescribing, which in potentially suicidal patients is patently dangerous. Unlike other categories of drug used in deliberate overdosage, the management of phenothiazine poisoning is difficult. ('Suicide attempts with psychotherapeutic drugs' *Archives of General Psychiatry* 17: 652-7, 1967.)

There are several individual compounds, and drug types, which ought not to be prescribed concomitantly with neuroleptics, or which, if absolutely necessary for the patient, may require very careful monitoring or adjustment in dosage. Major tranquillizers greatly increase the central depressant effects of barbiturates, other hypnotics and sedatives, opiates, and alcohol, so due allowance should be made if any of these are prescribed. Antipsychotics must not be used at the same time as the antiparkinsonian drug levodopa (l-dopa, Larodopa), although other drugs used in this condition (e.g. orphenadrine, Disipal) are compatible. Combination of neuroleptics with the anti-manic agent lithium carbonate (see below p. 363) is controversial, but is likely to complicate treatment with either. Reports have appeared which suggest that high doses of haloperidol (Serenace, Haldol) taken concurrently with lithium may produce brain damage. Antipsychotics are incompatible with a number of drugs used in cancer therapy (cyclophosphamide, vincristine, vinblastine), and also with diuretics (drugs to promote emptying of the kidneys): water retention and intoxication are special hazards in the latter case. Concomitant use of phenothiazines with antidepressants has been described (see Essay II). If these are combined, troublesome anticholinergic and CNS-depressant effects may arise: fixed-dose combinations, e.g. perphenazine + amitriptyline (Triptafen, Etrafon), have doubtful therapeutic benefits. Great care must be exercised if major tranquillizers are taken with antidiabetic drugs, including insulin; the anti-hypertensive guanethidine (Ismelin); antidepressants of the MAO-inhibitor type (see Essay II), such as tranylcypromine (Parnate) and isocarboxazid (Marplan); the anticonvulsant phenytoin (Epanutin); and curare-type skeletal muscle relaxants of the kind used in anaesthesia. Oral contraceptive pills which contain oestrogens may in conjunction with phenothiazines cause hypertrophy (overgrowth) of the breasts and galactorrhoea, or abnormal flow of milk. Injectable depôt preparations of fluphenazine, flupenthixol and other long-acting neuroleptics, if mixed in the same syringe, inactivate penicillin and the anticoagulant heparin (Pularin).

Newer Antipsychotic Drugs

Of the major tranquillizers already described, more recent introductions are two thioxanthenes – flupenthixol (Depixol) and *cis*-clopenthixol (Clopixol) – the two diphenylbutylpiperidine compounds pimozide (Orap) and fluspirilene (Redeptin), and lithium carbonate. None but the last-named drug is as yet available in the USA, but it is probable that one or more of these will be so within a short time. Flupenthixol is confusingly presented under two brand names from the same manufacturer: Fluanxol for a mild tablet formulation (0.5 mg), Depixol for a stronger tablet (3 mg) and for a long-lasting injection. Whereas this compound is intended to alleviate apathy, inertia, paranoid delusions, hallucinations, and anxiety in the schizophrenic patient (and at much smaller oral doses to control non-psychotic anxiety and tension), its close chemical analogue clopenthixol is indicated for management of schizophrenic states in which hyperagitation and aggressiveness are a major feature. Both drugs are prepared as depôt injections, one dose of which will act for between 2 and 4 weeks. Fluspirilene, too, is a long-acting antischizophrenic agent but with a duration of action of only one week. Its chemical relative pimozide, which is offered for the treatment of withdrawn and apathetic psychotic states, must be taken orally and is available in several tablet strengths. Contra-indications and special precautions for these newer compounds are generally as for the phenothiazines. It seems that pimozide may actually provoke hostile, violent symptoms in some schizophrenics. Injection of fluspirilene may, according to a recent paper, cause hard nodules at the injection site: this suggests that individual doses may be incompletely absorbed from the tissues and that formulation of the drug could possibly be improved.

The almost absurdly simple compound lithium carbonate was used as a salt substitute during the 1940s. This practice was discontinued quickly on account of severe toxic effects. An Australian psychiatrist, John Cade, first proposed that lithium was effective in mental illness as early as 1949, but nobody took any notice. Then in the late 1960s Mogens Schou and his colleagues in Denmark performed a series of controlled trials in which the substance was compared with standard antipsychotics. The results obtained by Schou's group and by other researchers have been questioned. Lithium has become established as a specific treatment for mania (especially in the manic phase of manic-depressive psychosis), although some workers have found it no more effective than chlorpromazine in controlling this intractable condition.

According to the authoritative *Medical Letter on Drugs and Therapeutics*: 'Lithium is the drug of choice for patients with mania and for prevention of recurrence of cyclic attacks of manic-depressive disorders . . . Lithium may take two to three weeks to have a therapeutic effect, and acutely manic patients often require temporary treatment with a phenothiazine or haloperidol [Serenace, Haldol] while awaiting the onset of action of lithium' (18: 91, 1976). During the depressive phase of manic-depression, a condition characterized by extraordinary mood-swings from the intensely euphoric to the most apathetically depressed, *Medical Letter* advocates the administration of antidepressants. Certain specialists recommend the drug also for hypomania, a type of abnormal excitement which does not quite reach the intensity of mania, and for recurrent depression, whether or not categorized as psychotic. Lithium's mechanism of action is unknown and not all psychiatrists admit its therapeutic usefulness.

The major problem with this drug is its very high toxicity: this is illustrated by the fact that 0.9–1.4 milli-equivalents (mEq) per litre of blood is the accepted level, while blood titres of 2.0 mEq/L are likely to be toxic. The dose is expressed in this way because of varying patient response to milligramme doses and also because, in order to prevent dangerous reactions, the blood lithium level must be monitored frequently in all patients under treatment with the drug. This should be done at least twice during the first week or two of therapy, and weekly thereafter. Because lithium can disturb the body's electrolyte (sodium and potassium) balance, and may be excreted erratically via the kidneys, this procedure is mandatory. Side-effects are common: fine tremor, nausea, diarrhoea, general lassitude and fatigue are typical. The drug's contra-indications are shown in Chart VI(B). Chief among these are impairment of kidney function, Addison's disease and hypothyroidism. Lithium is incompatible with a large number of other medicaments, including diuretics, corticosteroids, and amphetamine and other stimulants and appetite-suppressants. The adverse reactions of other neuroleptic agents are often enhanced by the drug.

In summary, lithium is not a drug which should ever be given routinely. Its use should be confined to that rather small number of patients who cannot be managed on other antipsychotic medication. Lately there has been a disturbing tendency for the compound to be prescribed by general practitioners (and others) to alleviate the symptoms of minor psychological disturbances, and failure in some cases to perform the necessary blood tests. There are special dangers in giving lithium for chronic or recurrent depression, since this may be intensified, and even small numbers of tablets can be lethal in patients who may be prone to attempt suicide.

Given all the risks attendant upon treatment with this substance, it is surprising that several different branded preparations of lithium are available: in the UK, Camcolit, Phasal and Priadel are now (1980) joined by Liskonum, while in the USA the listed formulations include Eskalith, Lithane, Lithonate, and Lithotabs. It has been suggested that if lithium is taken during pregnancy, cardiac abnormalities in the foetus may result. In view of the hazards of lithium, and the high incidence of negligent prescribing of psychotropic drugs, it may perhaps not be too much to suggest that the compound be restricted for hospital use only, as is the case with some other particularly dangerous or expensive medicaments (e.g. injectable CNS stimulants, such as amphetamine and methylphenidate; some cytotoxic agents).

The late 1970s saw the appearance of yet further drugs indicated to control the symptoms of schizophrenia. In the United States, loxapine (Loxitane, Daxolin) and molindone (Moban, Lidone) have been made available. Both belong to quite discrete chemical classes and are not related to the phenothiazines or their principal analogues, although loxapine's molecular structure is rather similar to that of the tricyclic antidepressants. In an already crowded, indeed glutted, market, it is not easy to see the rationale: clinical studies indicate that molindone and loxapine do effectively control psychotic symptoms, but it is by no means clear whether either offers any advantage over established neuroleptics. Side-effects are apparently similar in type, and perhaps in severity. One must await the results of further research before any legitimate claim can be made that these new drugs are therapeutically superior to the phenothiazines.

A few words might appropriately be added on alternative chemical treatments of psychotic states. Several experimental approaches have recently been tried. According to one study, thyrotropin-releasing hormone (TRH) proved beneficial in controlling schizophrenic symptoms, but an attempt to replicate these findings indicated that TRH exacerbated them. Precursors or analogues of dopamine, imbalance of which appears to produce psychotic states, have been tried: a Japanese team found low doses of the anti-parkinsonian drug levodopa helpful in schizophrenia, but again other work suggests that this aggravates the condition or that it has no effect. Megavitamins (i.e. vast doses of vitamins) are used by some psychiatrists, whose enthusiasm for these 'natural' substances seems boundless. The B vitamin niacin in particular has been claimed to produce remarkable benefits, while ascorbic acid (vitamin C) and pyridoxine have their advocates. The most stringently controlled clinical studies, however, have yielded negative results in each case.

Conclusion

In the above pages a description has been provided of the actions and uses of neuroleptic drugs, as if the conditions which these drugs may mitigate or 'cure' objectively existed. This has been quite deliberate. Having drawn attention to the looseness of diagnostic criteria for mental illness, and pointed out that such definitions are to some extent culturally conditioned, we seem to be accepting the diagnostic labels which are the common currency of Western psychiatry. In fact we do this for the sake of convenience and comprehensibility, since this is not the proper place for in-depth philosophical argument. The purpose of our remarks on the nature of psychological illness is principally to draw the reader's attention to the subjective and relativistic views which prevail today among specialists in the subject; and perhaps also to suggest to a prospective mental patient that, whatever the condition from which he is told he is suffering, it may be wise to question not only the diagnosis but also the means of treatment.

It is platitudinous to state that psychotropic drugs, even the most potent of them, are being heavily overprescribed. Not by all practitioners, certainly; but by a large number. We note with disquiet a tendency (which we do not consider illusory) among some GPs to prescribe either phenothiazines or antidepressants for patients who earlier were receiving diazepam (Valium) and similar 'minor' tranquillizers and sedatives. 'No abuse or dependence potential' is the Siren song which physicians seem increasingly to hear: thus they are more willing to prescribe a neuroleptic than a benzodiazepine, because the latter can be abused. Dangers associated with chlorpromazine and other major tranquillizers are different, but just as real, and these have been recounted in some detail. If chemical treatment of anxiety, or depression, or psychosis, is indicated, as almost all would agree is sometimes the case, then careful consideration should be given about which drug is to be prescribed. And the patient should also be encouraged to exercise some thought on the subject.

Suggestions for Further Reading

There is no completely non-technical work on the subject of these two types of drug which we feel able to recommend. Some popular accounts exist but none is adequate so far as the details of tranquillizing agents are concerned. However, one or more of the following books may be found useful:

Baldessarini, R. L., 'Drugs in the treatment of psychiatric disorders' in Goodman and Gilman, *op.cit.*, pp. 391-447.   .
    An authoritative account from the standpoint of contemporary psychiatric practice.

Garattini, S., Mussini, E. and Randall, L. O. (ed.): *The Benzodiazepines.* New York/Milano, 1973 (Monographs of the Mario Negri Institute for Pharmacological Research)
    This reports a most detailed symposium on the diazepam (Valium) type of tranquillizer. While much of this concerns the results of animal experiments, the clinical studies and summaries are interesting: the latter should be intelligible to the non-specialist.

Gordon, Maxwell (ed.): *Psychopharmacological Agents*, vol.3. New York, 1974 (Monographs in Medicinal Chemistry)

The several authors who have contributed to the third (updated) volume of this important work, while chiefly concerned with chemical matters such as the structure/activity relationship of psychotropic drugs, devote some space to reviews of a more general nature. Useful for the reader with some scientific knowledge.

Hollister, Leo H.: *Clinical Pharmacology of Psychotherapeutic Drugs*. Edinburgh/New York, 1978, pp. 131–226.

Although this book is intended for the working physician, a good deal of the material is presented clearly and without excessive technicality. Like all the author's work, this reads well and is refreshingly literate. It does, however, reflect Hollister's individualistic views.

Crammer, J., Barraclough, B. and Heine, B.: *The Use of Drugs in Psychiatry*. London, 1978.

Published under the auspices of the Royal College of Psychiatrists, this work provides a summary of the subject. In places it is inappropriately dogmatic, and some important information, e.g. on phenothiazines, is omitted.

Valzelli, L.: *Psychopharmacology: an introduction to experimental and clinical principles*. Flushing, NY, 1973.

For the reader who is interested in how mood-modifying drugs are tested, and how experiments are carried out to assess their effects, this book is fascinating.

Marks, J.: *The Benzodiazepines: use, overuse, misuse, abuse*. Lancaster, 1978.

An excellent study, in which clinical experience and literature are carefully reviewed. The author's conclusions about benzodiazepines must, however, be set against more recent evidence.

CHART VIA: TRANQUILLIZERS, ANXIETY RELIEVING

NOTE: These drugs are prescribed chiefly to alleviate states of anxiety, tension, and stress, whereas the 'major' tranquillizers (this Chart, section B) are used primarily to relieve symptoms associated with very profound psychological disturbances, such as schizophrenia. The Benzodiazepines are virtually identical chemically and pharmacologically and may be used interchangeably: they have effects other than as tranquillizers (see Essay), e.g. as anti-convulsants. Hydroxyzine is also given in Ménière's disease, chlormethiazole in alcoholic delirium, and propranolol principally to reduce high blood-pressure and in cardiovascular disorders: for details, see alphabetical entries for individual drugs.

Drug Name	Brand Name(s)	Usual Oral Dosage Range*	Number of Daily Doses (see text)
1: Benzodiazepines			
DIAZEPAM	UK: Valium, Atensine, Evacalm, Sedapam	4 – 40 mg	1–2
	US: Valium	(10–30 mg)*	
CHLORDIAZEPOXIDE	UK: Librium, Tropium	10–80 mg	1–3
	US: Librium, Libritabs, A-poxide, SK-Lygen		
CLOBAZAM	UK: Frisium	10–60 mg	1–2
CLORAZEPATE MONO- or DI-POTASSIUM	UK: Tranxene	15–60 mg	1
	US: Tranxene, Azene		
KETAZOLAM	UK: Anxon	15–60 mg	1
LORAZEPAM	UK: Ativan	1–6 mg	1–2
	US: Ativan	(3.5–8 mg)*	
MEDAZEPAM	UK: Nobrium	10–40 mg	1–2
OXAZEPAM	UK: Serenid-D, Serenid-Forte	20–120 mg	2–3
	US: Serax		
PRAZEPAM	US: Verstran	20–60 mg	1–2

ADVERSE EFFECTS: drowsiness, confusion, unsteadiness, psychological dependency (common); headache, vertigo, hypotension, Parkinsonism, jaundice, blood disorders, loss of libido, hyperactivity & other paradoxical effects, enhanced depression (less common or rare).

INTERACTIONS WITH OTHER DRUGS: Action of alcohol and all other central depressants (e.g. sleeping pills, narcotics) enhanced. Caution if digoxin + warfarin are to be given concurrently. Action of thyroxine may be increased, that of the anti-epileptic drug phenytoin reduced.

WARNINGS & CONTRA-INDICATIONS: Benzodiazepines should be avoided during pregnancy and lactation; in myasthenia gravis; for children (except to stop somnambulism); severe respiratory disease; known hypersensitivity. Caution in all respiratory disorders, impaired liver and kidney function, concurrent administration of other CNS depressants. Dosage should be halved for the elderly.

ALL THESE COMPOUNDS MAY IMPAIR REFLEXES: therefore, utmost caution in driving, operating machinery etc.

TOLERANCE AND PSYCHOLOGICAL (SOMETIMES PHYSICAL) DEPENDENCY OCCUR READILY: therefore benzodiazepines should not be prescribed on a continuous basis unless there are compelling reasons.

NOTE: Benzodiazepine compounds which are prescribed specifically to control insomnia are described in Chart IIIB: these are nitrazepam (Mogadon), flurazepam (Dalmane), temazepam (Euhypnos, Normison), triazolam (Halcion) and lormetazepam (Noctamid)

Drug Name	Brand Name(s)	Usual Oral Dosage Range*	Number of Daily Doses (see text)
2: Others			
CHLORMETHIAZOLE	UK: Heminevrin	0.5–1 G	2–4

ADVERSE EFFECTS: Tingling in nose, sneezing, irritation of eyes, gastric disturbances, confusion.
WARNINGS etc. Action of chlormethiazole is potentiated by all other central depressants; not advised in severe liver complaints. Reflexes may be impaired and physical/psychological dependency may follow regular use.

HYDROXYZINE	UK: Atarax	50–300 mg	3–4
	US: Atarax, Vistaril	(25–100 mg)*	

ADVERSE EFFECTS: Dry mouth, confusion, Parkinsonism; convulsions, tremor (rare and following high doses)
WARNINGS etc. Impaired reflexes, tolerance/dependency. Effect of other CNS depressants is enhanced. Contra-indicated in pregnancy and in cases of known hypersensitivity.

MEPROBAMATE	UK: Equanil, Miltown, Milonorm	200–800 mg	2–3
	US: Equanil, Miltown, Meprospan etc.		

ADVERSE EFFECTS: Common – as for benzodiazepines; less often, seizures, blood disorders, syncope (see Text)
WARNINGS etc. Interactions: as for other tranquillizers. Avoid in alcoholism, epilepsy, porphyria, caution in kidney or liver disorders. Dependency common.

PROPRANOLOL	UK: Inderal, Berkolol	80–160 mg	2
	US: Inderal		

ADVERSE EFFECTS: Nausea, insomnia, lethargy, diarrhoea, skin rashes, dry eyes (transient at low dosages)
INTERACTIONS: verapamil, clonidine, levodopa, oral anti-diabetic drugs, some bronchodilators (see Text)
WARNINGS etc: Caution – poor cardiac reserve; contra-indicated: diabetes, pregancy, after prolonged fasting, bronchospasm, heart block

*Figures given in parentheses refer to injected doses, which may be prescribed to control severe anxiety states, to control convulsions etc. (see Text).

CHART VIB: TRANQUILLIZERS, ANTIPSYCHOTIC

NOTE: These compounds are chiefly employed to mitigate the symptoms of schizophrenia and other severely disturbed states. Other actions include control of nausea/vomiting (promethazine, prochlorperazine), antihistaminic (anti-allergic: methotrimeprazine, trimeprazine), and the enhancing of opiate analgesics. Some of these drugs are given for specific conditions, e.g. benperidol for antisocial sexual deviancy, lithium to control mania in manic-depressive psychosis. All are more or less likely to provoke Parkinsonian effects, for which prophylactic medication should probably be given (see Text).

Drug Name	Brand Name(s)	Range of Daily Doses (Oral) Outpatient	Inpatient
1: **Phenothiazines**			
CHLORPROMAZINE	UK: Largactil US: Thorazine, Promapar, Sonazine	50–400 mg	200–1500 mg
METHOTRI- MEPRAZINE	UK: Veractil US: Levoprome	25–60 mg	–
PROMAZINE	UK: Sparine US: Sparine	25–75 mg	25–300 mg
PROMETHAZINE	UK: Phenergan US: Phenergan, Remsed	25–100 mg	–
TRIFLUPROMAZINE	US: Vesprin	20–50 mg	30–150 mg
TRIMEPRAZINE	UK: Vallergan	30–100 mg	–

aliphatics

Adverse Effects
Common: Sedation, hypotension, apathy, Parkinsonism, anticholinergic effects (e.g. dry mouth), sensitivity to light, mental depression, tardive dyskinesia
Less common: Jaundice, impotence & libido changes, slowed ejaculation, weight gain, blood disorders
Uncommon: Pigmentation of lens of eye, changes of cardiac rhythm (ECG), menstrual disturbances

ACETOPHENAZINE	US: Tindal	40–80 mg	60–100 mg
BUTAPERAZINE	US: Repoise	10–30 mg	10–100 mg
CARPHENAZINE	US: Proketazine	50–150 mg	75–400 mg
FLUPHENAZINE	UK: Moditen, Modecate US: Permitil, Prolixin	1–5 mg (25–50 mg/month)*	2–60 mg
PERPHENAZINE	UK: Fentazin	8–24 mg	12–64 mg
PROCHLORPERAZINE	UK: Stemetil, Vertigon US: Compazine	20–60 mg	60–200 mg
THIOPROPAZATE	UK: Dartalan	10–30 mg	30–100 mg
TRIFLUOPERAZINE	UK: Stelazine US: Stelazine	4–10 mg	10–60 mg

piperazines

Adverse Effects
Common: Parkinsonism, anticholinergic effects (dry mouth, blurred vision etc), apathy, mental depression
Less common: Hypotension, light sensitivity, changes in libido, impotence, inhibited ejaculation, tardive dyskinesia
Uncommon: Jaundice, blood dyscrasias, skin rashes, variations in cardiac (ECG) rhythm

Drug Name	Brand Name(s)	Range of Daily Doses (Oral) Outpatient	Inpatient
MESORIDAZINE	US: Serentil	25–200 mg	100–400 mg
PERICYAZINE	UK: Neulactil	5–25 mg	10–90 mg
PIPERACETAZINE	US: Quide	10–40 mg	20–160 mg
THIORIDAZINE	UK: Melleril US: Mellaril	50–400 mg	200–800 mg

(left margin label: piperidines)

Adverse Effects
Common: Sedation, hypotension, apathy, anticholinergic effects, mental depression
Less common: Parkinsonism, pigmentary retinopathy, impotence & retarded ejaculation, tardive dyskinesia, changes in cardiac rhythm
Uncommon: Jaundice, blood dyscrasias

2: Butyrophenones

HALOPERIDOL	UK: Haldol, Serenace US: Haldol	2–6 mg	4–100 mg
BENPERIDOL	UK: Anquil	0.25–1.5 mg	–
DROPERIDOL	UK: Droleptan	–	5–20 mg

Adverse Effects
Common: Parkinsonian reactions, mental depression, lethargy, sedation, changes in libido etc
Less common: Hypotension, rapid heartbeat, blood dyscrasias, tardive dyskinesia
Uncommon: Jaundice, skin rashes, light sensitivity

FLUSPIRILENE	UK: Redeptin	–	(2–12 mg/week)*
PIMOZIDE	UK: Orap	2–10 mg	2–16 mg

Adverse Effects
Similar to Phenothiazines but less severe
Fairly common: Hard subcutaneous nodules at site of injection (fluspirilene)

3: Thioxanthenes

CHLORPROTHIXENE	UK: Taractan	30–45 mg	45–400 mg
CLOPENTHIXOL	UK: Clopixol	–	(200–400 mg/2–4 weekly)*
FLUPENTHIXOL	UK: Depixol, Fluanxol	2–3 mg	3–18 mg (100–400 mg/2–4 weekly)*
THIOTHIXENE	US: Navane	6–30 mg	10–120 mg

Adverse Effects
Common: Drowsiness, lethargy
Less common: Anticholinergic effects, hypotension, Parkinsonism, tachycardia, libido changes
Uncommon: Blood dyscrasias, jaundice

ALL PHENOTHIAZINES, BUTYROPHENONES AND THIOXANTHENES:

INTERACTIONS WITH OTHER DRUGS:
Antipsychotic drugs enhance the sedative effects of all other central depressants, such as sleeping pills, powerful analgesics, and alcohol. Potentially serious interactions may occur with anticoagulants (e.g. warfarin), amphetamine-type drugs, lithium, MAO-inhibitor and tricyclic antidepressants, antidiabetic agents, guanethidine, oral contraceptives, phenytoin, and curare-like muscle relaxants. Fluspirilene and pimozide specifically block the effects of amphetamines and related stimulants.

CONTRA-INDICATED in semi-coma from barbiturate or alcohol overdosage, severe liver disease, bone-marrow depression; disorders of blood metabolism immediately following hepatitis; during pregnancy and for children unless reason are compelling; severe heart disease and atherosclerosis, liver or kidney failure, geriatric confusion, phaeochromocytoma, history of convulsive disorders (e.g. Parkinsonism). Caution in glaucoma and urinary retention. The elderly are especially susceptible to antipsychotic agents. *PHENOTHIAZINES and BUTYROPHENONES may induce, or exacerbate, severe psychological depression.*

ALL ANTIPSYCHOTIC DRUGS TEND TO SLOW REFLEXES, THUS NECESSITATING GREAT CAUTION IN DRIVING OR PERFORMING SKILLED TASKS.

SINCE THESE DRUGS PROVOKE PARKINSONIAN REACTIONS (MOTOR/MUSCULAR DISCO-ORDINATION, INVOLUNTARY MOVEMENTS, RIGIDITY etc), IN SOME PATIENTS EVEN AT RELATIVELY LOW DOSAGE, MEDICATION TO PREVENT SUCH EFFECTS MAY BE GIVEN CONCURRENTLY WITH THE TRANQUILLIZER: the most effective anti-parkinsonian agents are orphenadrine (Disipal), procyclidine (Kemadrin) and benzhexol (trihexiphenidyl; Artane).

N.B.: THE EFFECTS OF ANTIPSYCHOTIC MEDICATION MAY OBSCURE SYMPTOMS AND SIGNS OF A NUMBER OF SEVERE ACUTE CONDITIONS, INCLUDING BRAIN TUMOUR AND INTESTINAL OBSTRUCTION.

Drug Name	Brand Name(s)	Range of Daily Doses (Oral) Outpatient	Inpatient
4: Others			
LITHIUM CARBONATE	UK: Camcolit, Phasal, Priadel, Liskonum US: Eskalith, Lithotabs, Lithonate	1.2–1.6 G (but see Text)	

Adverse Effects
Common: Trembling, urinary frequency, nausea & other gastro-intestinal disturbances, disorientation
Less common: Muscular & motor disco-ordination, reversible goitre, changes in heart rhythm, renal damage
Uncommon: Many side-effects – see Text

INTERACTIONS: these include acetazolamide (Diamox), thiazine diuretics, aminophylline, barbiturates, methyldopa, phenothiazines, sodium chloride & sodium bicarbonate. Lithium blocks stimulant effects of amphetamines;
CONTRA-INDICATED in cardiac failure, impaired kidney function, low salt diets. BECAUSE LITHIUM IS EXTREMELY TOXIC, BLOOD-LEVELS MUST BE REGULARLY MONITORED (see Text)

LOXAPINE	US: Daxolin, Loxitane	15–40 mg	40–160 mg

Adverse Effects
Sedation, dizziness, faintness, weakness, confusion, Parkinsonism, tardive dyskinesia, weight gain, dermatitis, hypo- and hypertension (see Text)

INTERACTIONS: not yet fully understood, but probably as for phenothiazines; effectiveness of adrenaline impaired
CONTRA-INDICATED in severe CNS depression, pregnancy, convulsive disorders, cardiovascular illness, glaucoma, urinary retention, inter alia

MOLINDONE	US: Lidone, Moban	15–60 mg	40–225 mg

Adverse Effects
Similar to those of loxapine; also menstrual changes, insomnia, restlessness, hyperactivity, euphoria, gynaecomastia (see Text)

INTERACTIONS: as for phenothiazines; drug increases toxicity of antiparkinsonian drugs, antagonizes tetrabenazine; may affect phenytoin and tetracycline metabolism
CONTRA-INDICATIONS: as for other antipsychotic agents

---

*These quantities refer to depôt injections, which contain the drug in esterified form, usually in a vegetable oil vehicle: such preparations, which may produce effects lasting weeks, are increasingly popular among psychiatrists, partly because of their obvious convenience and also because of poor patient compliance with tablet regimens.

372

Annexes

ANNEX 1:
Conversion of Imperial and Metric Units

Rather surprisingly, since the Metric System is thought to have been standardized in medicine, a few prescribers in the UK continue to use Imperial (Apothecaries') Measures (grains, minims, etc). In the USA many drug preparations listed in *American Drug Index 1980* have constituents quoted in Imperial units, including difficult fractions: in some cases a product with several ingredients gives one in Metric and others in Imperial. This is a source of confusion to practitioners and patients alike. In prescription writing, the abbreviations g (G or gramme) and gr (grain) are so similar that serious mistakes have occurred in dispensing. The following Tables and suggested mathematical formulae for converting one type of measure into another should prove helpful.

IMPERIAL SYSTEM

Mass

	Metric equivalent (approximate)
1 grain (gr)	= 60 milligrammes (mg)
1 drachm (dr or ℈) = 60 grains	= 1.2 grammes (G)
1 ounce (℥) = 480 grains = 8 drachms	= 30 G

Volume

1 minim (m or ♏)	= 0.06 millilitres (ml)
1 fluid drachm (fl dr or ℈) = 60 minims	= 3.55 ml
1 fluid ounce (fl oz or ℥) = 8 fluid drachms	= 30 ml

METRIC SYSTEM

Mass

1 microgramme (μg or mcg)	= 1/6000 grain (gr)
1 milligramme (mg or mgm) = 1000 microgrammes	= 1/60 gr
1 centigramme (cg)* = 100 milligrammes	= 1½ gr
1 gramme (G or Gm) = 1000 milligrammes	= 15 gr

Volume

1 millilitre (ml)	= 15 minims (m)
1 litre (L)	= 30 fluid ounces (fl oz)

Note: The size of a 'teaspoonful' of liquid medicine has now been standardized to 5 millilitres, which is rather more than the capacity of the average teaspoon: therefore plastic 5-ml spoons are usually dispensed with the medication.

*The centigramme (cg) unit is not used in the UK or USA but is often found in continental Europe.

CONVERSION FROM METRIC TO IMPERIAL MEASURES (approximate)

Mass

1 microgramme (μg)	= 1/6000 grain (gr)
1 milligramme (mg)	= 1/60 gr
10 mg	= 1/6 gr
15 mg	= ¼ gr
20 mg	= ⅓ gr
30 mg	= ½ gr
50 mg	= ¾ gr
60 mg	= 1 gr
100 mg	= 1½ gr
150 mg	= 2⅓ gr
200 mg	= 3 gr
500 mg	= 7½ gr
750 mg	= 11½ gr
1 gramme (G)	= 15 gr

Note: To convert milligrammes to grains, multiply by 0.0154
to convert grammes to grains, multiply by 15
to convert grammes to ounces, multiply by 0.0311
to convert grammes to drachms, multiply by 0.257

Volume

0.1 millilitre (ml)	= 1⅔ minims (m)
0.5 ml	= 8½ m
1 ml	= 17 m
2 ml	= 34 m
5 ml	= 85 m
10 ml	= 169 m
15 ml	= 253 m
20 ml	= 338 m

30 ml	= 1 fluid ounce (fl oz)
50 ml	= 1⅔ fl oz
100 ml	= 3 fl oz
1 litre (L)	= 30 fl oz

Note: To convert millilitres to minims, multiply by 16.7
to convert millilitres to fluid ounces, multiply by 0.033

CONVERSION FROM IMPERIAL TO METRIC MEASURES (approximate)

Mass

1/6000 grain (gr)	= 0.01 milligramme (mg) = 1 μg
1/600 gr	= 0.1 mg
1/400 gr	= 0.15 mg
1/120 gr	= 0.5 mg
1/80 gr	= 0.75 mg
1/60 gr	= 1 mg
1/40 gr	= 1.5 mg
1/30 gr	= 2 mg
1/25 gr	= 2.5 mg
1/10 gr	= 5 mg
1/6 gr	= 10 mg
1/4 gr	= 15 mg
1/3 gr	= 20 mg
2/5 gr	= 25 mg
1/2 gr	= 30 mg
3/4 gr	= 50 mg
1 gr	= 60 mg
1½ gr	= 100 mg
2½ gr	= 150 mg
3 gr	= 200 mg
5 gr	= 300 mg
7½ gr	= 450 mg
10 gr	= 600 mg
11½ gr	= 750 mg
15 gr	= 1000 mg = 1 gramme (G)

Note: To convert grains into grammes, divide the number of grains by 15

Volume

1 minim (m)	= 0.06 millilitre (ml)
5 m	= 0.3 ml
10 m	= 0.6 ml
15 m	= 1 ml

25 m	= 1.5 ml
35 m	= 2 ml
85 m	= 5 ml
169 m	= 10 ml
250 m (½ fluid ounce)	= 15 ml
1 fl oz	= 30 ml
3 fl oz	= 100 ml
30 fl oz	= 1000 ml = 1 litre (L)

Note: To convert minims to millilitres, multiply by 0.06

ANNEX 2:
Prescription Writing

ABBREVIATIONS

Many abbreviations are used by practitioners in prescription-writing: usually these are employed for the purpose of saving time, for convenience, and out of tradition. Occasionally a prescription may be written in such a way as deliberately to make it difficult for the patient to understand what is being ordered and why. Drugs may be prescribed under their chemical name or as a branded preparation. Thus a physician may order 'trifluoperazine' rather than Stelazine, the proprietary form in which the medicament is available. The cross-indices in this book are designed so that the reader is able to track down details of the material prescribed, whether this is named as a generic, or official, formulation or a branded tablet, capsule etc. In the case of directions, the following list of abbreviations should render virtually all prescriptions comprehensible.

a.c.	*ante cibos*	= before meals
ad	*ad*	= to make (a total)
ad lib.	*ad libitum*	= as much as required
Amps.	Ampoules/Ampuls	
aq. dest.	*aqua destillata*	= distilled water
aq. pro inj.	*aqua pro injectionibus*	= water for injections
b.d.	*bis in die sumendum*	= twice daily
b.i.d.		
b.d.s.		
c. or c̄.	*cum*	= with
Caps.	Capsules	
c.m.	*cras mane sumendum*	= take tomorrow
c.m.s.		morning
c.n.	*cras nocte*	= take tomorrow
		evening
d.	*detur*	= give
det.		
e.m.p.	*ex modo prescripto*	= as directed
f.	*fiat*	= make up
ft.		

g. or G, Gm	*grammum*	= gramme
gr.	*granum*	= grain (NB difference from g,G)
Gtt.	*Guttae*	= Drops
Haust.	*Haustus*	= Draught
h.n.	*hac nocte*	= tonight
hor. decub.	*hora decubitus*	= at bedtime
h.s.	*hora somnii*	= at bedtime
Liq.	*Liquor*	= Solution
M, misce	*misce*	= mix
m. ⎫ m̄. ⎬ mitte ⎭	*mitte*	= dispense
m. et n.	*mane et nocte*	= morning and evening
mane	*mane*	= in the morning
m.d. ⎫ m.d.u. ⎭	*more dicto utendum*	= take as directed
mg., mgm.	*milligrammum*	= milligramme(s)
Mist.	*Mistura*	= Mixture
ml.		= millilitre(s)
mor. sol.	*more solito*	= as usual
nocte	*nocte*	= at bedtime
noct. maneq.	*nocte maneque*	= night and morning
n.r. ⎫ non rep. ⎭	*non repetatur*	= do not repeat
o.m.	*omni mane*	= each morning
o.n.	*omni nocte*	= each night
p.c.	*post cibos*	= after meals
p.p.a.	*phiala prius agitata*	= shake the bottle
p.r.n.	*pro re nata*	= as required
Pulv.	*Pulvis*	= Powder
q.h.	*quaque hora*	= every hour
q.6. h. etc	*quaque 6 hora*	= every six hours
q.d. ⎫ q.i.d. ⎬ q.d.s. ⎭	*quater in die sumendum*	= four times a day
q.s.	*quantum sufficiat*	= as much as necessary
℞	*recipe*	= supply
rep.	*repetatur*	= repeat
s. ⎫ sig. ⎭	*signetur*	= let it be labelled
ss.	*semi-*	= half
s.o.s.	*si opus sit*	= when required
stat.	*statim*	= at once

Syr.	*Syrupus*	= Syrup
Tabs.	*Tabellae*	= Tablets
t.d.	*ter in die sumendum*	= three times a day
t.d.s.		
t.i.d.		
Ung.	*Unguentum*	= Ointment
ut dict.	*ut dictum*	= as directed

(cf also symbols used in weights and measures: Annex 1)

PRESCRIPTIONS FOR CONTROLLED DRUGS

In recent years the rules governing the writing of prescriptions for
Controlled Drugs, such as morphine, pethidine, methadone and other
narcotic pain-killers, have been considerably tightened up: the object of
these provisions, as set out in the Misuse of Drugs Act 1971 and Misuse of
Drugs Regulations 1973, has been presumably to make it more difficult
for prescriptions to be altered by the patient or forged. The example
overleaf illustrates the legal requirements.

The entire prescription must be in the prescriber's own handwriting and
signed by him. It must be written in ink or be otherwise indelible.

Name and Address
of Patient

Physician's
Address* & date in writing

Type and Number of
Dosage Units to be
Dispensed

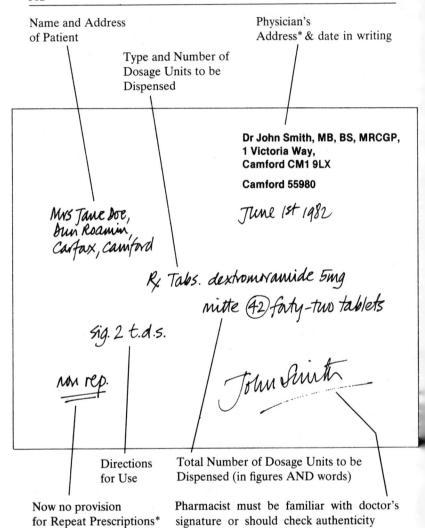

Directions
for Use

Total Number of Dosage Units to be
Dispensed (in figures AND words)

Now no provision
for Repeat Prescriptions*

Pharmacist must be familiar with doctor's
signature or should check authenticity

*In the case of a National Health Service prescription, the physician's address does not need to be written, as it will already be stamped on the form (FP10). The handwriting requirement is waived in respect of certain designated psychiatrists who work at Drug Dependency Clinics (DDCs): multiple prescriptions for narcotic addicts, to be dispensed daily, must then be prepared, and rubber stamps indicating the drug, dosage form, etc., are used.

ANNEX 3:
Dangerous Drugs: An International Directory

The following is a directory of prescription drugs and preparations which are subject to national and international restriction, under the UK Misuse of Drugs Act, the US Controlled Substances Act and corresponding legislation in other countries. The listing is in two parts: I for narcotic analgesics of the morphine type, II for powerful central stimulants such as amphetamine. Abbreviations for the countries concerned: UK = United Kingdom; US = United States; CA = Canada; GR = West Germany; FR = France; IT = Italy; AUS = Austria; SW = Switzerland; BEL = Belgium.

I : OPIATES (Narcotic Analgesics)

US,CA: ALPHAPRODINE Hydrochloride Injection USP (*Nisentil* amps, vials)

US,CA: ANILERIDINE Hydrochloride Tablets USP (*Leritine*)
ANILERIDINE Phosphate Injection USP (*Leritine* amps, vials)

BEL: BEZITRAMIDE (*Burgodin* tabs)

UK,US: CODEINE Phosphate Tablets BPC, USP (unbranded preps)†
CODEINE Sulfate Tablets USP (unbranded preps)
CODEINE Phosphate Injection USP (unbranded amps, vials)

CA *Paveral* (drops)
IT *Tebasolo** (amps)

UK: DEXTROMORAMIDE Tartrate Tablets BPC (*Palfium* tabs)
DEXTROMORAMIDE Tartrate Injection BPC (*Palfium* amps)

GR,FR: *Palfium* (tabs, amps, suppos)

GR: *Jetrium* (tabs, amps)
IT: *Narcolo* (tabs, amps, suppos)

UK: DIAMORPHINE Hydrochloride (Heroin) Injection BPC
           (unbranded)
           DIAMORPHINE Hydrochloride Linctus BPC (unbranded)
           DIAMORPHINE and COCAINE Elixir BPC ('Brompton
           Cocktail': unbranded)
           Diamorphine Hydrochloride Hypodermic Tabs (unbranded)

UK: DIETHYLTHIAMBUTENE Hydrochloride Injection BPC
           (*Themalon*: for veterinary use only)

UK: DIHYDROCODEINE Tartrate Tablets BPC (*DF–118*)†
           DIHYDROCODEINE Tartrate Injection BPC (*DF–118*)

UK: DIPIPANONE (*Diconal** tabs)

UK: ETORPHINE Hydrochloride Injection BPC (*Immobilon**:
           for veterinary use only)

UK,US: FENTANYL Citrate Injection BPC,USP (*Sublimaze,
           Thalamonal*, Innovar** amps, vials)

GR,AUS: *Sublimaze* (amps, vials), *Thalamonal** (amps, vials)
FR: *Fentanyl Le Brun* (vials)
IT: *Fentanest* (vials), *Leptofen** (vials)

US: HYDROCODONE Bitartrate Tablets USP (*Dicodid,
           Codone*)
           (also many compound formulations, not restricted in USA)

UK: *Dimotane-DC** (linctus)
CA: *Hycodan* (tabs, syrup)
GR: *Dicodid* (tabs, amps)

US: HYDROMORPHONE Hydrochloride Tablets USP
           (*Dilaudid*)
           HYDROMORPHONE Sulfate Injection USP (*Dilaudid*
           amps)

US: *Dilaudid Cough Syrup*, Dilocol* (syrup)

CA,GR,
SW: *Dilaudid* (tabs, amps, vials, suppos)

GR,SW: *Dilaudid-Atropin** (amps, suppos)
SW: *Scolaudol** (amps)

GR,AUS: KETOBEMIDONE (*Cliradon* tabs, drops, amps, suppos)

UK,US: LEVORPHANOL Tartrate Tablets BPC,USP (*Dromoran, Levo-Dromoran*)
           LEVORPHANOL Tartrate Injection BPC,USP (*Dromoran, Levo-Dromoran* amps)
GR: *Dromoran* (tabs, amps, suppos)

UK,US: METHADONE Hydrochloride Tablets BPC, USP (*Physeptone, Dolophine, Methadone Diskets, Westadone, Nodalin**)
UK: METHADONE Hydrochloride Linctus BPC (*Physeptone* and unbranded)
UK,US: METHADONE Hydrochloride Injection BPC,USP (*Physeptone* amps, *Dolophine* amps, vials)

GR,AUS: *L-Polamidon* (tabs, drops, amps, vials, suppos)
GR,AUS: *L-Polamidon-C** (tabs, drops, amps, vials, suppos)
AUS: *Heptadon* (tabs, amps), *Ultradon** (tabs, amps, suppos)
IT: *Mephenon* (amps), *Eptadone* (amps), *Physeptone* (tabs, amps)
SW: *Heptanal* (amps), *Ketalgin* (suppos)

UK,US: MORPHINE Sulphate Tablets BPC,USP (unbranded preps.; *MST-1* SR tabs)
           MORPHINE Sulphate Injection BPC,USP (unbranded amps, vials, *Duromorph* amps, *Cyclimorph** amps)
UK: MORPHINE Hydrochloride Solution BPC (unbranded)
UK: MORPHINE Hydrochloride Suppositories BPC (unbranded)
UK: MORPHINE Sulphate Suppositories BPC (unbranded)
UK: MORPHINE & Atropine Injection BPC (unbranded amps)
UK: *Nepenthe* (amps, soln)

CA: *Hyperduric Morphine* (amps)
GR: *Morphin-Thilo* (amps), *Morphin-Atropin-Thilo** (amps), *Amphiolen Morphinum Hydrochloridum* (amps), *Amphiolen Morphinum Hydrochloridum cum Atropino Sulfurico** (amps), *Amphiolen Morphinum Hydrochloricum cum Scopolamino Hydrobromico** (amps)
AUS: *Modiscop** (tabs, amps), *Theba-Intran* (amps), *Theba-Intran cum Atropino Sulfurico** (amps), *Thebametten* (tabs)

| CA,FR: | *Sédol** (amps) |
| IT: | *Cardiostenol** (amps), *Sedo-Corywas** (drops, amps), *Sedolo** (amps) |

| AUS: | NICOMORPHINE (*Vilan* tabs, amps, suppos) |

| CA: | NORMETHADONE (*Cophylac** tabs, soln, expectorant) |
| AUS: | *Ticarda** (tabs, drops) |

| AUS: | NORPIPANONE (*Orfenso** tabs, suppos) |

UK,US:	Powdered OPIUM BPC, USP (unbranded) also s.v. PAPAVERETUM
UK,US:	OPIUM Tincture (Laudanum) BPC,USP (unbranded)
UK,US:	Camphorated OPIUM Tincture BPC (= Paregoric USP; unbranded)†
UK:	Concentrated Camphorated OPIUM Tincture BPC (unbranded)

| US: | *Laudacin* (syrup), *B&O Supprettes** (suppos) |
| GR: | *Paverysat* (drops) |

UK:	OXYCODONE (*Proladone* suppos)
US:	*Percobarb** (tabs), *Percocet** (tabs), *Percodan** (tabs), *Tylox** (tabs)
GR:	*Eubine* (tabs, amps, suppos), *Eukodal* (tabs, amps), *Scophedal** (amps)
FR:	*Eubine* (amsp, suppos), *Pancodone-Retard* (amps, suppos)

| US: | OXYMORPHONE Hydrochloride Injection USP (*Numorphan* & unbranded preps) OXYMORPHONE Hydrochloride Suppositories USP (*Numorphan*) |

| UK: | PAPAVERETUM (TOTAL OPIUM ALKALOIDS) Tablets BPC (*Omnopon*) PAPAVERETUM Injection BPC (*Omnopon* amps, *Omnopon-Scopolamine** amps) *Aspirin & Papaveretum* (unbranded sol tabs)† |

US:	*Pantopon* (amps)
CA,FR:	*Spasmalgine** (amps)
GR,AUS:	*Pantopon* (tabs, drops, amps, suppos)
AUS:	*Tutopon* (tabs, drops, amps)

IT: *Morfalgin** (amps), *Preanest** (amps)
SW: *Spasmosol** (tabs, drops, suppos)

UK,US: PETHIDINE (MEPERIDINE) Hydrochloride Tablets
         BPC,USP (*Demerol* & unbranded)
UK,US: PETHIDINE (MEPERIDINE) Hydrochloride Injection
         BPC,USP (unbranded amps in UK, unbranded amps, vials,
         Demerol amps, vials)
US: PETHIDINE (MEPERIDINE) Hydrochloride Syrup USP
         (*Demerol* & unbranded)

UK: *Pamergan-P100** (amps), *Pamergan-AP** (amps),
         Pethilorfan* (amps)
US: *Demerol-APAP** (tabs), *APC + Demerol** (tabs),
         Mepergan* (vials), *Mepergan Fortis** (caps)
CA: *Demerol* (tabs, amps, vials), *AC-Demerol** (tabs), *Demer-Idine* (amps), *Pamergan** (caps, amps), *Pemadine** (amps), *Pethidine-Co-007** (tabs), *Sparidol** (vials)
GR: *Dolantin* (tabs, drops, amps, suppos), *Dolantin-Spezial** (amps), *Psyquil-Compositum** (amps)
FR: *Dolosal* (amps), *Suppolosal* (suppos)
AUS: *Alodan* (tabs, amps, suppos), *Alodan-Compositum** (amps), *Alodan-Atropin** (amps), *Alodan-Atropin-Promethazin** (amps)
IT: *Dolantin* (amps), *Dolosina* (amps), *Mefedine* (amps)

UK: PHENAZOCINE Hydrobromide Tablets BPC (*Narphen*)

UK: PHENOPERIDINE (*Operidine* amps)
FR: *R.1406* (vials)

UK: PIRITRAMIDE (*Dipidolor* amps)
GR,AUS: *Dipidolor* (amps, vials)

GR: THEBACON (*Acedicon* tabs)

        † in UK exempt from restriction
        * Compound preparations

II : STIMULANTS

UK,US: AMPHETAMINE Sulphate Tablets BPC,USP (unbranded
                tabs) also s.v. DEXAMPHETAMINE
US: AMPHETAMINE Sulfate Injection USNF 1970 (unbranded
                vials)

US,CA: *Benzedrine* (tabs, SR caps)
FR: *Orténal** (tabs)

UK,US: COCAINE Hydrochloride BPC, USP (unbranded crystals or
                powder)
UK: COCAINE Hydrochloride Eye-Drops BPC (unbranded)
UK: COCAINE and Homatropine Eye-Drops BPC (unbranded)
US: COCAINE Hydrochloride Tablets for Local Solution USP
                (unbranded)

UK,US: DEXAMPHETAMINE (DEXTROAMPHETAMINE)
                Sulphate Tablets BPC,USP (*Dexamed, Dexedrine*)
UK: *Durophet** (SR caps), *Durophet-M** (SR caps)
US: *Daro* (tabs, caps), *Dexampex* (tabs, caps), *Diphylets* (caps),
                Ferndex (tabs), *Oxydess* (tabs), *Robese-Forte* (tabs, vials),
                Spancap (caps), *Tidex* (tabs), *Dexamyl** (tabs, caps),
                Biphetamine* (caps), *Dextrobar** (tabs), *Eskatrol** (caps),
                Ro-Trim* (caps), *Trimex** (caps), *Obotan** (tabs)
CA: *Dexedrine* (tabs, caps), *Synatan* (tabs), *Dexamobarb** (caps),
                Dexamyl* (tabs, caps), *Seco-Synatan** (caps)
SW: *Dexedrine* (tabs), *Amphaetax* (tabs), *Obesit** (tabs)

UK,US: METHYLAMPHETAMINE (METHAMPHETAMINE)
                (*Methedrine* tabs, amps**)
US: *Desoxyn* (tabs), *Dee-10* (tabs), *Methampex* (tabs), *Obedrin*
                (tabs), *Aridol** (tabs), *Obe-Slim** (tabs), *Span-RD** (tabs),
                Mediatric* (tabs, caps)
CA: *Neodrine* (tabs), *Buta-Neodrine** (tabs)
GR,IT: *Pervitin* (tabs)

US: METHYLPHENIDATE Hydrochloride Tablets USP
                (*Ritalin*)
                METHYLPHENIDATE Hydrochloride Injection USP 1970
                (*Ritalin***)
UK: *Ritalin* (tabs, amps**)
CA: *Methidate* (tabs), *Ritalin* (tabs, amps**)
GR etc: *Ritalin* (tabs)

US: PHENMETRAZINE (OXAFLUMEDRINE)
                    Hydrochloride Tablets USP (*Preludin*)
UK: *Filon** (tabs)
CA: *Preludin* (tabs)
GR etc: *Cafilon** (tabs)

*indicates compound preparations   **injectable preparations for hospital use only

Note: In the UK, the above drugs and preparations are restricted under Schedule 2 of the Misuse of Drugs Regulations, along with the narcotics. Schedule 3, to which fewer constraints apply, lists only five drugs (benzphetamine, chlorphentermine, mephentermine, phendimetrazine, and pipradol): these are stimulants of moderate potency. While all are marketed in the USA, where they are not under special control, none of the five is available in the UK.

Apart from (1) Morphine and analogues, with a few exemptions, (2) Amphetamine and other powerful stimulants, and (3) Psychedelics (eg LSD) and Cannabis, none of the widely abused barbiturates are yet controlled in the UK, while the hypnotic methaqualone (*Mandrax**) is the only restricted soporific.

In the UK, according to the Misuse of Drugs (Notification of and Supply to Addicts) Regulations 1973, physicians are not permitted to prescribe diamorphine or cocaine to addicts, and may supply these drugs only for relief of organic illness or injury.

WEST GERMANY: SPECIAL CONTROLS

According to the *Betäubungsmittel-Verschreibungs-Verordnung* (Prescription of Narcotics Regulations) 1974, as amended 1978, maximum permitted daily dosages of Controlled Drugs have been instituted, as follows:

I: OPIATES (Narcotic Analgesics)

DRUG NAME	MAXIMUM DAILY DOSE	FORM IN WHICH AVAILABLE
DEXTRO-MORAMIDE*	100 mg	Jetrium (tabs 6.9 mg) Palfium (tabs 6.9 mg)
HYDROCODONE	200 mg	Dicodid (tabs 5 & 10 mg, amps 15 mg)
HYDRO-MORPHONE*	30 mg	Dilaudid (tabs 2.5 mg, amps 2 mg, suppos 2.5 mg) Dilaudid-Atropin (amps 4 mg, suppos 4 mg)

KETOBEMIDONE*	100 mg	Cliradon (tabs 5 mg, drops 10 mg/ml, amps 7.5 mg, vials 75 mg, suppos 10 mg)
LEVORPHANOL*	30 mg	Dromoran (tabs 1.5 mg, amps 2 mg)
MORPHINE*	200 mg	Amphiolen-Morphinum (amps 10 & 20 mg) Morphin-Thilo (amps 20 mg) Amphiolen-Morphinum (+ atropine: amps 10 & 20 mg) Morphin-Atropin-Thilo (amps 20 mg) Amphiolen-Morphinum (+ scopolamine: amps 20 mg) Paverysat (drops 2.25 mg/ 15 ml)
NORMETHADONE	200 mg	Ticarda (drops 15 mg/ml)
OPIUM/ PAPAVERETUM*	400 mg ($\equiv$ 200 mg morphine) $\equiv$ 200 mg morphine	Pantopon (tabs 10 mg, amps 20 mg, drops 20 mg/ml, suppos 20 mg) Opium Tincture
OXYCODONE*	200 mg	Eukodal (tabs 5 mg, amps 10 & 20 mg) Scophedal (amps 10 mg) Scophedal-Forte (amps 20 mg)
PETHIDINE*	1000 mg	Dolantin (tabs 25 mg, drops 50 mg/ml, amps 50 & 100 mg, suppos 100 mg) Dolantin-Spezial (amps 50 & 100 mg) Psyquil-Compositum (amps 50 mg)
PIRITRAMIDE*	200 mg	Dipidolor (amps 20 mg)

THEBACON	200 mg	Acedicon (tabs 5 mg)
FENTANYL**	5 mg	Fentanyl (amps 0.2 mg, vials 0.8 mg)

*may be doubled in particularly severe illnesses
**only for use in hospital or physician's practice

II: STIMULANTS

DRUG NAME	MAXIMUM DAILY DOSE	FORM IN WHICH AVAILABLE
AMPHETAMINE	for local application to eye 500 mg all other purposes 200 mg	
COCAINE	100 mg	as eye-drops or eye-ointment up to a concentration of 2%; for other purposes permitted concentration maximum of 1% with 0.1% atropine
	in practice	In ENT surgery, solution up to 20%
	1000 mg	As Lamellae or eye-ointment up to 2%
METHYL-AMPHETAMINE	100 mg	Pervitin (tabs 3 mg, amps 15 mg)
METHYLPHENI-DATE	200 mg	Ritalin (tabs 10 mg)
PHENMETRAZINE	600 mg	Cafilon (tabs 30 mg)

Source: *Rote Liste 1980: Verzeichnis von Fertigarzneimitteln der Mitglieder des Bundesverbandes der Pharmazeutischen Industrie e.V.* Aulendorf/Württ., 1980, pp. 12–17.

Similar regulations have come into force in Scandinavian Countries, with maximum permitted daily dosages similar to the above. See, for example, *Felleskatalog over farmasøytiske spesialpreparater registrert i Norge.* Oslo, 1981, pp. 259–79.

RESTRICTED DRUGS AVAILABLE ONLY ON SPECIAL LICENCE

According to the UK *Misuse of Drugs Act* 1971 and *Misuse of Drugs Regulations 1973* (SI 1973 no. 797) and corresponding legislation in other countries, certain Controlled Drugs have been placed in a special category: these may be legally possessed and prescribed only under a Licence for the purpose from the Home Office (or, in the USA, the National Institutes of Health). The compounds concerned are principally psychedelics or 'hallucinogens' of the lysergide (LSD) type, but also included are cannabis and its derivatives. The US list of such specially restricted agents is long and contains many substances which are abstruse and not used, even experimentally. That provided in the Misuse of Drugs Regulations (Schedule 4) is more concise and comprises the following 'substances and preparations':

Bufotenine
Cannabinol
Cannabinol derivatives (e.g. THC)
Cannabis and cannabis resin
Coca leaf
Concentrate of poppy-straw
Lysergamide
Lysergide (LSD) and other N-alkyl derivatives of lysergamide
Mescaline
Raw opium
Psilocin
N,N-Diethyltryptamine (DET)
N,N-Dimethyltryptamine (DMT)
2,5-Dimethoxy-α,4-dimethylphenethylamine (DOM)

The restriction extends to salts, isomers, esters, ethers etc of the above drugs. The scheduled substances are all dealt with in this book: CANNABIS, TETRAHYDROCANNABINOL (THC), LYSERGAMIDE, LYSERGIDE (LSD), MESCALINE, OPIUM, PSILOCIN, DET, DMT and DOM (STP) as separate individual entries and in the relevant Essays and Charts (Psychedelics; Potent Analgesics). Coca leaf is scheduled because it contains high concentrations of COCAINE, and concentrate of poppy-straw because this yields a considerable proportion of OPIUM. The penalties for illicit possession and sale of drugs on Schedule 4 are extremely severe (except in the case of small amounts of cannabis): more so, indeed, in many instances than for offences involving heroin and other narcotics. The following is a specimen of a Home Office Licence in respect of a Schedule 4 drug:

MISUSE OF DRUGS ACT 1971

In pursuance of the Misuse of Drugs Act 1971 (hereinafter called 'the Act') the Secretary of State hereby grants to Dr C O Jones DM FRCPsych the Professor of Therapeutics at the University of Mercia Medical School, Oxminster Infirmary, Tyneside TN1 5QQ (hereinafter called 'the Licensee'), a LICENCE to supply, offer to supply and to have in his possession not more than 10.00 milligrams of Lysergide (hereinafter called 'the Drug'), subject to the following conditions:–

1. The drug shall be used by the Licensee for the sole purpose of research, and may be supplied only in the course of administration under the direct personal supervision of Professor C O Jones or Dr E Coli to patients who are suffering from terminal and intractable carcinoma.

2. The licensee may not obtain during the period of validity of this licence more than 10.00 milligrams of the drug.

3. The licence must be produced to any person or firm in the United Kingdom from whom any supply of the drug is obtained and must be endorsed with the amount and form of the drug supplied and be signed and dated by such person or firm at the time when the transaction is effected in the form annexed hereto. In the event of a supply of the drug being obtained from a person or firm outside the United Kingdom, these details shall be entered thereon together with the number and date of issue of the licence under which authority the drug was imported.

4. All stocks of the drug shall at all times be in the charge of the licensee or some responsible person appointed by him for the purpose.

5. The licensee shall keep a complete record of all amounts of the drug coming into his possession in pursuance of this licence showing in respect of each amount the date when received, the form in which received and the name and address of the person or firm from whom received. Likewise, the licensee shall keep a complete record of all amounts of the drug administered and the quantity and form in which used. These entries shall be made on the day on which the drug is received or administered, as the case may be, or, when that is not reasonably practicable, on the following day. This record shall be preserved for a period of two years from the date of the last entry therein.

6. The licensee shall furnish to the Secretary of State such returns of the amounts of the drug in his possession or coming into his possession in pursuance of this licence, and the use of the drug, as may from time to time be required.

7. The licence is valid only for the licensee, and in respect of the address named herein. In the event of Professor C O Jones ceasing to be employed or otherwise engaged at this address, he shall return the licence immediately to the Secretary of State.

8. The licensee may not supply or offer to supply any of the drug, otherwise than by way of administration as aforesaid.

9. The licensee shall inform the Secretary of State as soon as practicable of any thefts or losses of the drug named herein.

10. The licence shall be produced for inspection when required by any person duly authorised under Section 23 of the Act by the Secretary of State.

The licence, unless sooner revoked, shall continue in force until 31 December 1980 or until the licensee has used all stocks of the drug held in pursuance of the licence, if that should occur sooner, and on expiry or revocation shall be surrendered to the Secretary of State.

(signed)

Assistant Under-Secretary of State

Home Office
50 Queen Anne's Gate
London
SW1H 9AT

1 January 1982

DANGEROUS DRUGS: INTERNATIONAL DIRECTORY

Index of Brand and Other Names

*indicates a compound preparation

BRAND NAME	MAIN COMPONENT	COUNTRY WHERE USED
AC-Demerol	pethidine*	CA
Acedicon	thebacon	GR
Alodan	pethidine	AUS

BRAND NAME	MAIN COMPONENT	COUNTRY WHERE USED
Alodan-Compositum	pethidine*	AUS
Alodan-Atropin	pethidine*	AUS
Alodan-Atropin-Promethazin	pethidine*	AUS
Amphaetax	dexamphetamine	SW
Amphiolen Morphinum hydrochloricum	morphine	GR
Amphiolen Morphinum hydrochloricum cum Atropino	morphine*	GR
Amphiolen Morphinum hydrochloricum cum Scopolamino	morphine*	GR
APC + Demerol	pethidine*	US
Aridol	methylamphetamine*	US
Aspirin & Papaveretum	papaveretum*	
B&O Supprettes	opium*	US
Benzedrine	amphetamine	US,CA
Biphetamine	dexamphetamine*	US
Brompton Cocktail	s.v. diamorphine*	
Burgodin	bezitramide	BEL
Buta-Neodrine	methylamphetamine*	CA
Cafilon	phenmetrazine*	GR,FR,IT
Cliradon	ketobemidone	GR,AUS
Codone	hydrocodone	US
Cyclimorph	morphine*	UK
Daro	dexamphetamine	US
Dee-10	methylamphetamine	US
Demer-Idine	pethidine	CA
Demerol	pethidine	US
Demerol-APAP	pethidine*	US
Desoxyn	methylamphetamine	US
Dexamed	dexamphetamine	UK
Dexamobarb	dexamphetamine*	CA
Dexampex	dexamphetamine	US
Dexamyl	dexamphetamine*	US,CA
Dexedrine	dexamphetamine	UK,US,SW
Dextrobar	dexamphetamine*	US
DF-118	dihydrocodeine	UK

BRAND NAME	MAIN COMPONENT	COUNTRY WHERE USED
Dicodid	hydrocodone	US,CA
Diconal	dipipanone*	UK
Dilaudid	hydromorphone	US,CA,GR
Dilaudid-Atropin	hydromorphone*	GR
Dilaudid Cough Syrup	hydromorphone	US
Dimotane-DC	hydrocodone*	UK
Diphylets	dexamphetamine	US
Dipidolor	piritramide	UK,GR
Dolantin	pethidine	GR
Dolantin-Spezial	pethidine*	GR
Dolophine	methadone	US
Dolosal	pethidine	FR
Dolosina	pethidine	IT
Dromoran	levorphanol	UK,GR
Duromorph	morphine*	UK
Durophet	dexamphetamine*	UK
Durophet-M	dexamphetamine*	UK
Eptadone	methadone	IT
Eskatrol	dexamphetamine*	US
Eubine	oxycodone	GR,FR
Eukodal	oxycodone	GR
Fentanest	fentanyl	IT
Fentanyl Le Brun	fentanyl	FR
Ferndex	dexamphetamine	US
Filon	phenmetrazine*	UK
Heptadon	methadone	AUS
Heptanal	methadone	IT
Heroin	s.v. diamorphine	
Hycodan	hydrocodone*	CA
Hyperduric Morphine	morphine	CA
Immobilon	etorphine*	UK
Innovar	fentanyl*	US,CA
Jetrium	dextromoramide	GR
Ketalgin	methadone	SW

BRAND NAME	MAIN COMPONENT	COUNTRY WHERE USED
Laudacin	opium	US
Laudanum	s.v. opium tincture	
Leptofen	fentanyl	IT
Leritine	anileridine	US,CA
Levo-Dromoran	levorphanol	US,CA
L-Polamidon	methadone	GR
L-Polamidon-C	methadone*	GR
Mediatric	methylamphetamine*	US
Mefedine	pethidine	IT
Mepergan	pethidine*	US,CA
Mepergan-Fortis	pethidine*	US
Meperidine	s.v. pethidine	
Mephenon	methadone	IT
Methadone Diskets	methadone	US
Methampex	methylamphetamine	US
Methedrine	methylamphetamine	UK
Methidate	methylphenidate	CA
Modiscop	morphine*	AUS
Morfalgin	papaveretum*	IT
Morphin-Thilo	morphine	GR
Morphin-Atropin-Thilo	morphine*	GR
Morphin-Atropin-Promethazin-Thilo	morphine*	GR
MST-1	morphine	UK
Narcolo	dextromoramide	IT
Narphen	phenazocine	UK
Neodrine	methylamphetamine	CA
Nepenthe	morphine	UK
Nisentil	alphaprodine	US,CA
Nodalin	methadone*	US
Numorphan	oxymorphone	US,GR
Obedrin	methylamphetamine	US
Obesit	dexamphetamine*	SW
Obe-Slim	methylamphetamine*	US
Obotan	dexamphetamine	US
Omnopon	papaveretum	UK
Omnopon-Scopolamine	papaveretum*	UK

BRAND NAME	MAIN COMPONENT	COUNTRY WHERE USED
Operidine	phenoperidine	UK
Orfenso	norpipanone*	AUS
Orténal	amphetamine*	FR
Oxydess	dexamphetamine	US
Palfium	dextromoramide	UK,GR,FR
Pamergan-P100	pethidine*	UK
Pamergan-AP	pethidine*	UK
Pancodone-Retard	oxycodone	FR
Pantopon	papaveretum	US,GR
Paregoric	s.v. opium tincture	
Paveral	codeine	CA
Paverysat	opium	GR
Pemadine	pethidine	CA
Percobarb	oxycodone*	US
Percocet	oxycodone*	US
Percodan	oxycodone*	US
Pervitin	methylamphetamine	GR,AUS
Pethidine-Co-007	pethidine*	CA
Pethilorfan	pethidine*	UK
Physeptone	methadone	UK,IT
Preanest	papaveretum*	IT
Preludin	phenmetrazine	US,CA
Proladone	oxycodone	UK
Psyquil-Compositum	pethidine*	GR
R.1406	phenoperidine	FR
Ritalin	methylphenidate	UK,GR,US
Robese-Forte	dexamphetamine	US
Ro-Trim	dexamphetamine	US
Scolaudol	hydromorphone*	SW
Scophedal	oxycodone*	GR
Seco-Synatan	dexamphetamine*	CA
Sedo-Corywas	morphine*	IT
Sédol	morphine*	FR
Sedolo	morphine*	IT
Span-Cap	dexamphetamine	US
Span-RD	methylamphetamine*	US
Sparidol	pethidine*	CA

BRAND NAME	MAIN COMPONENT	COUNTRY WHERE USED
Spasmalgine	papaveretum*	CA,FR
Spasmosol	papaveretum*	SW
Sublimaze	fentanyl	UK
Suppolosal	pethidine	FR
Synatan	dexamphetamine	CA
Tebasolo	codeine*	IT
Thalamonal	fentanyl*	UK,GR,AUS
Theba-Intran	morphine	AUS
Theba-Intran-cum Atropino	morphine*	AUS
Thebametten	morphine	AUS
Themalon	diethylthiambutene	UK
Ticarda	normethadone*	GR,AUS
Tidex	dexamphetamine	US
Trimex	dexamphetamine*	US
Tutopon	papaveretum	AUS
Tylox	oxycodone*	US
Ultradon	methadone*	AUS
Vilan	nicomorphine*	AUS
Westadone	methadone	US

REFERENCES

UK: *Misuse of Drugs Act 1971*
    Misuse of Drugs Regulations 1973 (SI no. 797)
    Misuse of Drugs (Notification of and Supply to Addicts) Regulations 1973 (SI no. 799)
    Medicines (Prescription Only) Order 1977 (SI no. 2127)
    Medicines (Prescription Only) Amendment (no. 2) Order 1978 (SI no. 987)
    Hay, C. E. & Pearce, M.E.: *Medicines and Poisons Guide*, ed. 2. Pharmaceutical Society: London, 1980
    Guide to the Misuse of Drugs Act 1971. DHSS: London, 1977
US: *Controlled Substances Act 1965* (with revisions 1973, 1978)
    United States Pharmacopeia, ed. 20. USP Commission: Rockville, Md., 1979, pp. 995–1017.

CONTINENTAL: *Rote Liste 1980: Verzeichnis von Fertigarzneimitteln.* Aulendorf, 1980

Dictionnaire Vidal 1980. Paris, 1980

Compendium of Pharmaceuticals and Specialties, ed. 15. Toronto, 1980

see also SELECT BIBLIOGRAPHY (Annex 6) and List of Sources (p. 435)

ANNEX 4:
How to Identify Tablets and Capsules: An Index of Markings

This Directory contains an index of imprints on tablets and capsules: branded and unbranded preparations of stimulants, tranquillizers, antipsychotics, anxiety-relieving tranquillizers, antidepressants and potent analgesics, which are currently available for prescription in the UK (and in some cases the USA also). The great majority of solid-dose formulations carry a distinguishing mark of some kind: this may be only the manufacturer's name or symbol or logo or code-letters or numbers. The British Pharmacopoeia lays down requirements for the size (in millimetres) of diameter for many preparations of drugs which are marketed only as generic, or unbranded, tablets or capsules: at the end of this Alphabetical Directory, a list is provided of BP specifications for unbranded products (e.g. phenobarbitone tablets of different strengths).

To save cumbersome cross-referencing, this Directory has been assembled as follows: when, as is the case with some preparations, the maker's name appears on one side of the tablet and some other marking on the reverse side, the manufacturer's name is given first. Thus a tablet marked *T 1* on one side and *JANSSEN* on the other is listed under *JANSSEN*. This identifies the preparation as *Triperidol* (trifluperidol tablets 1 mg). Unless otherwise stated, tablets are round and capsules bullet-shaped (made in two sections).

Tab = Tablet   SR Tab = Sustained-release Tablet
Cap = Capsule   SR Cap = Sustained-release Capsule

An asterisk (*) indicates that the preparation is restricted under the UK Misuse of Drugs Act, which applies to morphine and other narcotic analgesics, to potent stimulants of the amphetamine type, and to one hypnotic (methaqualone). A Statutory Instrument is shortly to go before Parliament similarly to restrict barbiturates (e.g. amylobarbitone, pentobarbitone), but at this writing these sleep-inducing agents are exempt from such control.

An oblique stroke (/) indicates that one imprint appears on the obverse, and another on the reverse, side of a tablet; or in the case of a capsule, on the cap and body respectively.

Preparations are identified first by their proprietary names and then by their official names in brackets: it is by these official or non-proprietary names that drugs are listed in the Alphabetical Entries. Several examples of makers' trade-marks or logos are shown: for those tablets or capsules which carry a pictorial design, see at the end of the alphabetical directory.

(Abbott Laboratories Ltd)		
A/ABBOTT	Nembutal (pentobarbitone sodium 100 mg)	yellow cap
(Allen & Hanburys Ltd)		
AH 1C	Fentazin 2 mg (perphenazine)	white tab
AH 1D	Triptafen-DA (amitriptyline co)	pink tab
AH 2C	Fentazin 4 mg (perphenazine)	white tab
AH 2D	Triptafen-Minor (amitriptyline co)	pink tab
AH 4C	Fentazin 8 mg (perphenazine)	white tab
AH 4D	Triptafen-Forte (amitriptyline co)	red tab
ANXON/15	Anxon 15 mg (ketazolam)	dark/light pink cap
ANXON/30	Anxon 30 mg (ketazolam)	dark/light pink cap
AVOMINE	Avomine (promethazine theoclate 25 mg)	white tab
(Berk Pharmaceuticals Ltd)		
BERK/D	Domical 10 mg (amitriptyline)	blue tab
BERK/D	Domical 25 mg (amitriptyline)	orange tab
BERK/D	Domical 50 mg (amitriptyline)	brown tab
BERK 2	Atensine 2 mg (diazepam)	white tab
BERK 5	Atensine 5 mg (diazepam)	yellow tab
BERK 1 N 4	Nitrados (nitrazepam 5 mg)	white tab
BERK 1 Z 1	Berkolol 10 mg (propranolol)	pink tab
BERK 2 Z 1	Berkolol 40 mg (propranolol)	pink tab
BERK 3 Z 1	Berkolol 80 mg (propranolol)	pink tab
BERK 4 Z 1	Berkolol 160 mg (propranolol)	pink tab
CAMCOLIT	Camcolit (lithium carbonate 250 mg)	white tab
CAMCOLIT S	Camcolit-S (lithium carbonate 400 mg)	white SR tab
C G	Cosalgesic (dextropropoxyphene co)	white oval tab
(Ciba Laboratories Ltd)		
CIBA / A B	*Ritalin (methylphenidate 10 mg)	white tab
CIBA / C O	Ludiomil 10 mg (maprotiline)	pink tab
CIBA / D P	Ludiomil 25 mg (maprotiline)	pale orange tab
CIBA / D Z	Ludiomil 150 mg (maprotiline)	orange tab
CIBA / E R	Ludiomil 50 mg (maprotiline)	orange tab
CIBA / F S	Ludiomil 75 mg (maprotiline)	dark orange tab
CIBA / G A	Doriden (glutethimide 250 mg)	white tab
CIBA / O L	Tacitin (benzoctamine 10 mg)	white tab
COX / C C	Cosalgesic (dextropropoxyphene co)	white oval tab
(DDSA Pharmaceuticals Ltd)		
DDSA	Remnos 5 mg (nitrazepam)	white tab
DDSA	Remnos 10 mg (nitrazepam)	yellow tab

(DDSA Pharmaceuticals Ltd *cont.*)		
DDSA	Tropium 5 mg (chlordiazepoxide)	green tab
DDSA	Tropium 5 mg (chlordiazepoxide)	yellow/black cap
DDSA	Tropium 10 mg (chlordiazepoxide)	green tab
DDSA	Tropium 10 mg (chlordiazepoxide)	green/white cap
DDSA	Tropium 25 mg (chlordiazepoxide)	green tab

(Duncan, Flockhart & Co Ltd)		
DF 118	DF-118 (dihydrocodeine 30 mg)	white tab
DF M T	Myanesin (mephenesin 200 mg)	white tab
DF O	Onadox-118 (dihydrocodeine co)	white tab
DF P	Paramol-118 (dihydrocodeine co)	white tab

D G	Distalgesic (dextropropoxyphene co)	white oblong tab
D G S	Distalgesic-Soluble (dextropropoxyphene co)	white octagonal tab
DISIPAL	Disipal (orphenadrine 50 mg)	orange tab
D N	Allegron 10 mg (nortriptyline)	yellow tab
D N D N	Allegron 25 mg (nortriptyline)	orange tab
D P	Napsalgesic (dextropropoxyphene co)	yellow oblong tab
E	Evidorm (hexobarbitone co)	white tab
E 10	Euhypnos 10 mg (temazepam)	green ovoid cap
E FORTE	Euhypnos 20 mg (temazepam)	green ovoid cap
ELAMOL	Elamol (tofenacin 80 mg)	orange/grey cap
FORTRAL 50	Fortral 50 mg (pentazocine)	grey/yellow cap
FRISIUM	Frisium (clobazam 10 mg)	pale blue cap

(Geigy Pharmaceuticals Ltd)		
GEIGY	Anafranil 20 mg (clomipramine)	brown/yellow cap
GEIGY	Anafranil 25 mg (clomipramine)	brown/orange cap
GEIGY	Anafranil 50 mg (clomipramine)	brown/blue cap
GEIGY	Insidon (opipramol 50 mg)	beige tab
GEIGY	Pertofran (desipramine 25 mg)	salmon-pink tab
GEIGY	Tofranil 10 mg (imipramine)	red-brown triangular tab
GEIGY	Tofranil 25 mg (imipramine)	red-brown tab

INDERAL 10	Inderal 10 mg (propranolol)	pink tab
INDERAL 40	Inderal 40 mg (propranolol)	pink tab
INDERAL 80	Inderal 80 mg (propranolol)	pink tab
INDERAL 160	Inderal 160 mg (propranolol)	pink tab
INDERAL L A	Inderal-LA (propranolol 160 mg)	mauve/pink SR cap
int	Integrin 40 mg (oxypertine)	white tab
INTEGRIN 10	Integrin 10 mg (oxypertine)	grey/green cap

(Janssen Pharmaceuticals Ltd)		
JANSSEN / A 0.25	Anquil (benperidol 0.25 mg)	white tab
JANSSEN / D 10	Droleptan (droperidol 10 mg)	yellow tab
JANSSEN / H 0.5	Haldol 0.5 mg (haloperidol)	white tab
JANSSEN / H 1.5	Haldol 1.5 mg (haloperidol)	yellow tab
JANSSEN / H 5	Haldol 5 mg (haloperidol)	blue tab
JANSSEN / H 10	Haldol 10 mg (haloperidol)	yellow tab
JANSSEN / H 20	Haldol 20 mg (haloperidol)	white tab
JANSSEN / O 2	Orap 2 mg (pimozide)	white tab
JANSSEN / O 4	Orap 4 mg (pimozide)	green tab
JANSSEN / O 10	Orap 10 mg (pimozide)	white tab

(Janssen Pharmaceuticals Ltd *cont.*)

JANSSEN / T 0.5	Triperidol 0.5 mg (trifluperidol)	white tab
JANSSEN / T 1	Triperidol 1 mg (trifluperidol)	white tab

(Thomas Kerfoot & Co Ltd)

K 2	unbranded Diazepam 2 mg	white tab
K 5	unbranded Diazepam 5 mg	yellow tab
K 5	unbranded Nitrazepam 5 mg	white tab
K 10	unbranded Diazepam 10 mg	blue tab
K 10	unbranded Amitriptyline 10 mg	white tab
K 25	unbranded Amitriptyline 25 mg	yellow tab
K 50	unbranded Amitriptyline 50 mg	orange tab
LARGACTIL 10	Largactil 10 mg (chlorpromazine)	white tab
LARGACTIL 25	Largactil 25 mg (chlorpromazine)	white tab
LARGACTIL 50	Largactil 50 mg (chlorpromazine)	white tab
LARGACTIL 100	Largactil 100 mg (chlorpromazine)	white tab

(Lederle Laboratories Ltd)

LEDERLE 4434	Artane 2 mg (benzhexol)	white tab
LEDERLE 4436	Artane 5 mg (benzhexol)	white tab
LEDERLE 4438	Artane-Sustets (benzhexol 5 mg)	green ovoid cap

(Eli Lilly & Co Ltd)

LILLY C 54	Dolasan (dextropropoxyphene co)	orange tab
LILLY F 23	Sodium Amytal 60 mg (amylobarbitone sodium)	blue cap
LILLY F 33	Sodium Amytal 200 mg (amylobarbitone sodium)	blue cap
LILLY F 40	Seconal Sodium 100 mg (quinalbarbitone sodium)	orange cap
LILLY F 42	Seconal Sodium 50 mg (quinalbarbitone sodium)	orange cap
LILLY F 65	Tuinal 100 mg (amylobarbitone co)	red/blue cap
LILLY F 66	Tuinal 200 mg (amylobarbitone co)	red/blue cap
LILLY H 03	Doloxene (dextropropoxyphene)	pale orange cap
LILLY H 17	Aventyl 10 mg (nortriptyline)	white/yellow cap
LILLY H 19	Aventyl 25 mg (nortriptyline)	white/yellow cap
LILLY H 91	Doloxene-Co (dextropropoxyphene co)	grey/red cap
LILLY T 32	Amytal 100 mg (amylobarbitone)	white tab
LILLY T 37	Amytal 50 mg (amylobarbitone)	white tab
LILLY T 40	Amytal 15 mg (amylobarbitone)	white tab
LILLY T 56	Amytal 30 mg (amylobarbitone)	white tab
LILLY U 13	Amytal 200 mg (amylobarbitone)	white tab
LILLY U 15	Sodium Amytal 200 mg (amylobarbitone sodium)	white tab
LILLY U 16	Sodium Amytal 200 mg (amylobarbitone sodium)	blue tab
LILLY U 36	Sodium Amytal 60 mg (amylobarbitone sodium)	blue tab
LILLY U 43	Sodium Amytal 60 mg (amylobarbitone sodium)	white tab
LOBAK	Lobak (chlormezanone co)	pink tab
LUM 15 / III	Luminal 15 mg (phenobarbitone)	white tab

LUM 30 / III	Luminal 30 mg (phenobarbitone)	white tab
LUM 60 / III	Luminal 60 mg (phenobarbitone)	white tab
(Lundbeck Ltd)		

LUNDBECK	Fluanxol (flupenthixol 0.5 mg)	red tab
LUNDBECK	Depixol (flupenthixol 3 mg)	yellow tab
m	Marsilid 25 mg (iproniazid)	pink tab
m	Marsilid 50 mg (iproniazid)	yellow tab
MEDOMIN	Medomin (heptabarbitone 200 mg)	white tab
MILONORM	Milonorm (meprobamate 400 mg)	white tab
(May & Baker Ltd)		
M & B	Vallergan (trimeprazine 10 mg)	blue tab
M & B	Phenergan 10 mg (promethazine)	dark blue tab
M & B / SU 50	Surmontil 50 mg (trimipramine)	green/white cap
MEL 10	Melleril 10 mg (thioridazine)	white tab
MELLERIL 25	Melleril 25 mg (thioridazine)	white tab
MELLERIL 50	Melleril 50 mg (thioridazine)	white tab
MELLERIL 100	Melleril 100 mg (thioridazine)	white tab
MERITAL	Merital 25 mg (nomifensine)	orange cap
MERITAL	Merital 50 mg (nomifensine)	orange/brown cap
(Merck Sharp & Dohme Ltd)		

MSD 23	Tryptizol 10 mg (amitriptyline)	light blue tab
MSD 26	Concordin 5 mg (protriptyline)	pink tab
MSD 45	Tryptizol 25 mg (amitriptyline)	yellow tab
MSD 47	Concordin 10 mg (protriptyline)	white tab
MSD 102	Tryptizol 50 mg (amitriptyline)	brown tab
MSD 649	Tryptizol 75 mg (amitriptyline)	orange SR cap
(Napp Laboratories Ltd)		
NAPP / MST 1	*MST-1 (morphine sulphate 10 mg)	brown SR tab
NEULACTIL	Neulactil 2.5 mg (pericyazine)	pale yellow tab
NEULACTIL 10	Neulactil 10 mg (pericyazine)	pale yellow tab
NEULACTIL 25	Neulactil 25 mg (pericyazine)	pale yellow tab
NOLUDAR	Noludar (methylprylone 200 mg)	white tab
NORVAL / 10	Norval 10 mg (mianserin)	orange tab
NORVAL / 20	Norval 20 mg (mianserin)	orange tab
NORVAL / 30	Norval 30 mg (mianserin)	orange tab
OPTIMAX	Optimax (1-tryptophan co)	white tab
OPTIMAX WV	Optimax-WV (1-tryptophan 500 mg)	white tab
(Organon Laboratories Ltd)		
ORGANON / CT 4	Bolvidon 10 mg (mianserin)	yellow tab
ORGANON / CT 6	Bolvidon 20 mg (mianserin)	white tab
ORGANON / CT 7	Bolvidon 30 mg (mianserin)	white tab
(Pharmax Ltd)		

P (in hexagon)	Phasal (lithium carbonate 300 mg)	white tab
P 9	Volital (pemoline 20 mg)	white tab
P 25	Prothiaden 25 mg (dothiepin)	red/brown cap
P 30	Prominal 30 mg (methylphenobarbitone)	white tab

P 60	Prominal 60 mg (methylphenobarbitone)	white tab
P 75	Prothiaden 75 mg (dothiepin)	red SR tab
P 200	Prominal 200 mg (methylphenobarbitone)	white tab

(Parke, Davis & Co Ltd)

PARKE DAVIS	Epanutin/Phenobarbitone (phenobarbitone co)	white cap
PCT 500	Pacitron (1-tryptophan 500 mg)	orange oblong tab

(Pfizer) **(Pfizer Ltd)**

PFIZER	Atarax 10 mg (hydroxyzine)	orange tab
PFIZER	Atarax 25 mg (hydroxyzine)	green tab
PFIZER / SQN 10	Sinequan 10 mg (doxepin)	orange cap
PFIZER / SQN 25	Sinequan 25 mg (doxepin)	orange/blue cap
PFIZER / SQN 50	Sinequan 50 mg (doxepin)	blue cap
PFIZER / SQN 75	Sinequan 75 mg (doxepin)	blue/yellow cap
PHENERGAN 25	Phenergan 25 mg (promethazine)	dark blue tab
PX / PA 60	Ponderax-PA (fenfluramine 60 mg)	blue/clear SR cap

(Riker Laboratories Ltd)

RIKER	*Durophet 7.5 mg (dexamphetamine co)	off-white cap
RIKER	*Durophet 12.5 mg (dexamphetamine co)	black/white cap
RIKER	*Durophet 20 mg (dexamphetamine co)	black cap
RIKER	*Durophet-M 12.5 mg (dexamphetamine co)	brown/green cap
RIKER	*Durophet-M 20 mg (dexamphetamine co)	brown/red cap
RIKER	Duromine 15 mg (phentermine)	grey/green cap
RIKER	Duromine 30 mg (phentermine)	grey/red cap
RIKER / N G	Norgesic (orphenadrine co)	white tab
RIKER / N X	Norflex (orphenadrine)	white tab
R 365 B	see under Pictorial Designs	
R 365 C	see under Pictorial Designs	

R / L **(Roussel Laboratories Ltd)**

R L / M x	*Mandrax (methaqualone 250 mg co)	white tab
R L / M X	*Mandrax (methaqualone 250 mg co)	dark/light blue cap

(Roche Products Ltd)

ROCHE	*unbranded Pethidine hydrochloride 25 mg	white tab
ROCHE	*unbranded Pethidine hydrochloride 50 mg	white tab
ROCHE	*Omnopon (papaveretum 10 mg)	buff tab
ROCHE	Marplan (isocarboxazid 10 mg)	pink tab
ROCHE	Libraxin (chlordiazepoxide co)	pale green tab
ROCHE	Taractan 15 mg (chlorprothixene)	pink tab
ROCHE	Taractan 50 mg (chlorprothixene)	brown tab
ROCHE /(two semicircles) see under Pictorial Designs		

(Roche Products Ltd *cont.*)

ROCHE /(two concentric circles) see under Pictorial Designs		
ROCHE 2	Valium 2 mg (diazepam)	white tab
ROCHE 2	Valium 2 mg (diazepam)	blue/white cap
ROCHE 5	Valium 5 mg (diazepam)	yellow tab
ROCHE 5	Valium 5 mg (diazepam)	blue/yellow cap
ROCHE 5	Librium 5 mg (chlordiazepoxide)	green tab
ROCHE 5	Librium 5 mg (chlordiazepoxide)	green/yellow cap
ROCHE 5	Limbitrol 5 mg (chlordiazepoxide co)	pink/green cap
ROCHE 5	Nobrium 5 mg (medazepam)	orange/ivory cap
ROCHE 5	Mogadon (nitrazepam 5 mg)	purple/black cap
ROCHE 10	Librium 10 mg (chlordiazepoxide)	light green tab
ROCHE 10	Librium 10 mg (chlordiazepoxide)	green/black cap
ROCHE 10	Limbitrol 10 mg (chlordiazepoxide co)	pink/green cap
ROCHE 10	Nobrium 10 mg (medazepam)	orange/black cap
ROCHE 10	Valium 10 mg (diazepam)	blue tab
ROCHE 15	Dalmane 15 mg (flurazepam)	grey/yellow cap
ROCHE 25	Librium 25 mg (chlordiazepoxide)	dark green tab
ROCHE 30	Dalmane 30 mg (flurazepam)	black/grey cap
RONYL	Ronyl (pemoline 20 mg)	white tab

(Searle Laboratories Ltd)

SEARLE	Lomotil (diphenoxylate co)	white tab
SEARLE	Lomotil/Neomycin (diphenoxylate co)	white tab
SEARLE	Dartalan 5 mg (thiopropazate)	white tab
SEARLE	Dartalan 10 mg (thiopropazate)	beige tab
SEARLE	Serenace 0.5 mg (haloperidol)	light/dark green cap
SEARLE 41	Serenace 1.5 mg (haloperidol)	white tab
SEARLE 12	Serenace 5 mg (haloperidol)	red tab
SEARLE 919	Serenace 10 mg (haloperidol)	pale pink tab
SEARLE 920	Serenace 20 mg (haloperidol)	deep pink tab
SEDAPAM 2	Sedapam 2 mg (diazepam)	white tab
SEDAPAM 5	Sedapam 5 mg (diazepam)	yellow tab
SEDAPAM 10	Sedapam 10 mg (diazepam)	blue tab

(Smith Kline & French Laboratories Ltd)

SK&F	*Dexedrine (dexamphetamine 5 mg)	yellow tab
SKF	Parnate (tranylcypromine 10 mg)	orange tab
SKF	Parstelin (tranylcypromine co)	dark green tab
SKF	Stelazine 1 mg (trifluoperazine)	dark blue tab
SKF	Stelazine 5 mg (trifluoperazine)	dark blue tab

(Smith & Nephew Pharmaceuticals Ltd)

SNP 2	*Narphen (phenazocine 5 mg)	white tab
SOLIS 2	Solis 2 mg (diazepam)	violet/green cap
SOLIS 5	Solis 5 mg (diazepam)	violet/mauve cap
SOMNASED	Somnased (nitrazepam 5 mg)	white tab
SONALGIN	Sonalgin (butobarbitone 60 mg co)	lilac tab
SONERGAN	Sonergan (butobarbitone 75 mg co)	mauve tab
SONERYL	Soneryl (butobarbitone 100 mg)	pink tab

(E R Squibb & Co Ltd)		
SQUIBB	Moditen 5 mg (fluphenazine)	white tab
SQUIBB 626	Noctec (chloral hydrate 500 mg)	red ovoid cap
SQUIBB 863	Moditen 1 mg (fluphenazine)	pink tab
SQUIBB 864	Moditen 2.5 mg (fluphenazine)	yellow tab
SQUIBB 877	Moditen 5 mg (fluphenazine)	white tab
STEMETIL 5	Stemetil 5 mg (prochlorperazine)	white tab
STEMETIL 25	Stemetil 25 mg (prochlorperazine)	white tab
SUREM 5	Surem (nitrazepam 5 mg)	mauve/grey cap
SURMONTIL 10	(trimipramine 10 mg)	white tab
SURMONTIL 25	(trimipramine 25 mg)	white tab
T R (as monogram) see under Pictorial Designs		

(Upjohn Ltd)		
UPJOHN	Halcion 0.125 mg (triazolam)	mauve oval tab
UPJOHN	Halcion 0.25 mg (triazolam)	blue oval tab
UPJOHN 10	Halcion 0.125 mg (triazolam)	mauve oval tab
UPJOHN 17	Halcion 0.25 mg (triazolam)	blue oval tab
VERACTIL 25	Veractil 25 mg (methotrimeprazine)	white tab
VIVALAN	Vivalan (viloxazine 50 mg)	yellow tab

(Wander Pharmaceuticals Ltd)		
WANDER	Noveril (dibenzepin 80 mg)	light orange tab
WANDER / J C	Teronac (mazindol 2 mg)	white tab

(Burroughs Wellcome: Wellcome Medical Division)		
WELLCOME F3A	*Diconal (dipipanone 10 mg co)	pink tab
WELLCOME F4A	*unbranded Pethidine hydrochloride 25 mg	white tab
WELLCOME H4A	*unbranded Pethidine hydrochloride 50 mg	white tab
WELLCOME L3A	unbranded Ephedrine sulphate 30 mg	white tab
WELLCOME L4A	*Physeptone (methadone 5 mg)	white tab
WELLCOME M3A	unbranded Ephedrine sulphate 60 mg	white tab
WELLCOME U2A	unbranded Cyclobarbitone 200 mg	white tab
WELLCOME Y3A	*Methedrine (methylamphetamine 5 mg)	white tab

(Carter-Wallace Ltd)		
W	Miltown 200 mg (meprobamate)	white tab
W	Miltown 400 mg (meprobamate)	white tab

(Wyeth Laboratories Ltd)		
W	Apisate (diethylpropion 75 mg co)	ochre tab
W	Equagesic (ethoheptazine 75 mg co)	white/yellow tab
W	Zactipar (ethoheptazine 75 mg co)	yellow tab
W / E E	Equanil 400 mg (meprobamate)	white tab
W / Z	Zactirin (ethoheptazine 75 mg co)	white tab
W / 10	Serenid-D 10 mg (oxazepam)	white tab
W / 15	Serenid-D 15 mg (oxazepam)	white tab
W / 30	Prondol 30 mg (iprindole)	ochre tab
W / 200	Equanil 200 mg (meprobamate)	white tab
W / 3263	Prondol 15 mg (iprindole)	yellow tab

(Wyeth Laboratories Ltd. *cont.*)

WYETH	Ativan 1 mg (lorazepam)	blue oblong tab
WYETH	Ativan 2.5 mg (lorazepam)	yellow oblong tab
WYETH	Serenid-Forte (oxazepam 30 mg)	red/green cap
WYETH	Normison 10 mg (temazepam)	yellow ovoid cap
WYETH 20	Normison 20 mg (temazepam)	yellow ovoid cap

Pictorial Designs

(Boehringer Ingelheim Ltd)

 Villescon (prolintane 10 mg co)　　orange tab

 / 15MG Tranxene (clorazepate　　grey/mauve cap
15 mg)

(Norgine Ltd)

 Somnite (nitrazepam 5 mg)　　white tab

(Pennwalt Pharmaceuticals Ltd)

 / 18–903 Ionamin 15 mg (phentermine)　　yellow/grey cap

 / 18–904 Ionamin 30 mg (phentermine)　　yellow cap

(Winthrop Laboratories Ltd)

 / FORTRAL Fortral 25 mg (pentazocine) yellow tab

 / FORTAGESIC Fortagesic　　white tab
(pentazocine co)

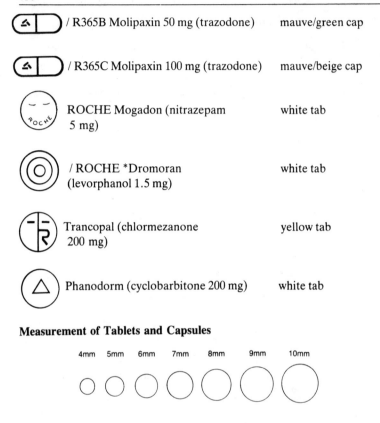

/ R365B Molipaxin 50 mg (trazodone)	mauve/green cap
/ R365C Molipaxin 100 mg (trazodone)	mauve/beige cap
ROCHE Mogadon (nitrazepam 5 mg)	white tab
/ ROCHE *Dromoran (levorphanol 1.5 mg)	white tab
Trancopal (chlormezanone 200 mg)	yellow tab
Phanodorm (cyclobarbitone 200 mg)	white tab

Measurement of Tablets and Capsules

4mm   5mm   6mm   7mm   8mm   9mm   10mm

Unmarked Tablets

Many preparations are marketed of standard drugs: these may be unbranded (generic) and lack any distinguishing markings. The following is a list of tablet diameters which in most cases have been laid down by *British Pharmacopoeia* specifications. Unless otherwise stated tablets are white in colour. The point of including such a list is to indicate that an unmarked white tablet of, say, 7.0 millimetres (mm) in diameter *may* be Codeine Phosphate BPC, i.e. if the tablet has a much larger or smaller diameter then it *cannot* be the preparation and strength named.

4 mm
Diamorphine Hydrochloride 10 mg   (hypodermic tabs)

5.0 mm
Codeine Phosphate 15 mg   –
Ephedrine Hydrochloride 7.5 mg   –

Ephedrine Hydrochloride 15 mg	–
Morphine Sulphate 10 mg	–
Morphine Sulphate 15 mg	–
Papaveretum 10 mg	buff (Omnopon)
Phenobarbitone 15 mg	–
Phenobarbitone Sodium 15 mg	–

5.5 mm

Amylobarbitone 15 mg	–
Amylobarbitone 30 mg	–
Amylobarbitone 50 mg	–
Codeine Phosphate 30 mg	–
Ephedrine Hydrochloride 30 mg	–
Morphine Sulphate 30 mg	–
Phenobarbitone 30 mg	–
Phenobarbitone Sodium 30 mg	–

6.5 mm

Amylobarbitone 60 mg	–
Butobarbitone 60 mg	pink
Dextromoramide 5 mg (*Palfium*)	white
Dextromoramide 10 mg (*Palfium*)	orange
Ephedrine Hydrochloride 50 mg	–
Morphine Sulphate 60 mg	–
Pethidine Hydrochloride 25 mg	–
Phenazocine Hydrobromide 5 mg	–
Phenobarbitone 60 mg	–
Phenobarbitone Sodium 60 mg	–
Prochlorperazine Maleate 5 mg	–
Propranolol Hydrochloride 10 mg	pink

7.0 mm

Codeine Phosphate 60 mg	–
Haloperidol 1.5 mg	–
Pentobarbitone 100 mg	–
Phenobarbitone 100 mg	–
Phenobarbitone Sodium 100 mg	–
Ephedrine Hydrochloride 60 mg	–

7.5 mm

Methadone Hydrochloride 5 mg	–
Methylamphetamine Hydrochloride 5 mg	–

8.0 mm

Amylobarbitone 100 mg	–
Benzhexol 2 mg	–

Diazepam 2 mg   –
Diazepam 5 mg   yellow
Diazepam 10 mg   blue
Dexamphetamine Sulphate 10 mg   yellow
Pethidine Hydrochloride 50 mg   –
Phenobarbitone 125 mg   –

8.5 mm
Amylobarbitone 200 mg   –
Butobarbitone 100 mg   pink
Dihydrocodeine Tartrate 30 mg   –
Meprobamate 200 mg   –
Orphenadrine Citrate 100 mg (Slow)   –
Prochlorperazine Maleate 25 mg   –
Propranolol Hydrochloride 40 mg   pink

9.5 mm
Amphetamine Sulphate 5 mg   yellow
Amylobarbitone Sodium 200 mg   –
Benzhexol 5 mg   –
Cyclobarbitone Calcium 200 mg   –
Ipecacuanha & Opium (Dover's Powder) 300 mg   brown

10.0 mm
Barbitone Sodium 300 mg   –
Carbromal 300 mg   –
Filon (Phenmetrazine 30 mg co)   yellow ovoid

11.0 mm
Barbitone Sodium 450 mg   –
Lithium Carbonate 250 mg   –
Propranolol Hydrochloride 80 mg   pink

12.0 mm
Nitrazepam 5 mg   –

12.5 mm
Lithium Carbonate 450 mg (Slow)   –

19.0 mm
Aspirin & Papaveretum (500 & 10 mg)   buff

ANNEX 5: Glossary of Medical Terms (including some slang terminology)

Note: SMALL CAPITAL LETTERS indicate cross-reference to other items in this Glossary, and *ITALICIZED CAPITALS* to the Alphabetical Entries.

ABSCESS	A pus-bearing area of tissue
ABSTINENCE REACTIONS	S.V. WITHDRAWAL SYNDROME
ACCUMULATION	The building up in organs and tissues of (perhaps toxic) quantities of a drug
ACID (slang)	*LYSERGIDE* (LSD)
ACTIVE PRINCIPLE	The principal active substance present in or isolated from a plant drug
ACUPUNCTURE	A Chinese technique of treating ailments by means of inserting needles into subcutaneous tissues in various parts of the body
ACUTE	Sudden or of short duration; opposite of CHRONIC
ADDICT, NOTIFIED	A person dependent upon a morphine-like drug (e.g. heroin) who has been notified (or 'registered') to the UK Home Office, and who receives legitimate supplies of drug
ADDICT, THERAPEUTIC	An individual who, in the course of medical treatment for a painful condition, has become dependent on a morphine-like drug
ADDICTION	A state of dependency on a drug, characterized by the onset of WITHDRAWAL SYMPTOMS if, following repeated use, supply of the substance concerned is abruptly discontinued. In this book the term is used only in this strict sense.
ADDISON'S DISEASE	A disorder resulting from deficiency in hormones normally produced by the adrenal glands and treated by replacement therapy (e.g. with cortisone)
ADRENALINE (EPINEPHRINE)	Hormone secreted by the adrenal glands: it stimulates the SYMPATHETIC NERVOUS SYSTEM by increasing heart and metabolic rate and other

reactions at times of excitement or fear; also used medicinally to reverse cardiac arrest and to treat other conditions

AETIOLOGY — The root cause of a disorder

AGONISTS, NARCOTIC — s.v. NARCOTIC AGONISTS

ALKALOID — Name given to a drug derived from a vegetable source (e.g. quinine, caffeine, morphine); not to be confused with *alkali*

ALZHEIMER'S SYNDROME — A form of senile dementia, characterized by forgetfulness, confusion and other symptoms

AMNESIA — Loss of memory

AMPHETAMINES — Potent stimulants of the central nervous system (see Essay I)

AMPHETAMINE PSYCHOSIS — A bizarre psychological state brought on usually by repeated abuse of large doses of *AMPHETAMINES* or similar powerful stimulants (see Essay I)

ANAEMIA — Deficiency of red blood-cells leading to debility of various kinds; may be caused by inadequate levels of vitamins, particularly iron, vitamin B_{12} (in the elderly) and folic acid (during pregnancy)

ANALEPTIC — Another term for central stimulant

ANALGESIA — Relief of pain

ANALGESIC, SIMPLE — Mild pain-relieving drug (e.g. aspirin, para-cetamol)

ANALGESIC, POTENT (or NARCOTIC) — Powerful pain-relieving agent, such as morphine and its derivatives and analogues

ANGEL DUST (slang) — *PHENCYCLIDINE*, a drug whose proper use is as a veterinary anaesthetic but large doses of which produce a state of excitement (see Chart V)

ANGINA PECTORIS — Chest pain which may be symptomatic of heart disease

ANOREXIA — Loss of appetite (anorexia nervosa is a specialized condition)

ANOREXIANT — Appetite-reducing; of drugs such as *AMPHETAMINES* and other central stimulants

ANTAGONIST, NARCOTIC — s.v. NARCOTIC ANTAGONIST

ANTIBIOTIC — Drug effective against bacterial infections

ANTICOAGULANT — Drug which slows blood clotting time; prescribed in certain forms of vascular disease

ANTICHOLINERGIC	Inhibiting release of acetylcholine, thereby reducing muscular actions of the digestive system (e.g. relieving nausea); cf ANTIHISTAMINE
ANTICONVULSANT	To prevent or treat convulsive states (e.g. epileptic fits)
ANTIDEPRESSANTS, MAO-INHIBITOR	Type of drug used to alleviate depression (see Essay II)
ANTIDEPRESSANT, TRICYCLIC	The most commonly prescribed class of antidepressant agents, e.g. *AMITRIPTYLINE* (see Essay II)
ANTI-EMETIC	To prevent or control nausea and/or vomiting
ANTIHISTAMINE	Medicament administered in allergic conditions (e.g. hay fever, bronchial asthma) to suppress release of histamine; an ingredient in many over-the-counter cough remedies
ANTIHYPER-TENSIVE	Agent to lower blood-pressure in HYPERTENSION
ANTI-PARKIN-SONIAN	Drug to control PARKINSON'S DISEASE, which may be provoked by most major tranquillizers or antipsychotic drugs
ANTIPSYCHOTIC	Drug given to relieve the symptoms of illness regarded as psychotic, i.e. severely disabling mental disorders
ANTITUSSIVE	To suppress cough
ANXIETY NEUROSIS	Ill-defined term denoting a type of anxious state involving irrational fear of physical illness, and covering various forms of psychosomatic complaint. Characterized by sense of inadequacy in facing up to commitments
ANXIOLYTIC	Anxiety- and tension-relieving
APNOEA, NEONATAL	Respiratory distress in the newborn baby; may be produced by administration of a narcotic to mother during labour
ARTERIO-SCLEROSIS	Thickening of the arteries, especially those surrounding the heart
ASEPTIC	Of sterile procedures (e.g. autoclaving instruments before surgery; use of sterile disposable injection equipment)
ASTHMA, BRONCHIAL	Allergic asthma, typified by intermittent difficulty in breathing
ATHEROSCLEROSIS	A form of ARTERIOSCLEROSIS, in which the arteries (especially coronary arteries) become clogged by fatty deposits

ATTENTION DEFICIT DISORDER	Another name for HYPERKINETIC SYNDROME
BARBS (slang)	Sleeping-pills of the barbiturate type
BARBEMETS	Tablets which contain, in addition to a barbiturate soporific, a small quantity of ipecacuanha: if more than the correct dose is taken, vomiting then occurs (see Essay III)
BARBITURATES	Class of sedative and anticonvulsant drugs (see Essay III)
BEFINDLICHKEITS-SKALA (BS)	A German rating scale for various symptoms of depression
BENNIES (slang)	Benzedrine (*AMPHETAMINE*) capsules
BENZODIAZEPINES	Class of anxiety-relieving and soporific drugs of the *DIAZEPAM* (Valium) type (see Essay VIA)
BENZOMORPHANS	Category of synthetic pain-relieving drugs of considerable potency, e.g. *PHENAZOCINE, PENTAZOCINE* (see Essay IV)
'BLIND'	S.V. DOUBLE-BLIND
BLOCKED (slang)	Considerably under the influence of *CANNABIS*; often to the point at which concentration may be impossible
BLOOD DYSCRASIAS	General old-fashioned term for disorders of blood function
BLUES (slang)	Tablets or capsules containing a mixture of *AMPHETAMINE* and a barbiturate, much liked by some drug abusers; also known as French blues, the colour reference is to a particular branded preparation (Drinamyl, Dexamyl)
BOMBERS, BLACK (slang)	Capsules which contain a high dose of dex- and laevo-*AMPHETAMINE* (Durophet, Biphetamine)
BRADYCARDIA	Slowed heart-rate
BROMIDES	Obsolete sedative drugs (cf Essay III)
BROMISM	Dangerous intoxication following repeated use of BROMIDES
BRONCHODILATOR	A substance which expands the main tubes of the lungs (e.g. *EPHEDRINE*)
BRUXISM	Involuntary gnashing of teeth; may occur after large doses of *AMPHETAMINES* or *COCAINE*
BUTYROPHENONES	Class of antipsychotic tranquillizers, of which the best-known example is *HALOPERIDOL* (see Essay VIB)

CARDIAC	Relating to the heart
CARDIOTOXICITY	Production of toxic effects on the heart; attribute of certain ANTIDEPRESSANTS (see Essay II)
CATAPLEXY	A kind of sudden stroke, in which one becomes immobilized through loss of muscle tone, while remaining conscious (may occur in NARCO-LEPSY)
CATECHOLAMINES	Naturally-occurring substances (e.g. ADRENALINE, 5-hydroxytryptamine) which affect the nervous system, the heart, body temperature and other functions
CENTRAL NERVOUS SYSTEM (CNS)	The system comprising the brain and spinal cord, together with nerve endings, which is responsible for changing mood and behaviour that is usually under control of the will
CHARAS	A type of hashish, or concentrated extract of *CANNABIS*, produced in India and Pakistan; characteristically very dark brown or almost black in colour and extremely potent
CHARLIE (slang)	*COCAINE*
CHINESE H (slang)	Adulterated *DIAMORPHINE* (heroin) found on the illicit market in the UK; believed to originate from China but more usually the product of other South-East Asian countries (e.g. Thailand)
CHIPPING (slang)	Occasional, rather than regular, injection of heroin, e.g. at weekends
CHRONIC	Of long duration, opposite of ACUTE
CIBAS (slang)	Tablets containing the hypnotic *GLUTETHIMIDE*, favoured by some drug abusers; so called because these bear the manufacturer's name, CIBA, on one side
COLIC, BILIARY	Very intense spasmodic pain in the abdomen, resulting from stones (calculi) lodged in the bile-duct
COLIC, RENAL	As biliary colic, but caused by kidney-stones (renal calculi); very sudden, often most intense loin pain
COMA	Complete unconsciousness, e.g. resulting from severe head injury, overdosage from certain drugs, in which the patient cannot respond to external stimuli
CONTRACEPTIVE	To prevent conception. Oral contraceptives ('the Pill') are tablets taken sequentially by women for

CONVULSION | A fit or seizure, which may occur in epilepsy or following overdosage from barbiturates and other drugs; a state of involuntary, alternating relaxation and expansion of the muscles

this purpose: these may contain the sex hormones progestogen and/or oestrogens or derivatives

CORTICOSTEROIDS Substances produced by the adrenal glands (e.g. cortisone); also derivatives of these, which are used medically for various indications (e.g. as anti-inflammatory agents in arthritis and other musculo-skeletal conditions)

CROSS-TOLERANCE Condition in which a patient, already habituated to drug A, if given drug B (A and B being of the same chemical or pharmacological group) will require comparably large doses of B: e.g. a person who has been taking *DIAZEPAM* (Valium) regularly will respond in the same way if switched to *CLORAZEPATE* or any other compound of the benzodiazepine class to which they both belong

COUMARIN ANTI-COAGULANT The most frequently prescribed medicaments for slowing blood clotting time, given orally (e.g. warfarin)

DELIRIUM A state of confusion and disorientation, which may be accompanied by fever, delusions or hallucinations

DELIRIUM TREMENS Popularly known as the DTs and alternatively called Korsakoff's syndrome: a chronic condition of disorientation and confusion, which may be provoked by chronic alcohol abuse or by certain infective and metabolic disorders

DELUSIONS Seeing, hearing or otherwise perceiving things which are not agreed to be there

DEPENDENCE LIABILITY The capacity of a drug to produce habituation, whether psychological or physical

DEPENDENCY Any state of habituation, psychological or physical, resulting from repeated use of a drug; not always synonymous with ADDICTION

DEPERSONALIZA-TION The sensation that one has lost one's identity; may be a phenomenon provoked by *LYSERGIDE* and other psychedelic substances (cf Essay V)

DEPRESSION, CENTRAL	Reduction in function of the central nervous system; may be produced by many types of drug, including alcohol
DEPRESSION, MENTAL	Psychological or mental depression is often typified by lowering of mood, listlessness, feelings of unworthiness etc (for the different, arbitrarily defined types, see Essay II)
DERMATITIS	Inflammation of the skin
DEX (slang)	Tablets or capsules of *DEXAMPHETAMINE* (Dexedrine)
DIABETES (MELLITUS)	Disorder in which the pancreas fails to metabolize carbohydrates (sugars etc) and which may require replacement therapy with insulin
DIPHENYLBUTYL-PIPERIDINES	A small class of recently-introduced antipsychotic drugs (see Essay VIB)
DISINHIBITION	Loss of usual social inhibitions; may be produced by excessive doses of alcohol, barbiturates, and certain tranquillizers. Can manifest as violent or antisocial behaviour
DISORIENTATION	Inability to 'keep one's bearings' in the psychological sense of appearing to be dissociated from one's surroundings
DIURETIC	Drug which increases flow of urine; may be effective in some forms of HYPERTENSION
DOPE (slang)	Often used of *CANNABIS*, but may refer to other drugs used in a non-medical setting
DOUBLE-BLIND	A technique of investigating drugs in which neither the patient nor the practitioner directly involved knows whether the compound, a standard drug, or a placebo has been administered
DOWNERS (slang)	Any drug which depresses the central nervous system; most commonly refers to BARBITURATES. Opposite of UPPERS
DRUG DEPEND-ENCY CLINIC	An institution attached to a psychiatric hospital where ADDICTS (NOTIFIED) are treated or, more commonly, receive repeat prescriptions for a narcotic drug. Such prescriptions are sent to designated pharmacies and dispensed on a daily basis
DYSKINESIA, TARDIVE	A form of PARKINSON'S DISEASE which is provoked by protracted use of antipsychotic drugs, most often in long-term psychiatric inpatients; associated with brain damage and may not be reversible (see Essay VIB)

DYSPHORIA	A feeling of unease, malaise, depressed mood; opposite of EUPHORIA
ECG (ELECTRO-CARDIOGRAM)	A device for recording electrical changes of the heart muscle
ECT (ELECTRO-CONVULSIVE THERAPY)	Technique for treating mental depression and other disorders considered within the psychiatrist's province, involving production of a fit similar to that which may occur in epilepsy; a still controversial procedure whose mode of action is unknown and whose efficacy is debatable
EEG (ELECTRO-ENCEPHALOGRAM)	Device for recording electrical impulses at various sites of the brain; not to be confused with either of the two preceding Entries
ENDORPHINS/ENKEPHALINS	Substances naturally produced which mimic the activity of morphine-like drugs (see Essay IV)
ENURESIS, NOCTURNAL	Bed-wetting: the passing of urine involuntarily, during sleep, as this occurs in children and adolescents
ENZYME INDUCTION	The acceleration of production of enzymes to break down a drug in the body. Some compounds, if taken regularly, induce their own metabolism (e.g. barbiturates) and that of other drugs
EPILEPSY	A condition characterized by convulsive seizures. The cause of most epileptic states is often not known and these may manifest in different ways, e.g. by grand mal, which is similar to CATAPLEXY, or petit mal, characterized by convulsions
EPINEPHRINE	Name given in the USA to the hormone ADRENALINE
EUPHORIA	Feeling of well-being which may be considered inappropriate to the situation
EUPHORIANT/EUPHORIGENIC	Producing euphoria
EXPECTORANT	A preparation, often a syrup or linctus, which facilitates the bringing up of sputum from the lungs and may suppress cough
EXTRA-PYRAMIDAL REACTIONS	s.v. PARKINSONISM
EYSENCK PERSONALITY INVENTORY (EPI)	A rating scale for psychological disorders, often used by contemporary psychiatrists

FLORID	Literally, flushed (of face); used of sudden, very marked appearance of symptoms considered to be psychotic
GABA (γ-aminobutyric acid)	A NEUROTRANSMITTER disturbances of which are believed to be associated with schizophrenic and other psychologically disturbed states
GANJA	West Indian name for dried flowering tops of *CANNABIS* herb
GANGRENE	Putrefaction of areas of tissue
GENERIC NAMES	Names of drugs which are official (as used in pharmacopoeias and other reference texts) as opposed to manufacturers' brand names
GILLES de la TOURETTE SYNDROME	Bizarre condition marked by inco-ordination of movement and involuntary use of foul language, parrot-like repetition and other signs
GLANDULAR FEVER	Properly known as infectious mononucleosis, a feverish ailment caused by Epstein-Barr virus, with enlargement and tenderness of the lymph glands and increased white blood-cell count
GLAUCOMA	One of a number of eye disorders in which the pressure within the eye is increased: certain types of drug (e.g. AMPHETAMINES) have this effect and are contra-indicated in such conditions
GOITRE	Enlargement of the thyroid gland, leading to sometimes gross swelling of the neck: may be caused by lack of iodine in the diet, infections, and other factors
GRASS (slang)	Cannabis in the form of dried flowering tops rather than resin (hashish); GANJA and KIF are different types of cannabis in this form
GYNAECOMASTIA	Enlargement of the breasts in men, sometimes very woman-like; may be a result of hormone treatment for cancers and sometimes occurs following repeated large doses of antipsychotic drugs
H (slang)	Heroin (*DIAMORPHINE*)
HABIT (slang)	State of physical dependency, usually on a morphine-like substance
HABITUATION	The condition produced by regular administration of a drug, in which the habitué requires very

HALF-LIFE (T½)

HALLUCINATION

HALLUCINOGEN

HAMILTON
RATING SCALE
HASH (slang)
HASHISH

HEPATITIS

HEARTS
HEROINIST
HIGH (slang)

HORMONE

HOSPICE

HORSE (slang)
HYDROXO-
COBALAMIN

large doses and may crave continued use; not necessarily synonymous with ADDICTION

The length of time (expressed in hours, days etc) for one-half of a given dose of a drug to be eliminated from the bloodstream (plasma half-life) or from the system (pharmacological half-life)

A perception (which may be auditory or visual) which is not shared by observers

A name applied to the PSYCHEDELIC class of compounds, suggesting that these provoke hallucinations: an inadequate and inaccurate term (cf also PSYCHOTOMIMETIC)

A questionnaire-type rating scale used in the diagnosis of depressive illnesses

Hashish

The dried, concentrated extract of *CANNABIS*. Unlike the herbal form, which consists of dried flowering tops, leaves and seeds, and resembles herbal tobacco, hashish appears in solid blocks, varying in colour from light brown to almost black (cf CHARAS)

A viral infection of the liver, which may manifest with fever, jaundice and a persistent feeling of weakness and debility; may be transmitted in several ways, particularly by use of unsterile injection equipment

S.V. PURPLE HEARTS

A habitué of diamorphine (heroin)

Used as adjective and noun to indicate a state of euphoria

A chemical produced by one gland or organ and carried to other parts of the body, stimulating them to special activity. An example is ADRENALINE, which is produced by the adrenal glands and increases heart-rate, alertness and other functions

An institution devoted to care of the dying, with particular emphasis on relief of pain and the psychological aspects of terminal illness

Heroin (diamorphine)

Vitamin B_{12b}: form of a vitamin often deficient in pernicious anaemia; given to correct this and in treatment of tobacco amblyopia, a visual disturbance caused by nicotine

HYPERAGITATION   A state of agitation considered inappropriate to the circumstances

HYPERKINETIC SYNDROME   A disorder or disorders of childhood and early adolescence marked by poor attention span, and excessive violent or unruly activity (see Essay I)

HYPERSENSITIVITY   The production of marked unwanted effects following even small doses of a particular drug or class of drugs; unusual individual susceptibility

HYPERTENSION   Raised blood-pressure; in its commoner forms this may be associated with heart disease, since the blood-pressure is dependent on cardiac output. May be associated with severe kidney disorder

HYPERTENSIVE CRISIS   A condition in which the blood-pressure rises uncontrollably (s.v. Essay II: MAO-INHIBITOR ANTIDEPRESSANTS)

HYPER-THYROIDISM   Overactivity of the secretions of the thyroid gland, characterized by increased appetite with weight loss, central excitation, insomnia

HYPNOTIC   To promote sleep

HYPODERMIC   Of an injection given shallowly into subcutaneous tissues

HYPODERMIC TABLETS   Extremely small tablets, which contain the minimum of filling and binding agents, for solution in sterile water or saline for injection. Hypodermic tablets may be useful formulations of drugs (e.g. *DIAMORPHINE*) which are unstable in solution

HYPOTENSION   Fall in blood-pressure; may occur when rising from a sitting or lying position

HYPOTHYROIDISM   Insufficiency of secretions from the thyroid gland

IATROGENIC   Term used to indicate illness produced by medical treatment

ILEUS, PARALYTIC   Intestinal obstruction due to muscular paralysis

ILEUM   That portion of the digestive tract which lies between the duodenum (which leads from the stomach) to the colon, or large intestine; otherwise known as the small intestine, it is important for food absorption

INGESTION   The taking of a substance via the alimentary tract or digestive system; usually applied to administration by mouth (oral)

INJECTION, INTRAMUSCULAR	Administration of a drug, normally in sterile solution, via a large-bore needle into the muscular tissues
INJECTION, INTRAVENOUS	Injection of a substance into one of the superficial veins, generally of the arm or hand, when very rapid effect is required
INJECTION, SUB-CUTANEOUS	Injection of a substance into the tissues beneath the skin surface, i.e. more shallowly than by the intramuscular route
INSOMNIA	Inability to sleep
INTOXICATION	(1) The condition arising from administration of toxic, i.e. dangerous, doses of a substance (2) More loosely, a state of inebriation or euphoria which a medicament may provoke
INTRA-CRANIAL PRESSURE	The pressure of the cerebro-spinal fluid in the space between the skull and the surface of the brain; may be raised following head injury
IPECACUANHA	A plant drug still considered valuable to produce vomiting: administration may be appropriate in certain cases of drug overdosage. Small quantities of ipecac have historically been given as an expectorant, in cough syrups
JACK UP (slang)	To inject into a vein
JOINT (slang)	A cigarette containing *CANNABIS*: in the UK this is commonly prepared by joining three cigarette-papers together and filling first with tobacco, then with herbal or resinous cannabis
KIF	Name given to the form in which *CANNABIS* is most often smoked in Morocco and elsewhere in North Africa; a fine, powdery green material composed of dried flowering tops
LABOUR	The period at the end of pregnancy culminating in expulsion of the foetus from the uterus (womb)
LACTATION	Secretion of milk by women suckling babies
LIBIDO	Sexual desire; not always synonymous with sexual capacity
LUDES (slang)	Abbreviated form of Quaalude, a US branded preparation of the much-abused soporific drug *METHAQUALONE*
LUDING OUT (slang)	The sensation obtained from consumption of excessive doses of methaqualone

MAINLINING (slang) — Injecting a drug, often a narcotic of the morphine type, into a vein

MAINTENANCE THERAPY — A somewhat euphemistic expression applied to the continuing prescription by psychiatrists of a drug (usually *METHADONE*) to opiate addicts (see Essay IV)

MALIGNANCY — Systemic disease caused by tumours (cancer)

MALIGNANCY, TERMINAL — State of inoperable cancerous illness in which death within a short period is anticipated

MANDIES (slang) — Abbreviation for the proprietary product Mandrax, which contains the highly habituating drug *METHAQUALONE*

MANIA — A condition described as psychotic and characterized by overactivity, an irrational superfluity of ideas, and sometimes delusions of grandeur

MANIC-DEPRESSIVE PSYCHOSIS — A psychological disorder marked by extraordinary alternating swinging of mood from energetic euphoria to deepest depression

MAO-INHIBITOR — A class of drugs which inhibit production of the enzyme monoamine oxidase, high levels of which are associated with mental depression; generally applied to a category of antidepressant drugs (see Essay II)

MEDULLA (OBLONGATA) — The lower portion of the brain-stem

MELANCHOLIA — An alternative term for mental depression (cf Essay II)

METABOLISM (OF DRUGS) — The process whereby substances are broken down, assimilated and excreted by the body

METABOLITE — A metabolic by-product

METH (slang) — Methedrine (*METHYLAMPHETAMINE*), a very potent stimulant

MICRODOT (slang) — An extremely small, coloured tablet containing *LYSERGIDE* (LSD)

MIGRAINE — A type of headache, often confined to one side, which may be accompanied by nausea, double vision, lights before the eyes

MIKES (slang) — Microgrammes (may be applied to *LYSERGIDE*)

MINIMAL BRAIN DYSFUNCTION — s.v. HYPERKINETIC SYNDROME

MMPI (MINNESOTA MULTIPHASIC PERSONALITY INVENTORY) — A type of questionnaire for assessing personality traits

MOLECULE	A chemical combination of two or more atoms to form a specific compound
MUCOSA	Mucous membranes (e.g. inside mouth, nose, rectum etc)
MUSCLE TONE	The normal condition of muscle, in which it contracts steadily and is able to resist pressure
MYOCARDIAL INFARCTION	Death of a portion of the heart muscle resulting from a thrombus (clot) of a coronary artery (coronary thrombosis); attended by intense chest pain and other symptoms
MYXOEDEMA	Disorder of thyroid or pituitary function with HYPOTHYROIDISM; may be caused by infection, surgical removal of thyroid gland or other factors
NARCOLEPSY	A chronic illness whose cause is not known, characterized by a tendency for the sufferer to fall asleep during the day despite normal nocturnal sleep; may be accompanied by CATAPLEXY (see also Essay I)
NARCOTICS	Term generally applied to potent pain-killers of the morphine type
NARCOTIC AGONISTS	These are drugs (including morphine, diamorphine, pethidine and the majority of potent analgesics) whose effects are reversed by administration of a narcotic antagonist
NARCOTIC ANTAGONIST	These may be partial antagonists (e.g. *PENTAZOCINE*) which are prescribed for pain relief but which may themselves be antagonized by pure antagonists (e.g. *NALOXONE*: see further Essay IV)
NAUSEA	Feeling that the stomach contents may be about to be regurgitated
NEBULIZER	A device for delivering individual doses of a drug, in the form of particles in a fine mist, such as a central stimulant (e.g. to relieve asthma), by inhalation
NEMBIES (slang)	Nembutal capsules, a branded preparation of the barbiturate *PENTOBARBITONE SODIUM*
NEUROLEPT-ANALGESIA	A technique, involving the use of a very short-acting narcotic (e.g. *FENTANYL*) with a neuroleptic or potent tranquillizer, used in anaesthetics: this enables the patient to remain conscious and co-operative although pain-free during short surgical procedures

NEUROLEPTIC — Another term for an antipsychotic drug or major tranquillizer of the *CHLORPROMAZINE* type (see Essay VIB)

NEUROTRANS- MITTERS — Chemicals released at nerve-endings which activate or stimulate adjacent nerves or muscle fibres (e.g. *ACETYLCHOLINE*)

NOCICEPTORS — Receptor sites, chiefly situated in the mid-brain, which are specific for pain stimuli (cf ENDORPHINS)

OBSTETRICS — The speciality of childbirth and the events in a woman's life which precede and succeed this

OPIATES — Strictly, drugs immediately derived from *OPIUM,* such as *MORPHINE* and *CODEINE*; more generally applied to other (including synthetic) compounds with comparably potent pain-relieving activity

OPIATES, NATURAL — The recently discovered chemicals isolated from brain tissue which are released when painful stimuli are experienced; term for ENDORPHINS and ENKEPHALINS

ORAL — By mouth

OVERDOSAGE — Administration of an excessive and often dangerous quantity of a drug or drugs

PARADOXICAL EFFECTS — This expression is aptly applied to reactions (predominantly psychological) which may occur following use of large doses of certain medicaments: for example, high doses of BARBITURATES and other sedatives may provoke states of stimulation and agitation. The mechanism whereby the phenomenon occurs is not known but this may obtain with several psychotropic agents, including *DIAZEPAM* (Valium) and similar tranquillizers, AMPHETAMINE-like stimulants, and alcohol

PARAESTHESIAE — Feelings of numbness at certain sites in the body, e.g. of the extremities in a variety of medical conditions

PARANOIA — One of the late great Emil Kraepelin's four types of SCHIZOPHRENIC illness, manifesting with thought disorders and fears that one is being persecuted or spied upon (considered to be irrational), as well as other DELUSIONS (cf Essay VIB)

PARENTERAL	Any mode of administration except via the gastro-intestinal system; in practice almost always refers to the different types of INJECTIONS
PARKINSONISM or PARKINSON'S DISEASE	A condition of disco-ordination which may manifest with muscle rigidity, involuntary movements of the limbs, trunk and/or eyes; a frequent early side-effect of treatment with antipsychotic drugs (also referred to as extra-pyramidal reactions); and insidious late form known as (TARDIVE) DYSKINESIA often occurs with prolonged use of antipsychotic tranquillizers
PEPTIDES	Substances consisting of two or more amino acids: the ENDORPHINS or natural opiates are peptides
PHAEOCHROMO-CYTOMA	Usually benign tumour of the adrenal glands, which may however provoke hypertension, fever and other reactions
PHARMACOPOEIA	An official, detailed listing of drugs, their chemical attributes, specifications for controlling the purity of preparations, means of identifying samples (e.g. from blood and urine) by colour tests, radioimmunoassay, infra-red spectrophotometry and other techniques. Such works are compiled by bodies (such as the Pharmacopoeia Commission) which are recognized by government and other institutions
PHENANTHRENES	In this case, a sub-class of synthetic pain-relieving drugs, whose prototype is the narcotic *METHADONE* (see Essay IV)
PHENOTHIAZINES	Numerically the largest classification of antipsychotic drugs related to *CHLORPROMAZINE* (see Essay VIB)
PHENTOLAMINE	A medicament given in heart failure and as an adjunct to treatment for PHAEOCHROMOCYTOMA; treatment of HYPERTENSIVE CRISES
PHENYL-PIPERIDINES	Potent synthetic analgesics of the *PETHIDINE (MEPERIDINE)* type
PITUITARY	Gland situated at the base of the brain, which secretes hormones responsible for growth, reproduction and other functions
POPPERS (slang)	Vitrellae, or glass capsules, of *AMYL NITRITE*, the short-acting cardiac and central stimulant
PORPHYRIA	One of three or four disorders in which abnormal quantities of porphyrins are secreted. Acute

intermittent porphyria (to which we principally refer) may manifest with abdominal pain, sensitivity to light, and disorders of nervous function; may be inherited or precipitated by excessive use of sulphonamides, BARBITU-RATES and some other drugs

POSTOPERATIVE | Following a (usually major) surgical procedure

POTENTIATION | Enhancing of the effects of one drug or drug type by another

PREMEDICATION | Medicament administered shortly before the beginning of surgery, to relax and/or render the patient unconscious

PROSTATE | A structure which is partly muscular and partly glandular, situated around the neck of the bladder and the urethra in males. It produces an opalescent liquid which is a constituent of semen

PSYCHEDELIC | Mind-revealing (of *LYSERGIDE*, or LSD, and other chemicals): see Essay V

PSYCHIC/ PSYCHOLOGICAL | Mental rather than physical

PSYCHOPATHY | A mental aberration (or series of them) in which the common factor is the individual's apparently total lack of conscience or other inhibition and behaviour (which may be antisocial) undertaken with no regard for the likely consequences

PSYCHO-PHARMACOLOGY | Now a recognized academic discipline, this is devoted to understanding of and research into drugs which affect mood or behaviour

PSYCHOSIS | One of various forms of severe psychological disturbance (see Essay VIB)

PSYCHOSIS, TOXIC | Psychosis precipitated by acute or chronic consumption of a toxic substance (e.g. AMPHETAMINE PSYCHOSIS)

PSYCHO-TOMIMETIC | Literally, 'psychosis-mimicking': a term inaptly applied to the class of chemicals otherwise known as HALLUCINOGENS or as PSYCHEDELICS (e.g. *LYSERGIDE* (LSD), *MESCALINE*)

PSYCHOTROPIC | Provoking changes in the central nervous system, especially of mood and behaviour. The expression 'psychotropic drugs' often relates in the clinical literature exclusively to those compounds used in psychiatry, despite the fact that others (e.g. HYPNOTICS, NARCOTIC ANALGESICS) are obviously mood-modifying

PUPIL   The circular aperture at the centre of the eye,
                                through which light passes; the pupils contract in
                                the presence of light under normal circumstances
PUPILS,   This state (miosis) may be seen following
CONSTRICTED   administration of certain drugs, particularly
                                morphine-type analgesics, and may be a useful
                                diagnostic sign
PUPILS, DILATED   Again this may be useful diagnostically: dilata-
                                tion of the pupils occurs with use of
                                amphetamine-like stimulants, high doses of bar-
                                biturates and other substances
PURPLE HEARTS   Preparations containing *DEXAMPHETAMINE*
(slang)   in combination with a BARBITURATE, usually
                                amylobarbitone; so called because of the original
                                colour and shape of a popular branded formula-
                                tion

RECEPTORS   Sites (notably in the mid-brain) which mediate
                                response to certain stimuli (e.g. pain; cf NOCICEP-
                                TORS)
REGIMEN   A programme or schedule (as for the administra-
                                tion of drugs)
REM (RAPID   Those alternating sections of sleep during which
EYE MOVEMENT)   rapid eye-movements occur and which are par-
SLEEP   ticularly characterized by dreaming. This func-
                                tion is suppressed by certain hypnotic drugs, such
                                as BARBITURATES
RESERPINE   Alkaloid from the Indian plant *Rauwolfia serpen-*
                                tina; historically used in psychiatry but now
                                almost exclusively in the treatment of HYPER-
                                TENSION
RETINOPATHY,   Degenerative condition of the cells of the retina
PIGMENTARY   at the back of the eye

SCAG (slang)   *DIAMORPHINE* (heroin)
SCHIZOPHRENIA   A so-called psychotic group of disorders involv-
                                ing altered ideas of reality, delusions, hallucina-
                                tions etc (for definitions, see Essay VIB)
SEDATION   Depressing of the central nervous system which
                                falls slightly short of complete unconsciousness;
                                thus, certain compounds normally prescribed to
                                promote sleep are given during the daytime for
                                their calming properties

SEPTICAEMIA	Poisoning of the bloodstream with pus-bearing material
SHIT (slang)	May be applied to almost any drug available on the illicit markets
SHOOT UP (slang)	To inject, usually intravenously, a drug in solution
SICK (slang)	Suffering from withdrawal reactions; in opiate addiction
SINUSITIS	Inflammation or blockage of the mucous membranes of the nose (sinusitis maxillaris) and throat
SKIN-POPPING (slang)	Injecting a substance into the tissues beneath the skin, rather than into a vein
SLEEPERS (slang)	Sleep-inducing drugs, particularly BARBITURATES
SMACK (slang)	*DIAMORPHINE* (heroin: from Yiddish *smeck* = taste)
SNOW (slang)	*COCAINE*
SOMNAMBULISM	Sleep-walking
SPASM	An involuntary, convulsive muscular action
SPEED (slang)	A powerful stimulant of the AMPHETAMINE type
SPEEDBALL (slang)	An injection consisting of a narcotic such as heroin together with a stimulant, generally cocaine
SPEED-FREAK (slang)	A person habituated to AMPHETAMINES
SPLIF (slang)	Alternative term for a cannabis cigarette or JOINT
STATUS EPILEPTICUS	A condition in which repeated seizures, or fits, occur
STEROIDS	S.V. CORTICOSTEROIDS
STONED (slang)	Experiencing euphoric effects from a drug
STROKE	Sudden loss of consciousness on account of brain haemorrhage, thrombosis (blood-clot) or other factors
SYMPATHETIC NERVOUS SYSTEM	That part of the nervous system which controls activity not under control of the will and governs metabolic function (pulse, heart-rate etc)
SYMPATHO-MIMETIC	Mimicking the function of the sympathetic nervous system (see Essay I)
SYNCOPE	Transient loss of consciousness caused by decrease in blood-supply to the brain
SYNTHETIC	Of a man-made material or substance, rather than one which occurs naturally

SYRINGE, HYPODERMIC	A device for administering injections, consisting of a barrel and a plunger, to which a hypodermic needle is attached
$T_{1/2}$	s.v. HALF-LIFE
TACHYCARDIA	Increased heart-rate
TETANUS	State of sustained muscular contraction with spasm; generally infectious in origin
TETRACYCLINES	Class of antibiotics effective against a wide range of bacteria
THIOXANTHENES	A category of antipsychotic drugs (see Essay VIB)
TINNITUS	Ringing in the ears
TOLERANCE	The process whereby an individual becomes accustomed to the effects of a drug
TOXICITY	Capacity for producing dangerous effects
TRACKS (slang)	Areas of scarred tissue which often follow the paths of superficial veins on the arms; e.g. in opiate addiction
TRANQUILLIZER, MAJOR	Term applied to compounds with chiefly antipsychotic effect (see Essay VI)
TRANQUILLIZER, MINOR	Anxiety-relieving rather than antipsychotic agents (see Essay VI)
TRAUMA	Injury, physical or psychological
TREMOR	State of involuntary trembling; may be associated with PARKINSONISM
TRIAL, CLINICAL	An experiment in which a drug or other treatment is administered to patients rather than laboratory animals
TRICYCLIC	Chemically, having three rings; e.g. of a class of ANTIDEPRESSANTS (see Essay II)
TRIP (slang)	An experience with *LYSERGIDE* (LSD) or another psychedelic substance
TUBERCULOSIS	Infectious disease caused by a bacterium (Mycobacterium), which principally but not exclusively damages the lungs
TURN ON (slang)	Also, to be turned on. Literally, to be STONED; more generally, to be an individual of the the new order
TYRAMINE	A chemical intermediate between tyrosine and ADRENALINE; an ingredient of certain foods and drinks (see Essay II)
ULCER, PEPTIC	Open sore or lesion of the mucous membrane of the stomach or duodenum

UPPERS (slang)	Stimulants, commonly of the AMPHETAMINE type
URETHRAL STRICTURE	Narrowing or closure of the narrow tube which runs from the bladder to the external urinary meatus; often due to bacterial infection
URINARY RETENTION	Retention of urine in the bladder; inability to pass urine
WITHDRAWAL SYNDROME	The signs and symptoms which follow abrupt discontinuation of a drug which has been taken repeatedly and to which physical dependency has developed

ANNEX 6: Select Bibliography

For recommended reading on each of the six principal categories of compounds to which this work is devoted, see lists at end of each Essay.

ABPI Data Sheet Compendium 1980–81. Association of the British Pharmaceutical Industry: London, 1980
AMA Council on Drugs: *Drug Evaluations,* ed.4. Littleton, Mass., 1981
Austria-Codex 1978/79. Österreichischer Apotheker-Verlag: Wien, 1978

BEECHER, H. K.: *Measurement of Subjective Responses: quantitative effects of Drugs.* New York, 1959
BENIGNI, R., CAPRA, C. and CATTORINI, P. E.: *Piante medicinali: chimica farmacologia e terapia.* Milano, 1962 & 1964. 2 vols.
BILLUPS, N. F. and BILLUPS, S. M.: *American Drug Index* 1980. Philadelphia, 1980
British National Formulary no. 1 British Medical Association/Pharmacopoeia Commission: London, 1981
[British] Pharmaceutical Codex, ed.11. British Pharmacopoeia Commission: London, 1979
British Pharmacopoeia Commission: *Approved Names 1977.* London, 1977
British Pharmacopoeia 1980; 2 vols, + Addendum, 1981. British Pharmacopoeia Commission: London, 1980
BROWN, W. R. L. and HADGRAFT, J. W.: *Drug Presentation and Prescribing.* Oxford, 1965

Chemist & Druggist Directory 1980. Tunbridge Wells, 1980
CLARKE, E. G. C.: *Isolation and Identification of Drugs in pharmaceuticals, body fluids and post-mortem material.* London, 1969 + Supplementary Volume (= vol. 2) 1975
CLARKE, E. H. (ed.): *How Modern Medicines Are Developed.* Mount Kisco, NY, 1977
Compendium of Pharmaceuticals and Specialties 1980. Canadian Pharmaceutical Association: Toronto, 1980
COOPER, P.: *An Index of Adverse Reactions to Drugs.* London, 1971

CRAMMER, J., BARRACLOUGH, B. and HEINE, B.: *The Use of Drugs in Psychiatry.* London, 1978

DAVIES, D. M.: *Textbook of Adverse Drug Reactions*, ed.2. Oxford, 1981
Drug and Therapeutics Bulletin vol.18 (London, 1980) et seq.

FALCONER, M. W., PATTERSON, H. R. and GUSTAFSON, E. A.: *Current Drug Handbook 1978–80.* Philadelphia, 1978
FOLCH JOU, G.: *Del Ópio a los modernos alucinógenos.* Real Academía de Farmacía: Madrid, 1969

GLATT, M. M.: *A Guide to Addiction and its Treatment.* Lancaster, 1975
GOODMAN, L. S., GILMAN, A., GILMAN, A. A. and KOELLE, G. B. (eds.): *The Pharmacological Basis of Therapeutics,* ed.6. New York, 1980
GORDON, M. (ed.): *Psychopharmacological Agents* vols. 3 & 4 (replacing vols. 1 & 2). New York, 1974 & 1976
Guide to the Misuse of Drugs Act 1971 and to certain Regulations under the Act. DHSS: London, 1977
GRIFFIN, J. P. and D'ARCY, P. F.: *A Manual of Adverse Drug Interactions,* ed.2. Bristol, 1979

HAY, C. E. and PEARCE, M. E.: *Medicines and Poisons Guide,* ed.2. London, 1980
HANSTEN, P. D.: *Drug Interactions,* ed.3. Philadelphia, 1977
HOLMSTEDT, B. and LILJESTRAND, G. (eds.): *Readings in Pharmacology.* Oxford, 1963
HOLLISTER, L. E.: *Clinical Pharmacology of Psychotherapeutic Drugs.* New York & Edinburgh, 1978

ISSEKUTZ, B.: *Die Geschichte der Arzneimittelforschung,* übersetzt von A Faragó. Budapest, 1971

KLINE, N. S. et al.: *Psychotropic Drugs: a manual for emergency management of overdosage.* New York, 1974
KORNETSKY, C.: *Pharmacology: Drugs affecting behavior.* New York, 1976

LEAKE, C. D.: *Historical Account of Pharmacology to the 20th Century.* Springfield, Ill., 1975
LEMBECK, F. and SEWING, K. F.: *Pharmakologie-Fibel.* Heidelberg, 1966

LEWIN, L.: *Phantastica: narcotic and stimulating drugs, their use and abuse,* tr. P. H. A. Wirth. London, 1931 (various reprints)
LEWIN, L.: *Gifte und Vergiftungen.* Berlin, 1929 (= *Lehrbuch der Toxikologie* ed. 4)
LEWIS, A. J. (ed.): *Modern Drug Encyclopedia and Therapeutic Index,* ed.15. New York, 1979

MacMAHON, F. G. (ed.): *Psychopharmacological Agents.* Mount Kisco, NY, 1975
MARINI, L. (ed.): *L'Informatore farmaceutico,* anno 1978. Milano, 1978
MARINI, L.: *Repertorio terapeutico: medicamenta: international index,* ed.5. Milano, 1976
Martindale's Extra Pharmacopoeia, ed.27 by A. Wade & J. E. F. Reynolds. London, 1977
Medical Letter on Drugs and Therapeutics. New Rochelle, NY, 1959–
The Merck Index: an encyclopedia of chemicals and drugs, ed.9. Rahway, NJ, 1976
MEYERS, F. H., JAWETZ, E. and GOLDFIEN, A. (eds.): *Review of Medical Pharmacology,* ed.5. Los Altos, Calif., 1976
MIMS (Monthly Index of Medical Specialties). London vol.18 (Jan 1980) et seq

Physicians' Desk Reference, ed.34. Oradell, NJ, 1980
PLEIN, J. N. and PLEIN, E. E.: *Fundamentals of Medications: a textworkbook of dosages, mathematics and introductory pharmacology.* Philadelphia [1967]

RICHARDS, D. J. and RONDEL, R. K. (eds.): *Adverse Drug Reactions: detection and assessment.* Edinburgh, 1972
Rote Liste 1980: Verzeichnis von Fertigarzneimitteln, ed. Bundesverband der deutschen Pharmazeutischen Industrie eV. Aulendorf/Württ., 1980

SCHNEIDER, W.: *Lexikon der Arzneimittelgeschichte: Pflanzliche Drogen.* Frankfurt aM, 1974. 5 vols.
SHADER, R. I. and DiMASCIO, A.: *Psychotropic Drug Side Effects: clinical and theoretical perspectives.* Baltimore, 1970
SILVERMAN, M. and LEE, P. R.: *Pills, Profits and Politics.* Berkeley, Calif., 1974
STOCKLEY, I. H.: *Drug Interactions and their Mechanisms.* London [1974]
STOCKLEY, I. H.: *Drug Interaction Alert.* Boehringer Ingelheim Ltd.: Bracknell, Berks, 1978 (Chart)
SZASZ, T. H.: *Ceremonial Chemistry: the ritual persecution of drugs, addicts and pushers.* London, 1975

United States Pharmacopeia, 20th revision/*National Formulary,* 15th ed. Rockville, Md., 1980

USDIN, E. and EFRON, D. H.: *Psychotropic Drugs and Related Compounds.* ed.2. Washington/Oxford, 1979

VIDAL, L. (ed.): *Dictionnaire Vidal 1980.* Paris, 1980

VALZELLI, L.: *Psychopharmacology: an introduction to experimental and clinical principles,* ed. W. B. Essman. Flushing, NY, 1973

WEIL, A.: *The Natural Mind.* London, 1973

Index of Brand Names and Alternative Names

This Index will enable the reader to locate any branded (proprietary) preparation of a drug which comes within the terms of reference of this book. Physicians more often prescribe by manufacturers' names than by official chemical names: thus the drug whose pharmaceutical name is CHLORDIAZEPOXIDE is usually prescribed as Librium, the Roche trade name for the compound. This index also lists alternative names: in the USA the official nomenclature may be different from that used in the UK (e.g. AMYLOBARBITONE is known as AMOBARBITAL in the United States). Sometimes the alternative names are entirely different: e.g. the drug called BENZHEXOL in Great Britain is referred to as TRIHEXYPHENIDYL in the USA. Such alternative names as cross-referenced here are indicated by capital letters; and proprietary names are given in lower case type.

NB: co indicates that the drug named is the principal, but not the only, ingredient in the preparation named.

The drugs below can be looked up under their pharmaceutical names in the Alphabetical Formulary on p. 25. More general information about the classes into which they fall can be found in the Essays and Charts starting on p. 207.

Trade name	Pharmaceutical name	
ACECARBROMAL	sv ACETYLCARBROMAL	
Adapin	doxepin	US
Adphen	phendimetrazine	US
Adipex-P	phentermine	US
Allegron	nortriptyline	UK
ALLYLBARBITURIC ACID	sv BUTALBITAL	
Allylgesic	allobarbitone co	US
Allylgesic/Ergotamine	allobarbitone co	US
Alurate	aprobarbitone	US
Amesec	amylobarbitone co	US
AMFEPRAMONIUM	sv DIETHYLPROPION	
Aminophylline/Amytal	amylobarbitone	US
Amitid	amitriptyline	US
Amitril	amitriptyline	US

Trade name	*Pharmaceutical name*	
Amobarbital D-Lay	amylobarbitone	US
Amodex	dexamphetamine co	US
Amosene	meprobamate	US
Amylomet	amylobarbitone co	UK
Amytal	amylobarbitone	UK,US
Amytal Sodium	amylobarbitone sodium	UK, US
Anafranil	clomipramine	UK
Andro-Medicone	yohimbine co	US
Anexsia-D	hydrocodone	US
Anquil	benperidol	UK
Anxon	ketazolam	UK
APB	amylobarbitone co	US
APC/Butalbital	butalbital co	US
APC/Meperidine	pethidine co	US
Apisate	diethylpropion co	UK
A-Poxide	chlordiazepoxide	US
Aquachloral	chloral	US
Arcoban	meprobamate	US
Aridol	methylamphetamine co	US
Artane	benzhexol	UK,US
Aspirin & Papaveretum	papaveretum	UK
Aspirol	amyl nitrite	US
Atarax	hydroxyzine	UK
Ataraxoid	hydroxyzine co	US
Atensine	diazepam	UK
Ativan	lorazepam	UK
Aventyl	nortriptyline	UK,US
Avomine	promethazine	UK
Azene	clorazepate	US
B&O Supprettes	opium.co	US
Bacarate	phendimetrazine	US
Bamate	meprobamate	US
Bamo	meprobamate	US
Banobese	phendimetrazine	US
Bar-8 etc	phenobarbitone	US
Barbipil	phenobarbitone	US
Barbita	phenobarbitone	US
BC-2605	nabilone	
Benadryl	diphenhydramine	UK,US
Benzedrex	propylhexedrine	US
Benzedrine	amphetamine	US
Berkolol	propranolol	UK

Berkomine	imipramine	UK
Beta-Chlor	chloral	US
Biphetamine	dexamphetamine co	US
Bolvidon	mianserin	UK
Bontril-PDM	phendimetrazine	US
Brigen-G	chlordiazepoxide	US
Brompton Cocktail	sv DIAMORPHINE	
Bromural	bromisovalum	US
Buff-A-Comp	butalbital co	US
Buta-Barb	secbutobarbitone	US
BUTABARBITAL	sv SECBUTOBARBITONE	US
Butal	secbutobarbitone	US
Butalan	secbutobarbitone	US
Butazem	secbutobarbitone	US
BUTETHAL	sv BUTOBARBITONE	
Buticaps	secbutobarbitone	US
Butisol	secbutobarbitone	US
Butomet	butobarbitone co	UK
Butte	secbutobarbitone	US
Cafergot	butalbital co	UK
Camcolit	lithium carbonate	UK
Carbrital	carbromal co	US
Carbropent	carbromal co	US
Cartrax	hydroxyzine co	US
Chlordiazeachel	chlordiazepoxide	US
Chlornidium	chlordiazepoxide co	US
Chlorophen	chlorphentermine	US
Chlorzine	chlorpromazine	US
Clairvan	ethamivan	UK
CLOMETHIAZOLE	sv CHLORMETHIAZOLE	
Clopixol	clopenthixol	UK
Coditrate	hydrocodone co	US
Codone	hydrocodone	US
Cohidrate	chloral	US
Colonil	diphenoxylate co	US
Combid	prochlorperazine co	US
Compazine	prochlorperazine	US
Comploment	pyridoxine	UK
Concordin	protriptyline	UK
Cosalgesic	dextropropoxyphene co	UK
CP 50, 556	sv LEVONANTRADOL	
Cyclimorph	morphine co	UK
Cyclomet	cyclobarbitone co	UK

Cylert	pemoline	US
Cystospaz	secbutobarbitone co	US
Dalmane	flurazepam	UK,US
Daro	dexamphetamine	US
Dartal	thiopropazate	US
Dartalan	thiopropazate	UK
Darvocet-N	dextropropoxyphene	US
Darvon	dextropropoxyphene	US
Darvon-Co	dextropropoxyphene co	US
Darvon-N	dextropropoxyphene	US
Darvon-N/ASA	dextropropoxyphene co	US
Da-Sed	secbutobarbitone	US
Daxolin	loxapine	US
Deaner	deanol	US
Delcobese	dexamphetamine co	US
Dee-10	methylamphetamine	US
Demerol	pethidine	US
Demerol-APAP	pethidine co	US
Depixol	flupenthixol	UK
Depronal-SA	dextropropoxyphene	UK
Desoxyn	methylamphetamine	US
DET	sv DIETHYLTRYPTAMINE & DIMETHYLTRYPTAMINE	
Dexamed	dexamphetamine	UK
Dexampex	dexamphetamine	US
Dexamyl	dexamphetamine co	US
Dexedrine	dexamphetamine	UK,US
DEXTROAM-PHETAMINE	sv DEXAMPHETAMINE	
Dextrobar	dexamphetamine co	US
DF-118	dihydrocodeine	UK
Dialog	allobarbitone co	US
Diazemuls	diazepam	UK
DICHLORAL-ANTIPYRENE	sv DICHLORALPHENAZONE	
Dicodid	hydrocodone	US
Dicodrine	hydrocodone co	US
Diconal	dipipanone co	UK
Didrex	benzphetamine	US
DIHYDRO-CODEINONE	sv HYDROCODONE	
Dilaudid	hydromorphone	US
Dilaudid Cough Syrup	hydromorphone co	US

Dilocol	hydromorphone co	US
Dimotane-DC	hydrocodone co	UK
Diphylets	dexamphetamine	US
Dipidolor	piritramide	UK
Disipal	orphenadrine	UK,US
Diskets Methadone	methadone	US
Distalgesic	dextropropoxyphene co	UK
Distalgesic-Soluble	dextropropoxyphene co	UK
DMT	sv DIMETHYLTRYPTAMINE	
Dolasan	dextropropoxyphene co	UK
Dolene	dextropropoxyphene co	US
Dolophine	methadone	US
Doloxene	dextropropoxyphene	UK
Doloxene-Co	dextropropoxyphene co	UK
Domical	amitriptyline	UK
Dopram	doxapram	US
Doraphen	dextropropoxyphene co	US
Doriden	glutethimide	UK,US
Dorimide	glutethimide	US
DOSULEPINE	sv DOTHIEPIN	
Dover's Powder	sv OPIUM	
Droleptan	droperidol	UK
Dromoran	levorphanol	UK
Duradyne-DHC	hydrocodone co	US
Duromine	phentermine	UK
Duromorph	morphine	UK
Durophet	dexamphetamine co	UK
Durophet-M	dexamphetamine co	UK
Ectasule	amylobarbitone co	US
Elamol	tofenacin	UK
Elavil	amitriptyline	US
Emesert	pentobarbitone co	US
Enarax	hydroxyzine co	US
Endep	amitriptyline	US
Epanutin/Phenobarbitone	phenobarbitone co	UK
Ephedrine/Amytal	ephedrine co	US
Ephedrine/Seconal	ephedrine co	US
Equagesic	ethoheptazine co	UK
Equanil	meprobamate	UK,US
ERGINE	sv LYSERGAMIDE	
Eskabarb	phenobarbitone	US

Eskalith	lithium carbonate	US
Eskatrol	dexamphetamine co	US
Etrafon	amitriptyline co	US
Euhypnos	temazepam	UK
Evacalm	diazepam	UK
Evadyne	butriptyline	UK
Evidorm	hexobarbitone co	UK
Ex-Obese	phendimetrazine	US
Expansatol	secbutobarbitone	US
Fastin	phentermine	US
Felsules	chloral	US
Fenarol	chlormezanone	US
Fentazin	perphenazine	UK
Ferndex	dexamphetamine	US
Filon	phenmetrazine co	UK
Fiorinal	butalbital co	US
Flexon	orphenadrine	US
Fluanxol	flupenthixol	UK
Fortagesic	pentazocine co	UK
Fortral	pentazocine	UK
Frisium	clobazam	UK
Gardenal	phenobarbitone	US
Gemonil	metharbitone	US
Halcion	triazolam	UK
Haldol	haloperidol	UK,US
Harmar	dextropropoxyphene	US
Heminevrin	chlormethiazole	UK
Henomint	phenobarbitone	US
HEROIN	sv DIAMORPHINE	
Hexyphen	benzhexol	US
HS-Need	chloral	US
Hycodan	hydrocodone co	US
Hypnette	phenobarbitone	US
Hypnorm	fentanyl co	UK
Hyzine	promazine	US
ICN-65	dextropropoxyphene	US
Imavate	imipramine	US
Immobilon	etorphine co	UK
Inapsine	droperidol	US
Inderal	propranolol	UK

Infadorm	phenobarbitone	US
Innovar	fentanyl co	US
Insidon	opipramol	UK
Intasedol	secbutobarbitone	US
Integrin	oxypertine	UK
Intraval	thiopentone	UK
Ionamin	phentermine	UK,US
Isomel	bromisovalum	US
Janimine	imipramine	US
Kalmm	meprobamate	US
Kethamed	pemoline	UK
Klorazine	chlorpromazine	US
Komazine	chlorpromazine	US
Lanabrom	potassium bromide co	US
Largactil	chlorpromazine	UK
Largon	propiomazine	US
LAUDANUM	sv OPIUM	
Lentizol	amitriptyline	UK
Leritine	anileridine	US
Levo-Dromoran	levorphanol	US
LEVOMEPRO-MAZINE	sv METHOTRIMEPRAZINE	
Levoprome	methotrimeprazine	US
Librax	chlordiazepoxide co	US
Libraxin	chlordiazepoxide co	UK
Libritabs	chlordiazepoxide	UK,US
Librium	chlordiazepoxide	UK,US
Lidone	molindone	US
LILLY 109514	nabilone	
Limbitrol	chlordiazepoxide co	UK,US
Liskonum	lithium carbonate	UK
Lithane	lithium carbonate	US
Lithobid	lithium carbonate	US
Lithonate	lithium carbonate	US
Lithonate-S	lithium citrate	US
Lithotabs	lithium carbonate	US
Lobak	chlormezanone co	UK
Lomotil	diphenoxylate co	UK,US
Lomotil/Neomycin	diphenoxylate co	UK,US
Lorfan	levallorphan	UK,US
Loryl	chloral hydrate	US

Lo Tense	chlordiazepoxide	US
Lotusate	talbutal	US
Loxitane	loxapine	US
LSD	sv LYSERGIDE	
Lucidril	meclofenoxate	UK
Ludiomil	maprotiline	UK
Luminal	phenobarbitone	UK,US
Mandrax	methaqualone co	UK
Marax	hydroxyzine co	US
Marplan	isocarboxazid	UK,US
Marsilid	iproniazid	UK
Maso-Bamate	meprobamate	US
Maso-Chloral	chloral hydrate	US
Maso-Pent	pentobarbitone	US
Mebaral	methylphenobarbitone	US
Mebroin	methylphenobarbitone	US
Medarsed	secbutobarbitone	US
Mediatric	methylamphetamine co	US
Medomin	heptabarbitone	UK,US
Megimide	bemegride	UK
Melfiat	phendimetrazine	US
Mellaril	thioridazine	US
Melleril	thioridazine	UK
Menrium	chlordiazepoxide co	US
Menta-Bal	methylphenobarbitone	US
Mentran	barbitone co	US
MEPERIDINE	sv PETHIDINE	
Mephoral	methylphenobarbitone	US
Meprocon	meprobamate co	US
Meprospan	meprobamate	US
Mequin	methaqualone	US
Merital	nomifensine	UK
Mervaldin	mephenesin	US
Methampex	methylamphetamine	US
METHAM-PHETAMINE	sv METHYLAMPHETAMINE	
Methedrine	methylamphetamine	UK
Methenex	methadone co	US
Midrid	dichloralphenazone co	UK
Midrin	dichloralphenazone co	US
Milonorm	meprobamate	UK
Milpath	meprobamate co	US
Milprem	meprobamate co	US

Percocet	oxycodone co	US
Percodan	oxycodone co	US
Permitil	fluphenazine	US
Pertofran	desipramine	UK
Pertofrane	desipramine	US
Pethilorfan	pethidine co	UK
Pfi-Lithium	lithium carbonate	US
Phanodorm	cyclobarbitone	UK
Phasal	lithium carbonate	UK
Phenergan	promethazine	UK,US
Phenobarbitone Spansules	phenobarbitone	UK
Phenomet	phenobarbitone co	UK
Pheno-Squar	phenobarbitone	US
Phentrol	phentermine	US
Phenzine	phendimetrazine	US
Phrenilin	secbutobarbitone co	US
Physeptone	methadone	UK
Pipanol	benzhexol	US
Placidyl	ethchlorvynol	US
Plegine	phendimetrazine	US
Plexonal	barbitone co	US
PMB	meprobamate co	US
Ponderax	fenfluramine	UK
Pondimin	fenfluramine	US
Potensan-Forte	yohimbine co	UK
Poxy Co-65	dextropropoxyphene co	US
Preludin	phenmetrazine	US
Presamine	imipramine	US
Pre-Sate	chlorphentermine	US
Priadel	lithium carbonate	UK
Progesic	dextropropoxyphene co	US
Proketazine	carphenazine	US
Proladone	oxycodone	UK
Prolixin Decanoate	fluphenazine decanoate	US
Prolixin Enanthate	fluphenazine enanthate	US
Prolixin Hydrochloride	fluphenazine hydrochloride	US
Promachel	chlorpromazine	US
Promachlor	chlorpromazine	US
Promapar	chlorpromazine	US
Promaz	chlorpromazine	US
Prominal	methylphenobarbitone	UK
Prondol	iprindole	UK
PROPERICIAZINE	sv PERICYAZINE	

Pro-Pox	dextropropoxyphene	US
Propoxychel	dextropropoxyphene	US
PROPOXYPHENE	sv DEXTROPROPOXYPHENE	
Prothiaden	dothiepin	UK
Proxagesic	dextropropoxyphene	US
Quaalude	methaqualone	US
Quide	piperacetazine	US
Quiebar	secbutobarbitone	US
Rapidal	cyclobarbitone	UK
Reactivan	fencamfamin co	UK
Rectules	chloral hydrate	US
Redeptin	fluspirilene	UK
Remnos	nitrazepam	UK
Renbu	secbutobarbitone	US
Repoise	butaperazine	US
Repro-Con	dextropropoxyphene co	US
Ritalin	methylphenidate	UK,US
Robese	dexamphetamine	US
Ro-Diet	diethylpropion	US
Rolaphent	phentermine	US
Rolathimide	phentermine	US
Romilar	dextromethorphan	US
Ronyl	pemoline	UK
Ropoxy	dextropropoxyphene	US
Ro-Trim	dexamphetamine co	US
Sanorex	mazindol	US
Saronil	meprobamate	US
Saroten	amitriptyline	UK
Screen	chlordiazepoxide	US
Scrip-Dyne-Co	dextropropoxyphene co	US
Sec-Kap	quinalbarbitone	US
SECOBARBITAL	sv QUINALBARBITONE	
Seco-8	quinalbarbitone	US
Seconal	quinalbarbitone	UK,US
Sedadrops	phenobarbitone	US
Sedamyl	acetylcarbromal	US
Sedapam	diazepam	UK
Serax	oxazepam	US
Serenace	haloperidol	UK
Serenid-D	oxazepam	UK
Serenid-Forte	oxazepam	UK

Serensil	ethchlorvynol	US
Serentil	mesoridazine	US
Sernylan	sv PHENCYCLIDINE	
Sinequan	doxepin	UK,US
SK-65	dextropropoxyphene	US
SK-65-Co	dextropropoxyphene co	US
SK-Amitriptyline	amitriptyline	US
SK-Bamate	meprobamate	US
SK-Diphenoxylate	diphenoxylate co	US
SK-Lygen	chlordiazepoxide	US
SK-Phenobarbital	phenobarbitone	US
SK-Pramine	imipramine	US
Slim-Tabs	phendimetrazine	US
Sodium Amytal	amylobarbitone sodium	UK
Soduben	secbutobarbitone	US
Solis	diazepam	UK
Solubarb	phenobarbitone	US
Sombulex	hexobarbitone	US
Somnased	nitrazepam	UK
Somnite	nitrazepam	UK
Sonalgin	butobarbitone co	UK
Sonazine	chlorpromazine	US
Sonergan	butobarbitone co	UK
Soneryl	butobarbitone	UK
Sopor	methaqualone	US
S-Pain-65	dextropropoxyphene	US
Span-Cap	dexamphetamine	US
Span-RD	methylamphetamine	US
Sparine	promazine	UK,US
SPRX	phendimetrazine	US
Stadol	butorphanol	UK,US
Statobex	phendimetrazine	US
Stelazine	trifluoperazine	UK,US
Stemetil	prochlorpereazine	UK
Stental	phenobarbitone	US
Sublimaze	fentanyl co	UK
Surem	nitrazepam	UK
Surmontil	trimipramine	UK,US
Synalgos-DC	dihydrocodeine co	US
Tacitin	benzoctamine	UK
Talwin	pentazocine	US
Taractan	chlorprothixene	UK
Temaril	trimeprazine	US

Temgesic	buprenorphine	UK
Tenavoid	meprobamate co	UK
Tenax	chlordiazepoxide	US
Tenuate	diethylpropion	UK,US
Tepanil	diethylpropion	US
Teramine	phentermine	US
Teronac	mazindol	UK
Thalamonal	fentanyl co	UK
THC	sv TETRAHYDRO-CANNABINOL	
Themalon	diethylthiambutene	UK
Thorazine	chlorpromazine	US
Tidex	dexamphetamine	US
Tindal	acetophenazine	US
Tofranil	imipramine	UK,US
Tofranil-PM	imipramine pamoate	US
Tora	phentermine	US
Trancopal	chlormezanone	UK
Tranmep	meprobamate	US
Tranquinal	bromisovalum co	US
Tranxene	clorazepate	UK,US
Tremin	benzhexol	US
Triavil	amitriptyline co	US
Triclos	triclofos	US
TRIHEXYPHENIDYL	sv BENZHEXOL	
Trilafon	perphenazine	US
Trimex	dexamphetamine co	US
Trimstat	phendimetrazine	US
Trimtabs	phendimetrazine	US
Triperidol	trifluperidol	UK
Triptafen	amitriptyline co	UK
Tryptizol	amitriptyline	UK
Tuinal	amylobarbitone co	UK,US
Tussend	hydrocodone co	US
Tussionex	hydrocodone co	US
Tybatran	tybamate	US
Tylox	oxycodone co	US
Ultrased	hexobarbitone	US
Valium	diazepam	UK,US
Valledrine	trimeprazine co	UK
Vallergan	trimeprazine	UK
Vallex	trimeprazine co	UK

Valmid	ethinamate	US
Vannor	bromisovalum co	US
Vaporole	amyl nitrite	US
Verstran	prazepam	US
Vertigon	prochlorperazine	UK
Vesprin	triflupromazine	US
Vicodin	hydrocodone co	US
Villescon	prolintane co	UK
Vistaril	hydroxyzine	US
Vistrax	hydroxyzine co	US
Vivactil	protriptyline	US
Vivalan	viloxazine	UK
Volital	pemoline	UK
Voranil	clortermine	US
WANS	pentobarbitone co	US
WDD	imipramine	US
Welldorm	dichloralphenazone	UK
Westadone	methadone	US
Wilpo	phentermine	US
Wilpowr	phentermine	US
Wyamine	mephentermine	US
Zactane	ethoheptazine	US
Zactipar	ethoheptazine co	UK
Zactirin	ethoheptazine co	UK,US
Zelmid	zimelidine	
Zetran	chlordiazepoxide	US

ADDENDA

While this book was in the press, a number of new preparations of drugs already described have been introduced. The most significant are:

BUPRENORPHINE (see p. 42)

A new presentation of buprenorphine has become available (1981). This is in the form of tablets for sublingual use, ie they should be held under the tongue until dissolved rather than swallowed. The manufacturers claim that this route of administration for the pain-reliever concerned is both convenient and effective. Latest research confirms that buprenorphine offers a markedly greater duration of action than most other analgesics of comparable potency. Data concerning the substance's abuse and dependence potential are equivocal, however: on the one hand, persons accustomed to morphine have found that buprenorphine provokes psychological effects that are not dissimilar, including in some cases euphoria. On the other hand, it is also suggested that even following protracted use any withdrawal reactions will be mild if these occur at all. Recent experiments conducted at Harvard indicate that, because opiate habitués find the drug euphoriant and because as a partial narcotic antagonist it 'blocks' the effects of heroin, buprenorphine might be a suitable candidate for the maintenance of addicts (see Essay IV, p. 283).

DIAZEPAM (see p. 77)

Two new types of formulation of this well-known tranquillizer are now marketed. *Valium* is available as suppositories (5 & 10 mg), in addition to the more usual preparations. Suppositories may be useful in all the medical indications for diazepam, for administration to patients who find difficulty in taking tablets or capsules. A different company has just made available *Diazemuls* (Amps 10 mg/2 ml). Injectable diazepam is useful for premedication, to relieve severe acute anxiety, and to treat convulsions. However, the standard *Valium* ampoule formulation contains diazepam (a water-insoluble drug) dissolved in 65% propylene glycol: the presence of such a large proportion of this viscous liquid is chiefly responsible for the fact that diazepam injection is often painful, and can lead to thrombosis of the vein used. As has already been noted, accidental arterial injection can be most dangerous. These problems are much less likely to arise with *Diazemuls*, which has been administered in Sweden for some years with great success: these ampoules contain the drug in an oil- and water emulsion, white in colour. In particular, injection is far less painful and venous complications are less likely to occur.

LORMETAZEPAM

This compound, a very close chemical analogue of TEMAZEPAM, has just been introduced under the brand name *Noctamid* (Schering): Tabs 0.5 & 1 mg for treatment of insomnia. Similar to other benzodiazepines (see Essay III).

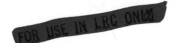

FOR USE IN LRC ONLY

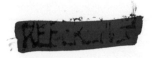